Unilateral Biportal Endoscopic Spine Surgery

Dong Hwa Heo
Cheol Woong Park • Sang Kyu Son
Jin Hwa Eum
Editors

Unilateral Biportal Endoscopic Spine Surgery

Basic and Advanced Technique

Springer

Editors
Dong Hwa Heo
Department of Neurosurgery
Seoul Bumin Hospital
Seoul, Korea (Republic of)

Cheol Woong Park
Department of Neurosurgery
Daejeon Woori Hospital
Daejeon, Korea (Republic of)

Sang Kyu Son
Department of Neurosurgery
PARK WEON WOOK Hospital
Busan, Korea (Republic of)

Jin Hwa Eum
Department of Neurosurgery
MEDREX Hospital
Seoul, Korea (Republic of)

ISBN 978-981-16-8203-2 ISBN 978-981-16-8201-8 (eBook)
https://doi.org/10.1007/978-981-16-8201-8

This Springer imprint is published by the registered company Springer Nature Singapore Pte Ltd.
The registered company address is: 152 Beach Road, #21-01/04 Gateway East, Singapore 189721, Singapore

Preface

The endoscopic spine surgery (ESS) has brought a new paradigm in the surgical treatment of spinal disorders about 20 years ago. Since then, there has been a remarkable development in technologies and the biomedical researches that many different approaches and instruments have been developed and applied. This is due to our colleagues, who, as experts in their fields, have dedicated their time and resources in research and shared their knowledge and experiences with others.

The unilateral biportal endoscopic (UBE) spine surgery has recently applied in ESS as well. Despite some skepticism, it has shown remarkable results and improvement of patients' quality of life after the surgery with significant other pros. UBE has proven to be very effective in certain situations with less hospital stay and postoperative complications leading to increase in the number of UBE performed, becoming one of the significant treatment of choice in recent years. This calls for the need of UBE textbook for those who want to learn the UBE to incorporate in their practice.

This book may give basic scientific knowledge and surgical skills as it has incorporated the advanced biomedical research and clinical practice in the interim. I do believe that this book is a milestone in ESS and definitely becomes a guiding light to many. ESS itself is an innovation and UBE as well, and this won't be the last. This book will provide continuous education to not only those who are new but also with well-established practice and skills.

I am honored to be part of this monumental project and being given the opportunity to endorse the first edition of UBE textbook in the world while I could serve as the third president of UBE research institute of Korea. I wish to express my appreciation to the authors who have dedicated their time and efforts for this book. This book could not have been edited without the dedicated help of our editor-in-chief, Dr. Dong Hwa Heo. My great respect to the editor-in-chief. Thank you.

Daejeon, Republic of Korea Cheol Woong Park

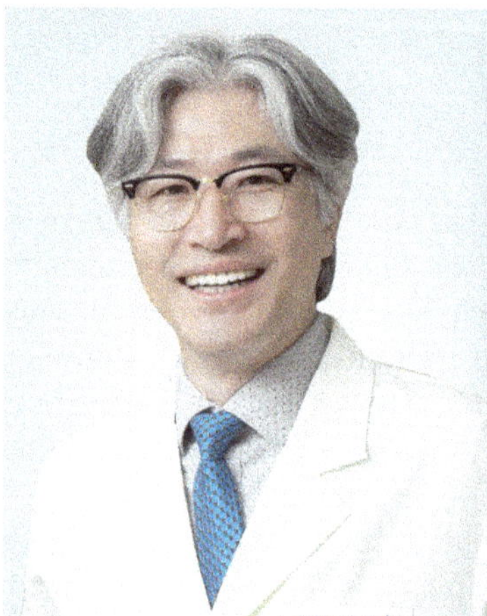
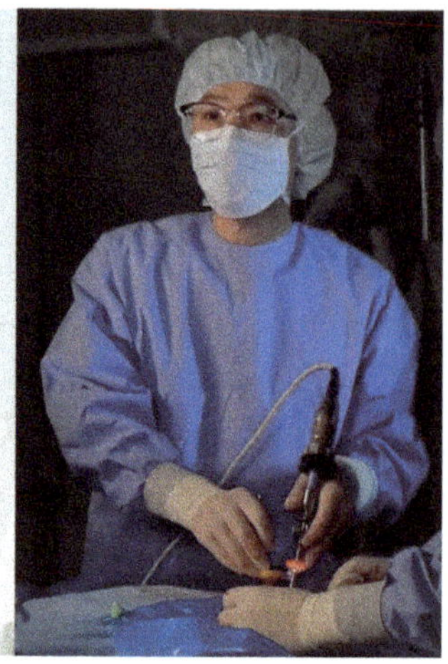

Preface

Unilateral Biportal Endoscopic Spine Surgery: A New Paradigm in Endoscopic Spine Surgery

Endoscopic spinal surgery is the most minimally invasive spine surgery.

Although the benefits of endoscopic surgery are well known, spine surgeons are difficult to learn because of the steep learning curve. In addition, due to unfamiliar surgical anatomy in endoscopic spine surgery and the possibility of incomplete decompression, it was even more difficult to attempt endoscopic spine surgery.

The basic surgical technique in unilateral biportal endoscopic (UBE) spine surgery is highly similar to microsurgery. Also, because UBE surgeries primarily entail a posterior spinal approach, the anatomical orientation is familiar to spinal surgeons. I believe that UBE is the easiest way to learn spinal endoscopic surgery.

Recently, many spinal surgeons performed UBE surgeries, and many UBE-related articles have been published worldwide. However, no textbook on UBE has been published. Accordingly, the Korean UBE Research Society has invited an expert on UBE to author and compile this textbook. I want to create the UBE textbook with a focus on practical content involving actual UBE surgery. We hope that this textbook published by the UBE Research Society in Korea will be of great help to spine surgeons interested in learning UBE surgery. Also, I would like to express my sincere thanks to the wonderful authors who authored the textbooks.

Seoul, Republic of Korea Dong Hwa Heo

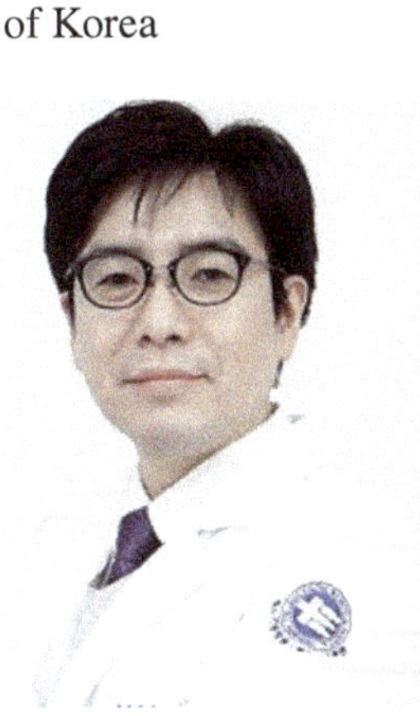

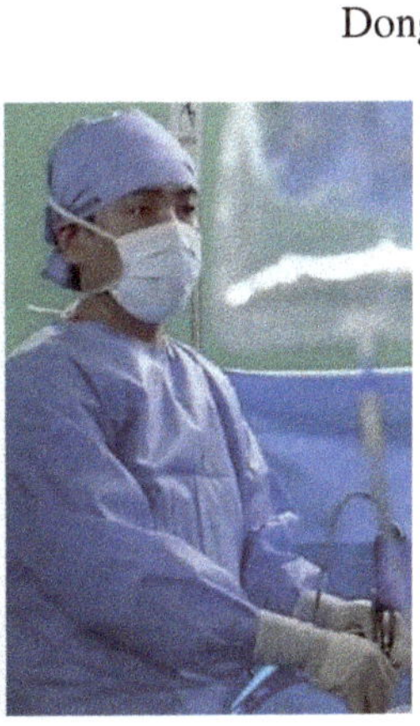

Preface

Once in a while, I recall one of my professors in medical school saying "Medical doctors exist because there are patients," which means that the health and happiness of the patients are the most important priority of doctors. While paying my respect to all my senior professors who are fully dedicated to patients in need, I always keep in mind that my utmost mission presently is to research and develop more advanced medical technology based on those valuable find-outs by my seniors of all ages.

The advancement of endoscopic spinal surgery, which embodies the minimal invasiveness including less muscle damage, is critical to preserving the integrity of the spine. The UBE technique combines the accessibility of open surgery, no visual or motion limitations, and the minimal invasiveness of endoscopic surgery. I believe that this harmonized UBE technique can make it happen, so called, the practical better-patient-care. UBE is the abbreviation of unilateral bi-portal endoscopy and it has a different surgical concept comparing the preceding transforaminal spine endoscopy. UBE makes two surgical ports in the same side of the spine, one for the endoscope and the other for the instruments. In the UBE technique, the endoscope and instruments move independently, so it achieves the same free movement that you might have in open surgery. UBE is a surgical technique that allows spine surgeons the freedom to use the same surgical indications as in open surgery while having no concerns that too much tissue damage might be done.

Spinal surgery techniques will be developed that replace the proven technical benefits and improve the shortcomings of our daily surgical routine. I personally hope that the present UBE can help many doctors and patients in need and be the initial manure to prepare for the quantum jump in the history of spinal surgery advancements. I hope this book helps you proceed on your long-term missionary journey for the better care of spine patients in need.

Busan, Republic of Korea Sang Kyu Son

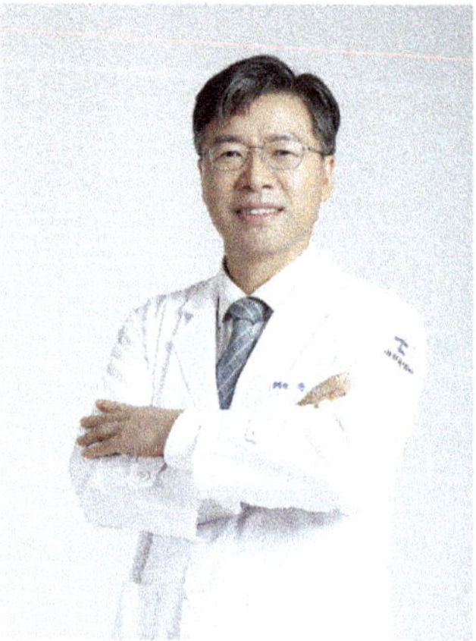
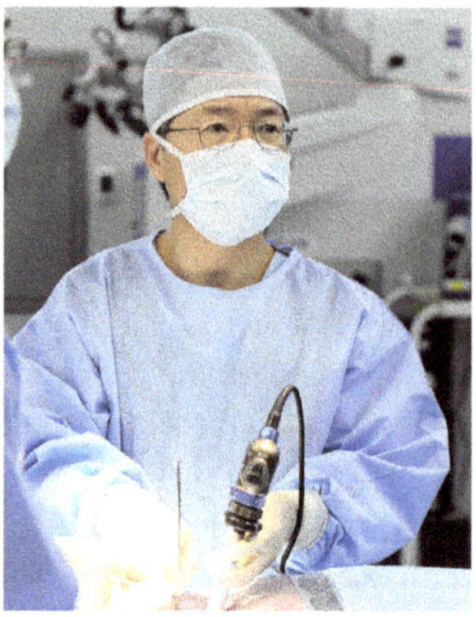

Preface

My name is Jin Hwa Eum, and it is my pleasure to introduce the UBE technique. Dr. Yeung Chul Choi and I first observed the biportal endoscopic spine surgery technique by Dr. Abdul Gaffar at AAOS, February 28, 2001. It was amazing and innovative, something we did not expect. Inspired, we discussed and studied it, trying to make the surgery easier. Now, the UBE technique has emerged as one of the most promising minimally invasive spine surgeries. During the past two decades, this technique was developed further by collaboration of many Korean spine surgeons. To encourage this teaching and outline the journey, this textbook will be a guide through the complex maze of endoscopic spine surgery.But most importantly, I would like to honor Dr. Choi, all the other authors, and young, ambitious spine surgeons. Finally, I sincerely appreciate all the patients who worked with surgeons to willingly undergo this surgery. Without everyone's endless effort and energy, the UBE technique as we know it wouldn't have been possible.

Al Ain, UAE

Jin Hwa Eum

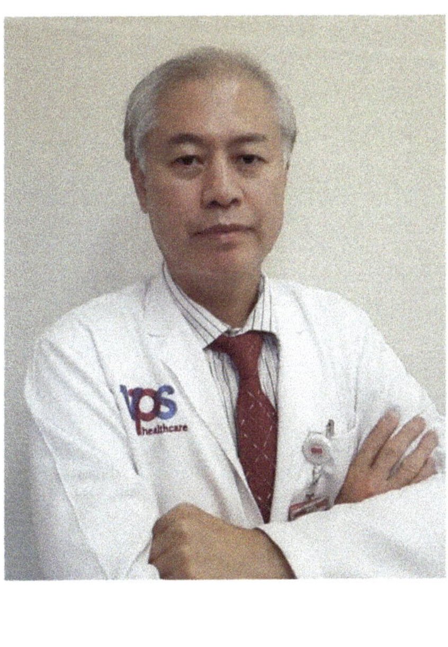

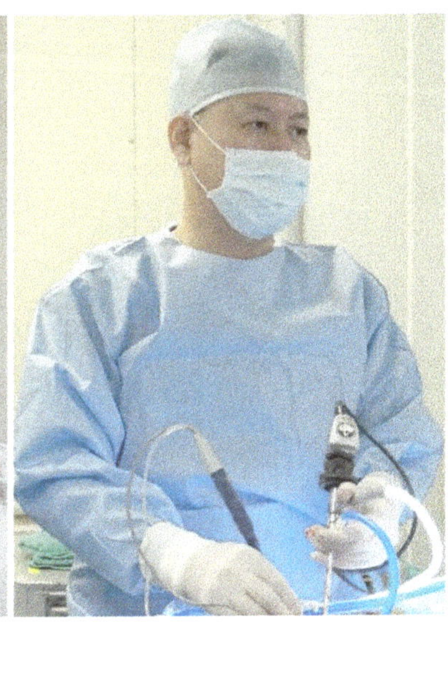

Congratulatory Address

In recent years, the field of endoscopic spinal surgery has witnessed remarkable advances and development, and endoscopic techniques are now taking their place as important methods for spinal surgery. Once again, I would like to thank the Korean spine surgeons who are leading the global development of endoscopic spinal surgery. I admire their efforts to organize and develop their passion and academic achievements through this textbook. Unilateral biportal endoscopy (UBE), which is considered to be the most innovative method of endoscopic spinal surgery and has recently been developed at a rapid pace, is a broadly-applicable surgical method that can be applied easily even by general spine surgeons. As the editor-in-chief of *Neurospine*, I am proud that many papers related to UBE have been published in *Neurospine* to help establish UBE as a surgical method used across the globe. In the future, we will continue our efforts to support endoscopic spine surgeons to publish many outstanding and innovative studies in *Neurospine*.

Again, as the editor-in-chief of *Neurospine*, I congratulate the authors on publishing this UBE textbook.

Ha Yoon

Department of Neurosurgery,
Severance Hospital, College of Medicine
Yonsei University, Seoul, South Korea

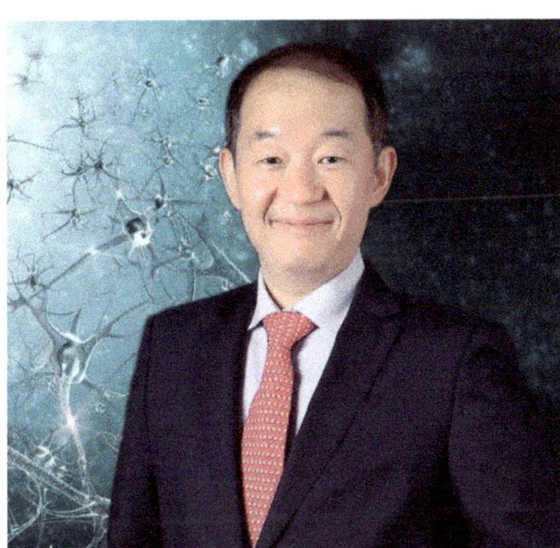

Publishing UBE Textbook

"Unilateral biportal endoscopy" has been the key phrase dominating clinical and scientific efforts in all surgical specialties over the last few years. Considering this aspect, a surgical textbook of UBE seemed useful. It has been a very great pleasure for us to review this magnificent textbook, which makes such an impression and contributes so much to its filed.

The editors have gathered experts in UBE and have presented them in a uniform way including the indications/contraindications, instruments, technical aspects of UBE, and complications. The contributors were chosen based on their expertise on a given topic. Each contributor was given the opportunity to describe their surgical techniques beyond that of a journal article or presentation; specifically, they were specifically asked to describe surgical techniques that they employed in performing the operative procedure that would achieve the maximum clinical outcome, while avoiding complications. An attempt was made to keep the text simple and to support it by operative images and video which are as easy to comprehend as possible.

We would like to express our deepest thanks to all authors who have contributed to this textbook and who have provided us with a tremendous amount of new information. We sincerely thank the staff of Springer publishers for their excellent constructive input and assistance with the book and the pleasant collaboration.

This book is a must for every spine surgeon who is contemplating the use of UBE, or has already some experience with them. It is our sincere hope that this book will contribute to the further understanding and acceptance of UBE philosophies in the emerging field of spinal surgery.

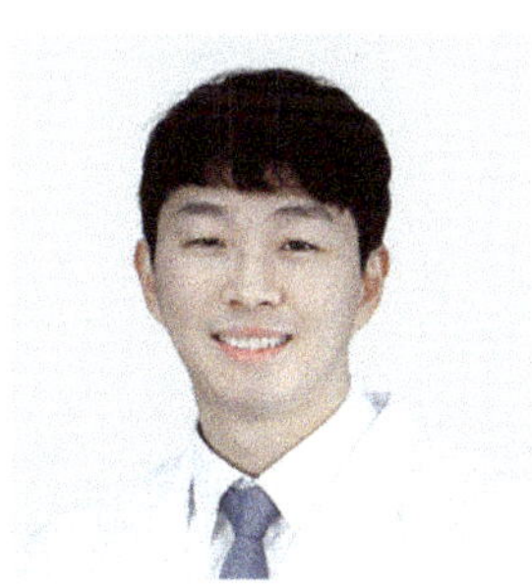

Man Kyu Park

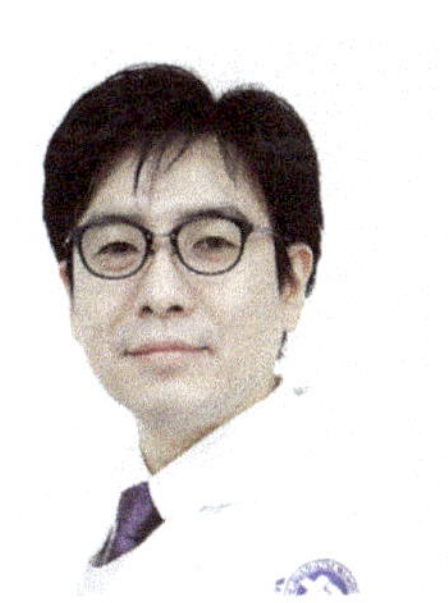

Dong Hwa Heo

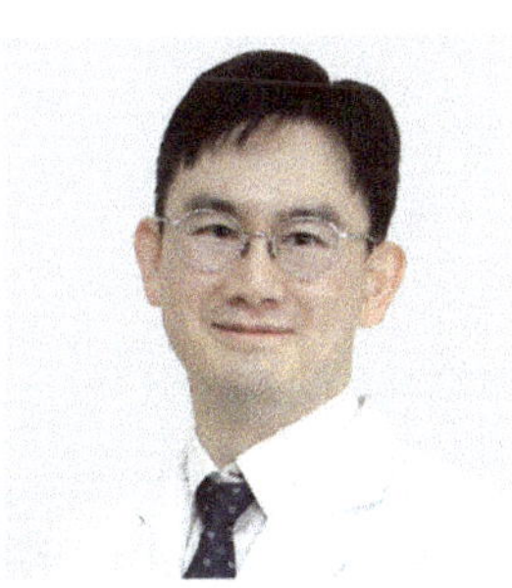

Ji Yeon Kim

Acknowledgement

This textbook was produced with the support of **the World UBE society, Korean minimally invasive spine surgery society (KOMISS)**, and **Neurospine**, the official journal of ASIA SPINE, the Neurospinal Society of Japan, Taiwan Neurosurgical Spine Society, and the Korean Spinal Neurosurgery Society.

Contents

Part I

Introduction

A Brief History of Unilateral Biportal Endoscopic Spine Surgery

1

Hee Seok Yang, Choon Keun Park, and Jeong Yoon Park

1.1 Introduction

Developments of endoscopy created a subfield of minimally invasive spine surgery that moves the point of visualization away from the surgeon's eye or microscope and puts it directly at the location of spine pathology [1]. Early endoscopic spine surgeons treated disc herniation instead of spinal stenosis and targeted repair of disc herniation that would be less invasive than traditional open techniques. Early endoscopic spine surgery was used primarily to treat disc herniation and proved to be less invasive than traditional open techniques. Surgeons now have the tools and knowledge to treat a myriad of spine pathologies beyond lumbar disc herniation.

The current position of the field of endoscopic spine surgery is the result of two directions of evolution: big-to-small and small-to-big [2]. Using as small as possible conventional incision, minimizing soft tissue damage, endoscopic spine surgery evolved to solve various spine pathologies.

Percutaneous one-portal endoscopic spine surgery has evolved from conventional spine surgery, and unilateral biportal endoscopic (UBE) spine surgery has been developed to overcome limitations of percutaneous one-portal endoscopic spine surgery. This article describes the history of UBE spine surgery and its major milestones and challenges that have resulted in a "powerful" minimally invasive spine surgical technology.

1.2 History

1.2.1 Innovations and the Initiation of UBE Spine Surgeries

In 1996, *De Antoni* et al. published the first technical note in which endoscope and instrument were inserted independently through two portals [3]. Two years later, they described the use of standard arthroscopic instruments for magnification, illumination, and irrigation and reported clinical results [4]. *Soliman* published surgical results for lumbar disc herniation and spinal stenosis in 2013 and 2015, using UBE techniques with independent portals, which is very similar to the current method [5, 6]. The surgical technique shown in Fig. 1.1 appears very similar to today's UBE technique.

H. S. Yang
Department of Neurosurgery, Seoul Barunsesang Hospital, Seoul, South Korea

C. K. Park
Department of Neurosurgery, Spine Center, The Leon Wiltse Memorial Hospital, Suwon, South Korea

J. Y. Park (✉)
Department of Neurosurgery, The Spine and Spinal Cord Institute, Gangnam Severance Hospital, Yonsei University College of Medicine, Seoul, South Korea
e-mail: spinepjy@yuhs.ac

D. H. Heo et al. (eds.), *Unilateral Biportal Endoscopic Spine Surgery*,
https://doi.org/10.1007/978-981-16-8201-8_1

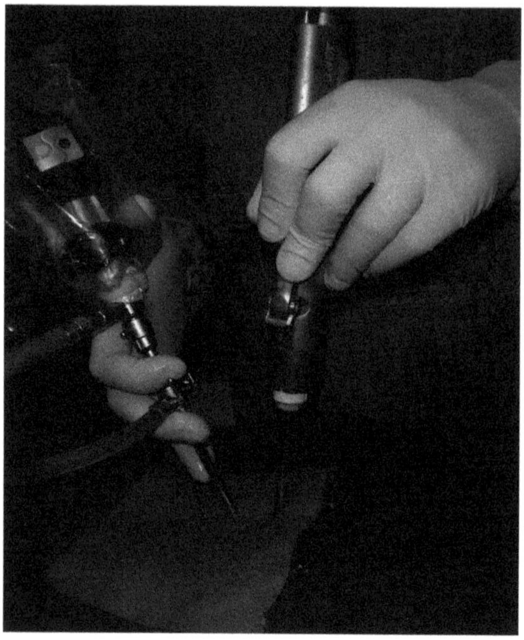

Fig. 1.1 Intraoperative image showing endoscope and arthroscopic shaver introduced through two separate portals. Figure from *Soliman*'s papers in 2013 and 2015

The term "biportal" was used first in 2016, and "UBE" was introduced in an article published in Korea [7–10]. Increased experience of endoscopic spine surgeons with UBE has led to an explosion of innovation, mainly in Korea. As a result, Korean surgeons were able to apply the UBE technique to various pathologies such as thoracic ossified yellow ligament and cervical approaches [11], which are considered challenging, as well as relatively common applications such as lumbar spinal stenosis [9], far-lateral disc herniation [12, 13], recurrent disc herniation [8], discitis, and abscess [14]. The biportal approach has enabled endplate preparation and foraminal decompression under direct visualization, which is vital for lumbar interbody fusion [15, 16]. All major UBE-related papers since 2016 have been published in Korea, which is attributed to Korea's independent history of UBE.

Based on various trials and clinical results of UBE, systematic reviews of literature and prospective randomized comparative studies have assessed the feasibility of spinal decompression [17, 18], and studies for maintaining stable water dynamics have been reported because it is an important step to a safer technique [19, 20]. Currently, UBE is recognized as the most important endoscopic surgery of the spine and can be applied in all areas of lumbar degenerative disease, including fusion, and can be applied to the cervical spine.

1.3 Brief UBE History in Korea

Abdul Gaffar presented the article, "Lumbar Disc Excision by Midline Extradural Endoscopy," at the 68th American Academy of Orthopedic Surgeons (AAOS) in 2001. Korean Dr. Young Chul Choi visited *Abdul Gaffar* in 2002, and began implementing UBE with *Uhm Jin-Hwa* for the first time in Korea (Fig. 1.2). In 2003, Jin Hwa Eum presented the article, "Endoscopic lumbar discectomy for far-lateral disc herniation," with biportal endoscope, at the 4th Biennial Korea-Japan Conference on Spine Surgery, in Japan. In 2013, Dr. Eum and another Korean UBE pioneer Sang Kyu Son presented, "Unilateral biportal endoscopic segmental sub-laminoplasty for lumbar central stenosis," at the International Society of Minimally Invasive Spine Surgery (ISMISS) in Japan. In 2013, Sang Kyu Son presented, "The endoscopic unilateral laminectomy and bilateral decompression (ULBD), foraminotomy and fusion using UBE," at the International Intradiscal Therapy Society (IITS) in Korea (Fig. 1.3). Workshops on UBE led by Sang Kyu Son were held for the first time in Korea in 2013 (Fig. 1.4).

In Korea, since 2002, independent trials and research of UBE have been conducted, and full-scale presentations of research results and related workshops have been held since 2013. Based on these achievements, The UBE Research Society was organized in 2017 and has contributed to the development and popularization of UBE procedures through its academic activities. The unique history of UBE in Korea includes a background that led to various research achievements and attempts related to UBE.

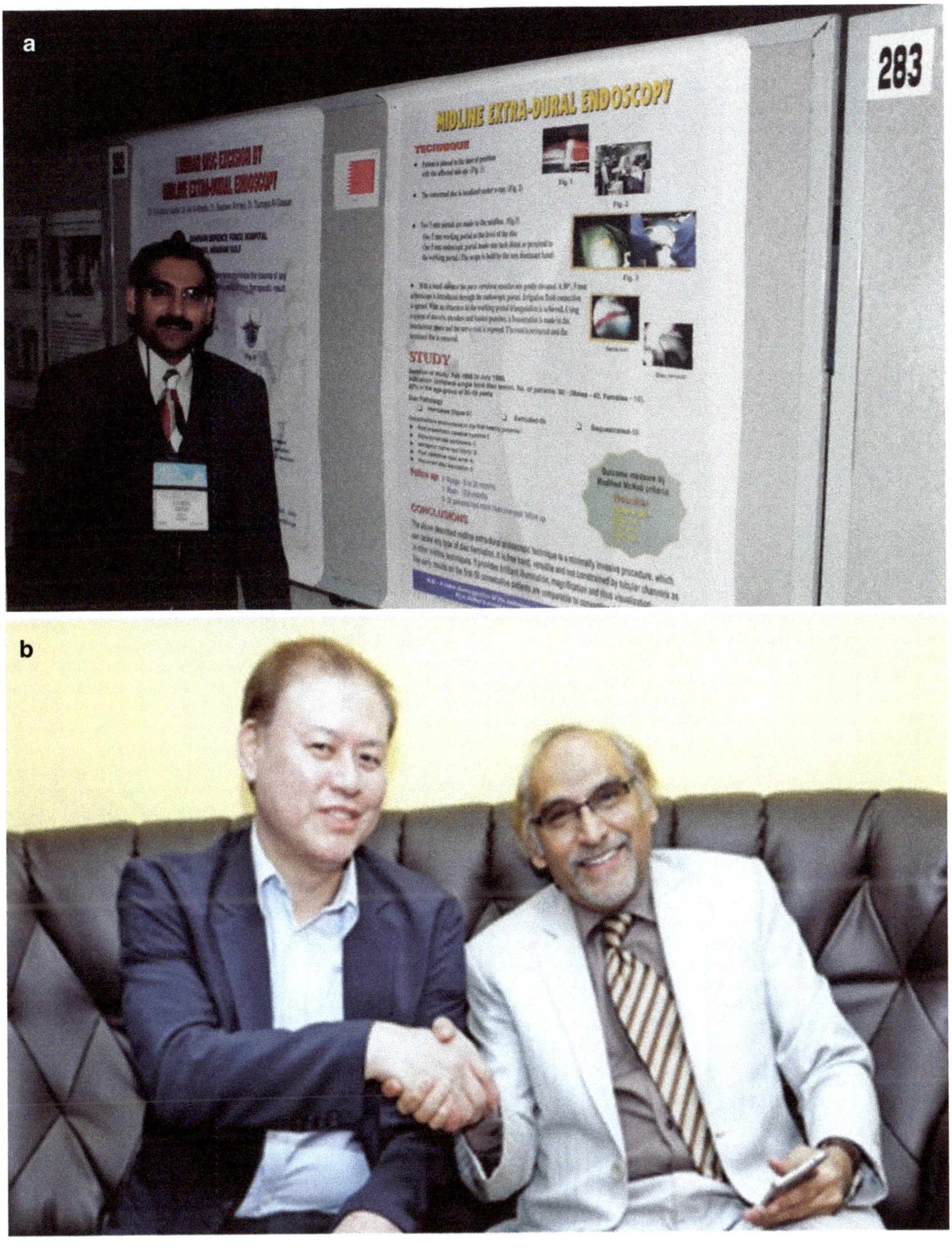

Fig. 1.2 (**a**) *Abdul Gaffar* presenting in 2001, and (**b**) Photograph of *Abdul Gaffar* (Rt) and Jin Hwa Eum (Lt) in 2018

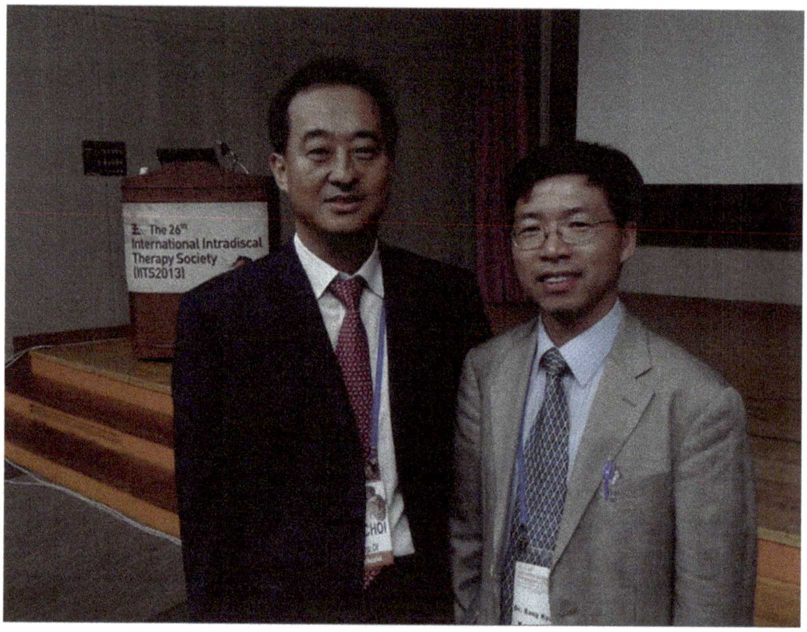

Fig. 1.3 Photograph of *Gun Choi* (Lt, President of International Intradiscal Therapy Society 2013) and Sang Kyu Son (Rt), in 2013

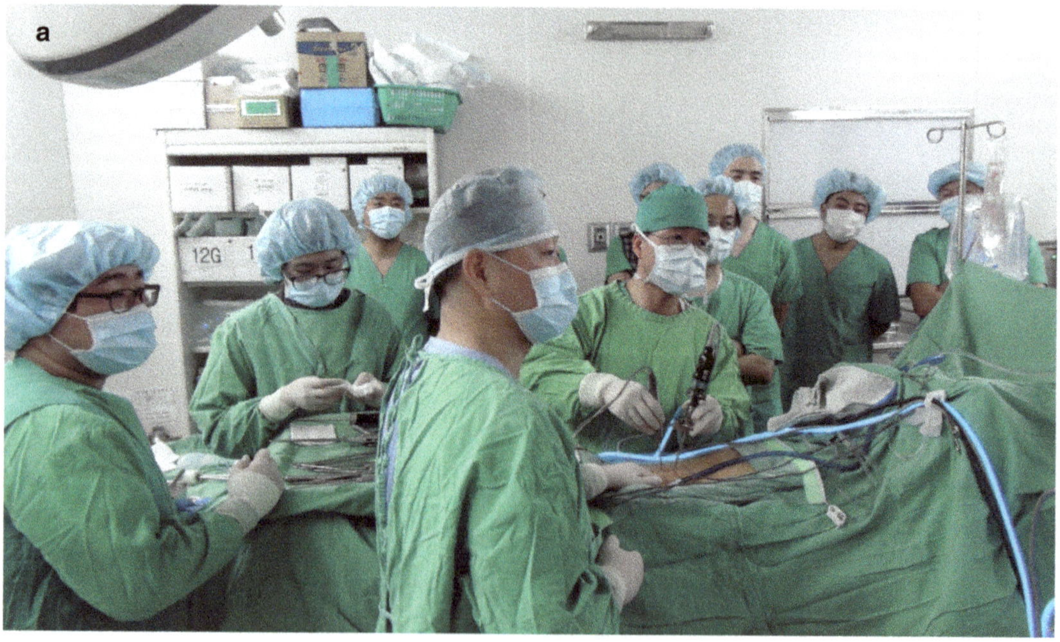

Fig. 1.4 UBE Korean live surgery (**a**) and seminar (**b**) in 2014

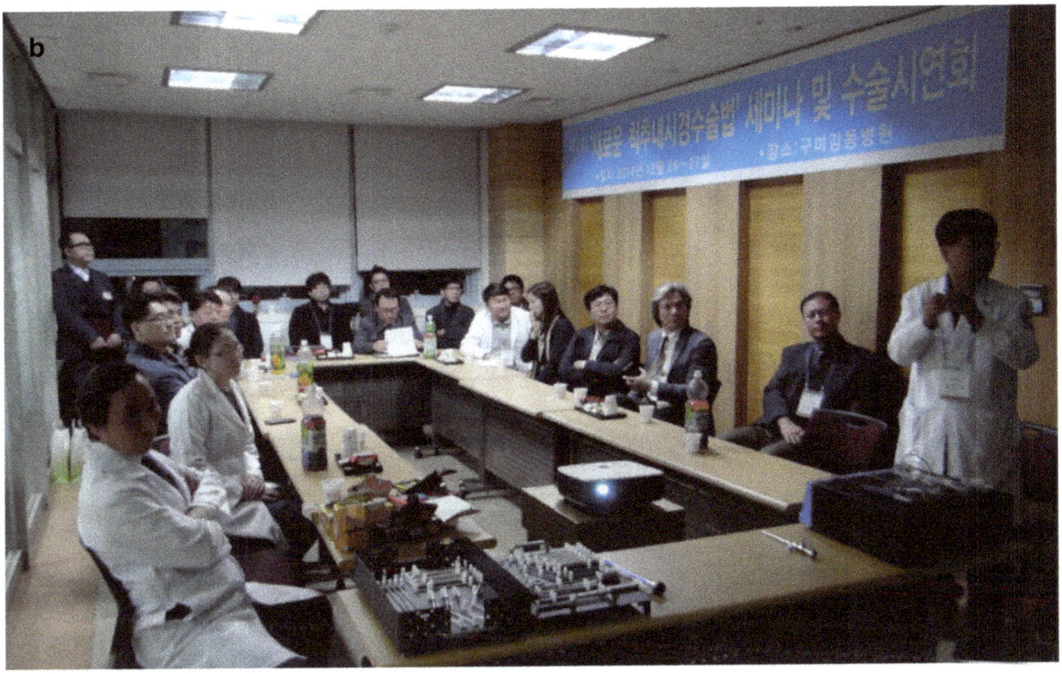

Fig. 1.4 (continued)

1.4 Future of UBE

The advantages of continuous irrigation (hemostasis, flushing of small bleeding, identification of the bleeding source, better identification of microanatomy, and separation of tissue layers by simple irrigation) and developments of instruments increased success rates and decreased recurrence rates of spinal surgeries using UBE. The indication spectrum of UBE spine surgery is expected to become wider and possibly cover all types of degenerative spinal pathologies.

References

1. Mayer HM. A history of endoscopic lumbar spine surgery: what have we learnt? Biomed Res Int. 2019;2019:4583943.
2. Telfeian AE, Veeravagu A, Oyelese AA, Gokaslan ZL. A brief history of endoscopic spine surgery. Neurosurg Focus. 2016;40(2):E2.
3. De Antoni DJ, Claro ML, Poehling GG, Hughes SS. Translaminar lumbar epidural endoscopy: anatomy, technique, and indications. Arthroscopy. 1996;12(3):330–4.
4. DeAntoni DJ, Claro ML, Poehling GG, Hughes SS. Translaminar lumbar epidural endoscopy: technique and clinical results. J South Orthop Assoc. 1998;7(1):6–12.
5. Soliman HM. Irrigation endoscopic discectomy: a novel percutaneous approach for lumbar disc prolapse. Eur Spine J. 2013;22(5):1037–44.
6. Soliman HM. Irrigation endoscopic decompressive laminotomy. A new endoscopic approach for spinal stenosis decompression. Spine J. 2015;15(10):2282–9.
7. Choi CM, Chung JT, Lee SJ, Choi DJ. How I do it? Biportal endoscopic spinal surgery (BESS) for treatment of lumbar spinal stenosis. Acta Neurochir. 2016;158(3):459–63.
8. Choi DJ, Jung JT, Lee SJ, Kim YS, Jang HJ, Yoo B. Biportal endoscopic spinal surgery for recurrent lumbar disc herniations. Clin Orthop Surg. 2016;8(3):325–9.
9. Hwa Eum J, Hwa Heo D, Son SK, Park CK. Percutaneous biportal endoscopic decompression for lumbar spinal stenosis: a technical note and preliminary clinical results. J Neurosurg Spine. 2016;24(4):602–7.
10. Eun SS, Eum JH, Lee SH, Sabal LA. Biportal endoscopic lumbar decompression for lumbar disk herniation and spinal canal stenosis: a technical note. J Neurol Surg A Cent Eur Neurosurg. 2017;78(4):390–6.

11. Park JH, Jun SG, Jung JT, Lee SJ. Posterior percutaneous endoscopic cervical foraminotomy and diskectomy with unilateral biportal endoscopy. Orthopedics. 2017;40(5):e779–e83.
12. Akbary K, Kim JS, Park CW, Jun SG, Hwang JH. Biportal endoscopic decompression of exiting and traversing nerve roots through a single interlaminar window using a contralateral approach: technical feasibilities and morphometric changes of the lumbar canal and foramen. World Neurosurg. 2018;117:153–61.
13. Park JH, Jung JT, Lee SJ. How I do it: L5/S1 foraminal stenosis and far-lateral lumbar disc herniation with unilateral bi-portal endoscopy. Acta Neurochir. 2018;160(10):1899–903.
14. Kang T, Park SY, Lee SH, Park JH, Suh SW. Spinal epidural abscess successfully treated with biportal endoscopic spinal surgery. Medicine (Baltimore). 2019;98(50):e18231.
15. Heo DH, Son SK, Eum JH, Park CK. Fully endoscopic lumbar interbody fusion using a percutaneous unilateral biportal endoscopic technique: technical note and preliminary clinical results. Neurosurg Focus. 2017;43(2):E8.
16. Heo DH, Eum JH, Jo JY, Chung H. Modified far lateral endoscopic transforaminal lumbar interbody fusion using a biportal endoscopic approach: technical report and preliminary results. Acta Neurochir. 2021;163(4):1205–9.
17. Lin GX, Huang P, Kotheeranurak V, Park CW, Heo DH, Park CK, et al. A systematic review of unilateral biportal endoscopic spinal surgery: preliminary clinical results and complications. World Neurosurg. 2019;125:425–32.
18. Park SM, Kim GU, Kim HJ, Choi JH, Chang BS, Lee CK, et al. Is the use of a unilateral biportal endoscopic approach associated with rapid recovery after lumbar decompressive laminectomy? A preliminary analysis of a prospective randomized controlled trial. World Neurosurg. 2019;128:e709–e18.
19. Kang MS, Park HJ, Hwang JH, Kim JE, Choi DJ, Chung HJ. Safety evaluation of biportal endoscopic lumbar discectomy: assessment of cervical epidural pressure during surgery. Spine (Phila Pa 1976). 2020;45(20):E1349–e56.
20. Hong YH, Kim SK, Hwang J, Eum JH, Heo DH, Suh DW, et al. Water dynamics in unilateral biportal endoscopic spine surgery and its related factors: an in vivo proportional regression and proficiency-matched study. World Neurosurg. 2021;149:e836–e43.

The Basics and Concepts of Unilateral Biportal Endoscopy

2

Sang-Kyu Son, Dong Han Kim, and Hayati Aygün

2.1 All Endoscopic Procedures Require a Working Space

In 1853, Antoine Jean Desormeaux of France developed an instrument specifically designed to examine the urinary tract and bladder. He named it an "endoscope," and it was the first time this term was used in history [1]. Kussmaul is generally credited as being the first to perform a gastroscopy in 1868 [1]. Laparoscopy or endoscopically examining the peritoneal cavity was first attempted in 1901 by Gorge Kelling [1]. Thereafter, much progress has been made, which also established the foundation for the development of robotic abdominal surgery. Professor Kenji Takagi in Tokyo has traditionally been credited with performing the first arthroscopic examination of a knee joint in 1918 [2]. Now, arthroscopic surgery is one of the main surgeries performed in orthopedics. Endoscopic spinal surgery began as percutaneous endoscopic discectomy. Kambin (1973) and Hijikata et al. (1975) attempted the earliest percutaneous nucleotomy in the 1970s [3]. However, endoscopic spinal surgery is still not considered a mainstream technique in the spinal surgical field.

S.-K. Son (✉) · D. H. Kim
Neurosurgery, Spine Center, Parkweonwook Hospital, Busan, South Korea

H. Aygün
Orthopedic Surgery, Spine Center, Medicabil Hospital, Bursa, Turkey

Endoscopic spinal surgery starts late compared to other surgical fields. The reason may be that the spine, from an anatomical point of view, has no working space for surgeons to perform surgery [4]. To acquire working space, gastroscopy uses the lumen of the stomach and laparoscopy utilizes the potential cavity which is made by CO_2 infusion to the abdominal space. Knee arthroscopy uses the joint cavity, which already exists anatomically, and shoulder arthroscopy is performed in the extra-cavitary area, which is secured after removing the subacromial bursa. In the spine, which has no anatomical working space, the important meaning of Kambin's triangle is to supply the corridor that allows the initial approach to the lumbar disc lesion in endoscopic surgery [4].

Unilateral biportal endoscopy (UBE) is endoscope-assisted spinal surgery, which requires making a series of working spaces with potential space around the spine. There could be a posterior or transforaminal approach depending upon the location of the pathologic region. "Son's space" is the important anatomical working space in the posterior approach (Fig. 2.1). There are two potential spaces in the posterior part, the interfascicular space, which is located between the two small muscles of the multifidus, and the other is the space containing fat and connective tissue located between the multifidus and the lamina. If these two potential spaces can be converted to an atraumatic working corridor and space, UBE

D. H. Heo et al. (eds.), *Unilateral Biportal Endoscopic Spine Surgery*,
https://doi.org/10.1007/978-981-16-8201-8_2

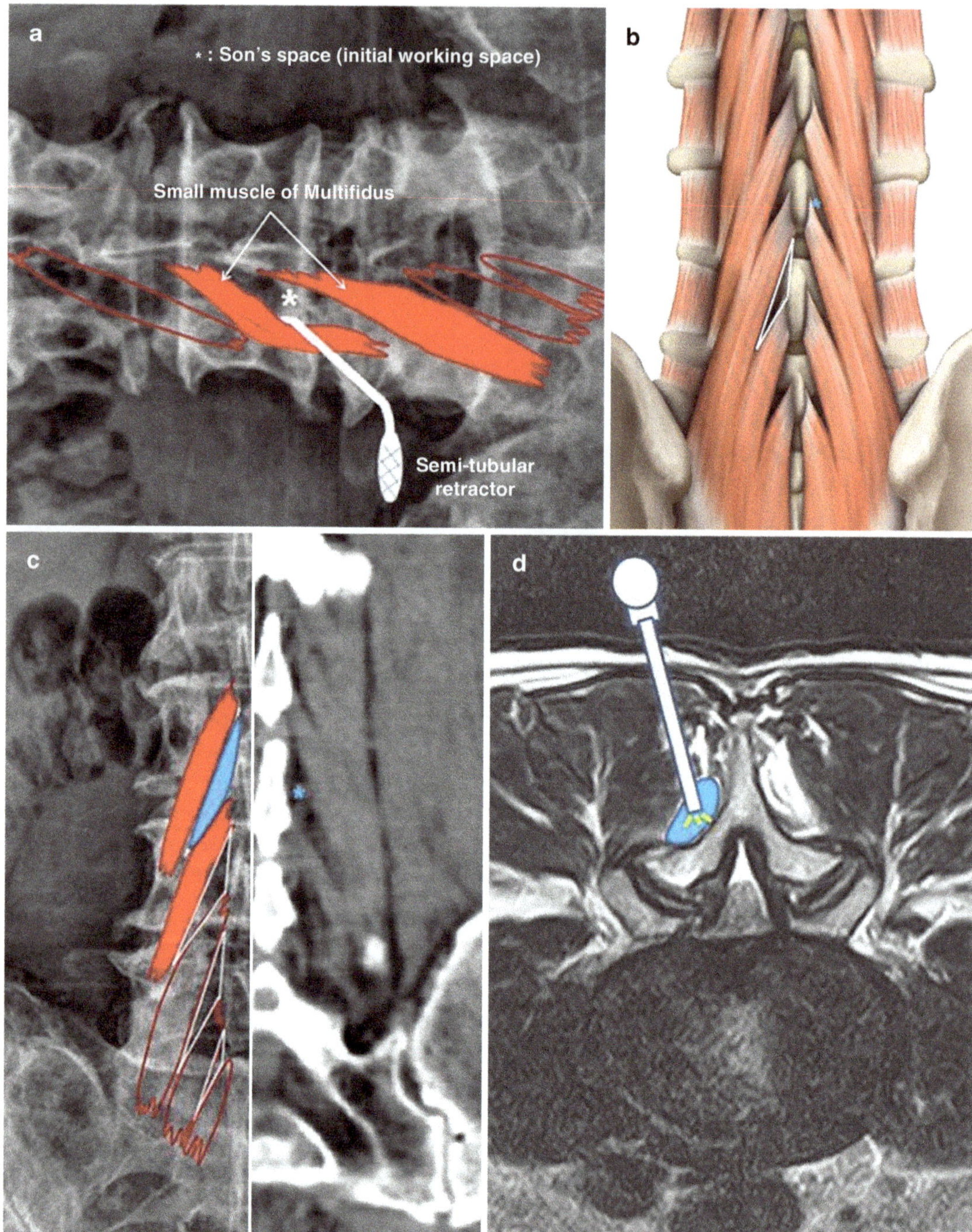

Fig. 2.1 (**a–d**). Son's space is a three-dimensional working space made by two main forces, mechanical retraction and hydrostatic pressure, which is planned and designed for less tissue damage

guarantees the same indications as conventional spinal surgery and achieves minimally invasive spinal surgery as in spinal endoscopy. In the transforaminal approach, the surrounding area of the foramen with fat and connective tissue acts as the working space.

Following are the steps for acquiring an atraumatic working corridor and space through the posterior approach:

1. Check the true anteroposterior view of the C-arm radiography.
2. The initial target point on the C-arm view is the junction of the spinous process and the lamina.
3. Make a skin incision for the working portal, which is roughly located on the medial margin of the lower pedicle.
4. Make a skin incision for the scopic portal, which is generally located 3-cm cranially from the working portal.
5. Incise 1-cm for two portals. The authors prefer transverse incision.
6. Insert the core dilator for the working portal under C-arm radiography. It is important that the core dilator is inserted through the interfascicular space without resistance. The direction of the core dilator is from the medial margin of the lower pedicle to the junction of the spinous process and the lamina. The upper small muscle of the multifidus anatomically attaches to the mamillary body of the lower superior articular process (SAP), which is slightly lateral to the medial wall of the lower pedicle.
7. Insert all serial dilators for the working portal and move them medio-caudally 2–3 times. This motion can separate the two small multifidus muscles to widen the working space with less muscle damage.
8. Remove the serial dilators from the working portal and insert the directional guide, which maintains the working portal tunnel.
9. Insert a serial dilator for the scopic portal to the initial target point and finally, make a triangulation between the working portal and the scopic portal.
10. Insert the sheath with an obturator through the scopic portal. The tip of the sheath must touch the lamina directly for less soft tissue in front of the lens.
11. Move the directional guide to remove some soft tissue in front of the tip of the sheath. This motion is called the "sleeve-up technique."
12. Insert the endoscope through the scopic sheath. Clear visibility of the lamina indicates proper placement. If the lamina is not visible, the scope should be touched to the bone, and the freer elevator through working portal help remove some of the soft tissue in front of the scope.
13. Insert the specially designed semi-tubular retractor through the working portal and retract the upper small multifidus muscle. This retraction can make a wider working space.
14. Check the output of the irrigating saline.
15. Finally, visualize the lamina with some fat and connective tissue. The space above the lamina is the initial working space. After drilling out some bone, there will be a clearer and wider space, which is called the true working space.

2.2 UBE Is Fluid-medium Surgery, Not Air-based

In open surgery, the surgical space is secured by clearing the soft tissue, which includes muscle, fat, and other tissue through many retraction movements with a self-retractor, and the space becomes filled with air. Because there is no influence or complication caused by the air filling the space, surgeons do not consider the air as an important clinical factor. Endoscopic spinal surgery is a fluid-medium surgery, which is similar to joint arthroscopic surgery that uses irrigating saline. UBE has an operational concept similar to that of joint arthroscopic surgery. In UBE surgery, two surgical portals are needed on the same side of the spine; one is for the endoscope and the other is for the instruments. Irrigating saline enters the endoscopic portal and leaves through the working portal (Fig. 2.2). Continuous and controlled circulation of the saline is the critical factor in performing successful UBE surgery.

Although UBE has a similar surgical concept as that of knee joint arthroscopy, the anatomy and anatomical circumstances are quite different. Therefore, to prevent fluid-related complications, which are the main stumbling block for beginners, it is important to understand the anatomical differences between the knee joint and the spine. The knee joint has a cavity with an envelope, but the spine does not enough have space for surgery. Therefore, UBE should use the secured working space, but the factitious space in UBE does not have an envelope and is very close to the epidural space without any separating structure. With a better understanding of the anatomical differences, care should be taken to control the saline pressure to not negatively affect the neural system while performing UBE surgery. Another point to remember is that the spine has a much greater anatomical distance from the skin to the lamina compared to the skin to the joint cavity in the knee. Thus, the outflow of the irrigating saline is not very smooth and there is a high risk of complications due to high hydrostatic pressure. To prevent the fundamental risk of complications in fluid-medium surgery, the standard use of the specially designed semi-tubular retractor, which functions as a control device for guaranteeing outflow and maintaining controlled pressure inside the working space, is recommended.

The optimal hydrostatic pressure is 30–50 mmHg, which varies according to the distance between the irrigating saline bag and the working space. Usually, the working space in the patient is fixed, and the height of the saline bag decides the pressure. The pressure (mmHg) is calculated by dividing the distance (cm) between the patient and the saline bag by 1.36. [height(cm) ÷

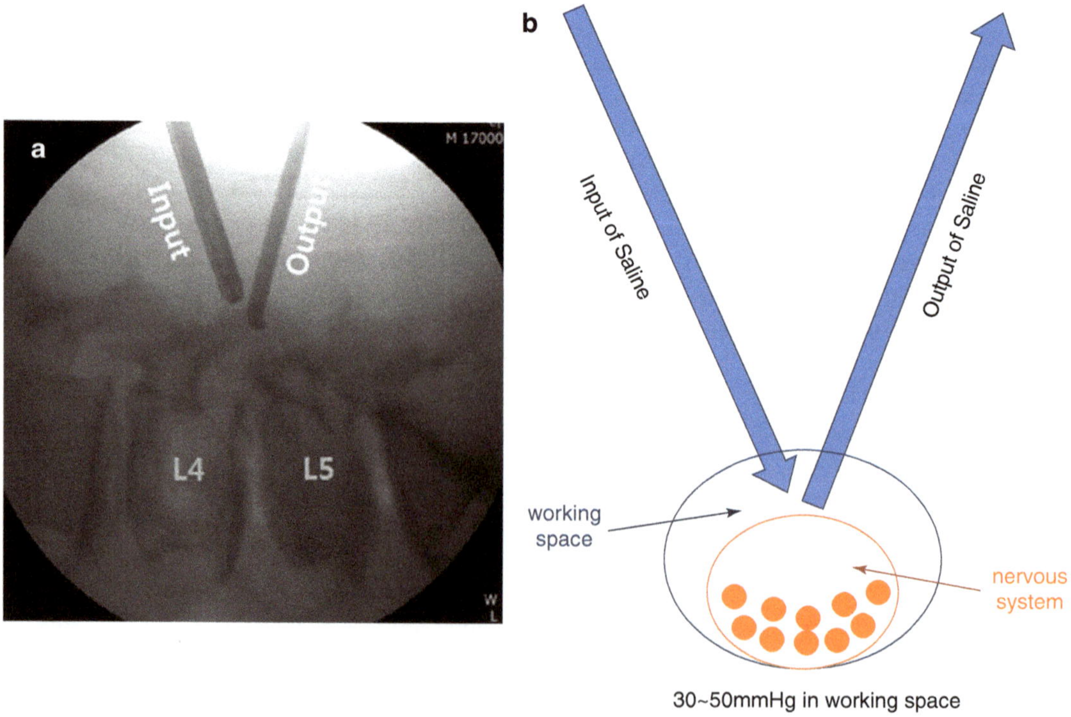

Fig. 2.2 UBE is fluid-medium surgery, with an input of irrigating saline through the endoscopic portal and an output through the working portal. The optimal pressure in the working space is 30–50 mmHg. (**a**) C-arm radiography. (**b**) Illustration of fluid input and output in UBE

1.36 = pressure (mmHg)] [5]. The authors prefer natural drainage than a pump-controlled system.

Three main factors are related to fluid-related complications. First, excessive saline pressure in the epidural space impacts the neural system. It causes a headache, nuchal pain, long-level epidural bleeding, delayed awakening from general anesthesia, seizure, intracranial hematoma, and blindness due to retinal bleeding [6, 7]. Second, although rare, a massive abdominal fluid collection could occur while performing the paraspinal approach. It is caused by massive damage to the intertransverse membrane and ligaments, which function as a barrier between the back and abdominal cavity. Third, the patient could experience hypothermia, which means low body temperature, caused by the prolonged use of cold saline. Therefore, tepid saline is recommended, and a heating pad on the surgical table can help prevent this complication.

2.3 The General UBE System

(A) The operating room setting (Fig. 2.3)

1. Operating team: surgeon (A), assistant (B), scrub nurse (C), circulating nurse, anesthesiologist, and radiological technician.
2. Equipment: endoscopic system (endoscope, camera, cable, and monitor) and drilling system (a), C-arm radiography and monitor (b), and radiofrequency system (RF), irrigating saline and pole, operating Table (O), anesthetic device and displays.

(B) The operation setting

1. Anesthesia

All common anesthesia methods such as local, epidural, spinal, and general anesthesia

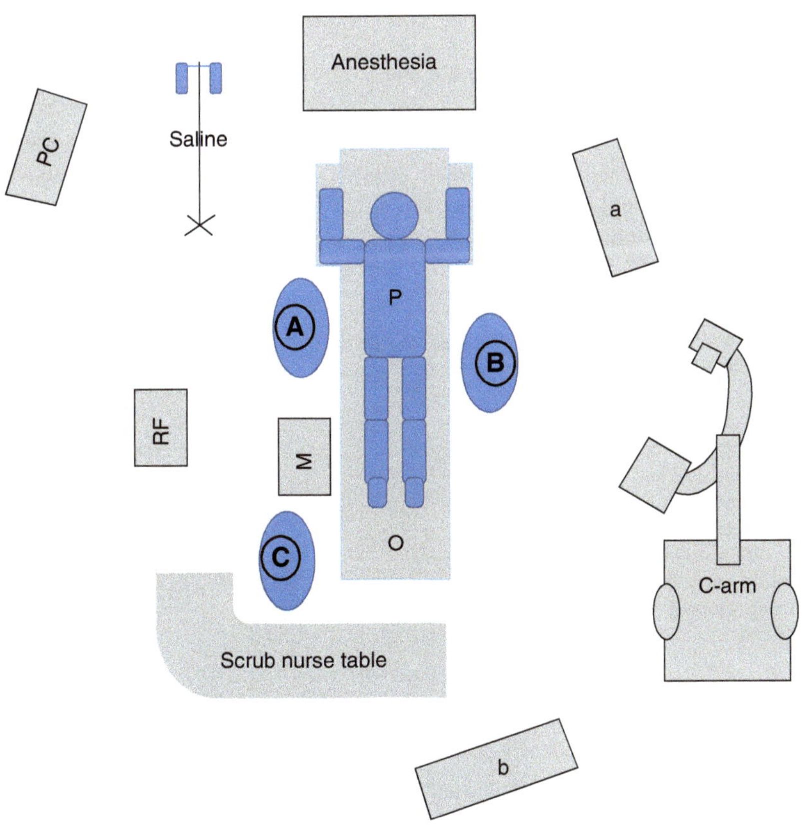

Fig. 2.3 Graphical illustration of the basic operating room setting in the author's hospital. A: surgeon, B: assistant, C: scrub nurse, P: patient, O: operating table, a: endoscopic and drilling systems, b: monitor for C-arm radiography, PC: computer, RF: radiofrequency device, M: Mayo table, Anesthesia: anesthetic device and displays

can be used in UBE surgery. In reality, general anesthesia or local anesthesia and sedation with midazolam and dexmedetomidine (Precedex) are usually applied.

2. Position

Generally, the prone position is applied. In the Knee-chest position, which is commonly used in open surgery, abdominal pressure would be increased, it could cause epidural bleeding. Thus, the authors commonly apply a flat rolling pad instead of the Wilson frame.

3. Drape

Considering that UBE surgery uses lots of irrigating saline during surgery, an endo-spine pack with a fluid-collecting bag should be applied. If a ready-made UBE specialized surgical drape is not available, try to make a hump around the operative site and attach a sterilized vinyl bag to collect the used saline.

4. Location of the surgical system and irrigating saline lines

In the case of a right-handed surgeon, the operator commonly stands on the left side of the patient. The left hand, which is the non-dominant hand, holds the endoscope, so the endoscope-related lines, camera cable, and irrigating saline line, should be tucked to the left side of the operator. The drilling system and RF system should be fixed at the right side of the surgeon. A rubber tube is attached to the drill handpiece for draining the used saline. Also, another rubber tube is attached to the RF wand, which functions as a drain for saline warmed by the RF firing (Fig. 2.4).

5. Bag of irrigating saline

Hydraulic pressure is important for a safe and smooth operation and it can be controlled by gravity. If the saline bag is placed at the height of the operator's head, it comes to be placed as high as 50–70 cm above the patient's back, and the water pressure inside stays around 37–51 mmHg. (Fig. 2.5).

(C) Surgical tools

1. Endoscope

The 0-degree endoscope is commonly used because it blocks any vision distortion that could be caused by an angled lens. In some exceptional cases, such as the ventral area of the thoracic dura matter, 30 degrees endoscope might help.

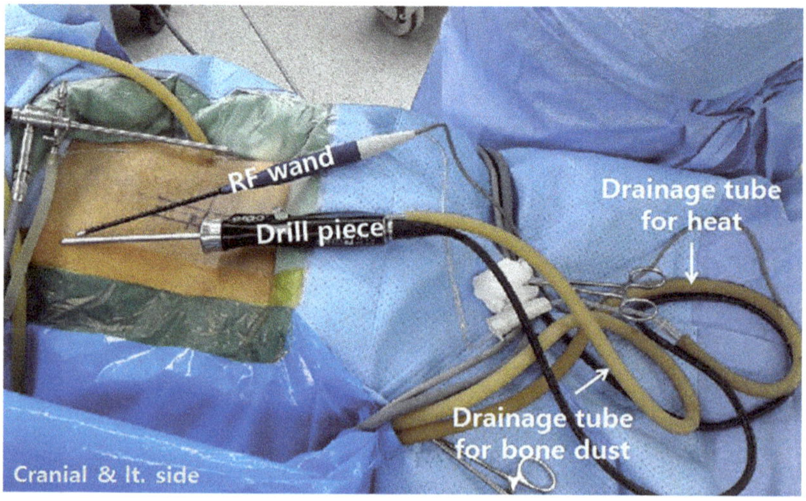

Fig. 2.4 Picture of the operating field setting. A rubber tube is attached to the drill handpiece for draining the used saline and bone dust and another tube is connected to the RF wand for draining the saline warmed by RF firing. Drainage occurs by gravity

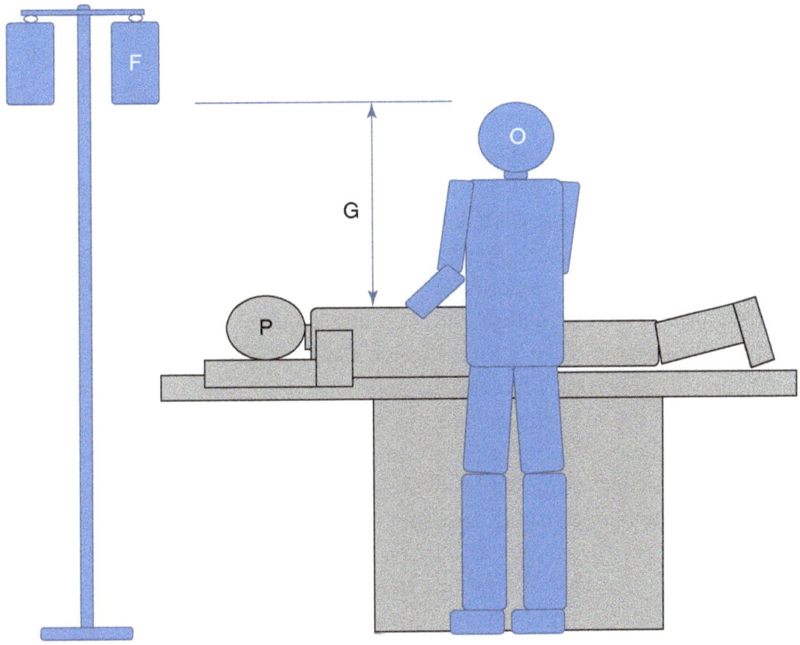

Fig. 2.5 Hydraulic pressure can be controlled by gravity. O: Operator, F: Fluid bag, P: Patient, G: Gab between Fluid bag and operating field. If the saline bag is placed at the height of the operator's head, it comes to be placed as high as 50–70 cm above the patient's back, and the water pressure inside stays around 37–51 mmHg

2. Drilling system

I use the drill burr with a sheath commonly used in arthroscopy. However, occasionally, a high-speed drill without a sheath is applied for areas near sensitive cord levels. A standard endoscopic drill burr with a sheath is effective for controlling the water pressure in the working space and for bone dust drainage, which can be accomplished by the interactive cooperation of an assistant. The assistant controls the flow of saline by crimping the rubber tube on and off. While the operator is drilling, the assistant closes the rubber tube by bending the tube, which helps to increase the saline pressure inside the operating field, and accordingly, the soft tissue and dura are pushed away to make a larger working space (Fig. 2.6). Finally, the assistant's action helps the UBE surgeon achieve safer drilling. While off-drilling, the rubber tube is in the open position and the bone dust inside comes to be drained smoothly by the difference in gravity between the end-tip attached to the drill handpiece and the other end-tip of the tube, which is placed in a bucket on the floor.

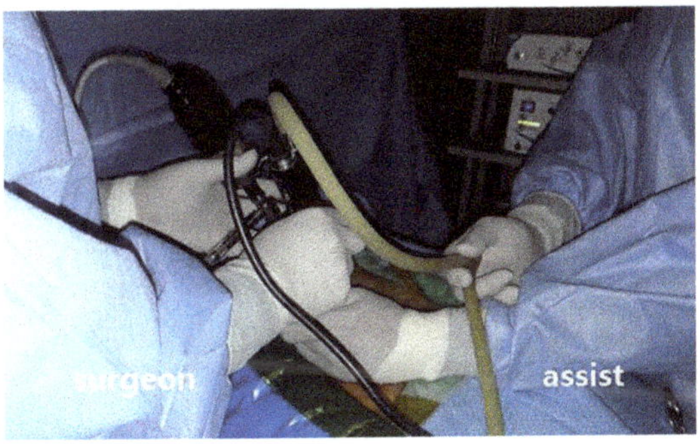

Fig. 2.6 The cooperation of the surgeon and assistant is very important in performing UBE. The assistant has a key role in controlling the flow of saline by crimping the rubber tube on and off and holding the semi-tubular retractor designed for controlling water circulation

3. RF system

RF plasma is a very effective energy source for coagulation and ablation in fluid situations. The heat generated by RF firing can vary depending upon the irrigation flow rate, the RF power level, and firing time. Commonly, operating field's temperature varies between 35 and 95 degrees Celsius [8]. According to an experiment that observed the tissue changes from an RF frequency of 42 degrees Celsius applied to the rat dorsal root ganglion and sciatic nerve, there were no histological changes and all clinical symptoms were recovered after a maximum of 21 days. However, 80 degrees Celsius heat caused permanent tissue damage [9]. Even low-temperature heat that is applied continuously can cause moderate-temperature burns, which could cause protein denaturation [10], and then it may be possible to be spinal muslce damage by using RF. The risk of tissue damage can be decreased by draining the heated saline through a rubber tube attached to the RF wand (Fig. 2.5) and frequent, short-term and brief use of the RF wand is recommended rather than one prolonged application.

Following are the energy parameters recommended for RF application (based on the Arthrocare® RF device): (Table 2.1).

4. Surgical instruments

There is a specially designed UBE toolset, which is comprised of devices for establishing the standard UBE surgical pathway and performing all surgical steps. Also, the Rotating Kerrison punch and the Curved Kerrison punch are essential for UBE surgery.

(D) Blood pressure

Optimal blood pressure (BP) is essential for a bloodless endoscopic view. The optimal systolic BP is 90–100 mmHg in general anesthesia and 120–130 mmHg in local anesthesia. This reference value is based on the author's vast personal experiences. Further randomized and systemized study is needed.

Table 2.1 The energy parameters recommended for RF application

	The energy parameter (based on the Arthrocare® RF device)	
	Ablation	Coagulation
The area above the bone	7	2
The epidural space	3	1
Near the dura matter	x	1

2.4 UBE Should Be Performed with a Complete Understanding of the Eight Basic Concepts

Most spine surgeons have varied experience with many different methods of spinal surgery. However, in most cases, surgeons perceive new surgical techniques based on their own knowledge and limited experiences. Therefore, it is natural to revert to their own routine surgical methods or just modify the new technique to fit their own routine method. Every surgical technique has pros and cons. Therefore, continuous efforts should be made to improve the weak points. Every surgical technique has its own distinct basic concepts. In the learning curve period of a new technique, trials to understand and utilize the new basic concepts should be ongoing. By doing so, a consistently desirable surgical outcome is guaranteed while minimizing the possibility of complications.

UBE has eight basic concepts as follows (Fig. 2.7)**:**

1. Unilateral biportal endoscopy

The very first use of the terminology "biportal" used in spinal endoscopy was in the "bilateral biportal approach" in the late 1990s, and it referred to the surgical approach to the transforaminal area in percutaneous endoscopic lumbar discectomy (PELD) [11]. UBE applies the knee arthroscopy surgical concept to the spine, and that is why UBE is simply explained as a biportal system. UBE is spinal endoscopy where two portals are made in the same (unilateral) side of the spine. One is used as the endoscopic portal and the other is used as the working portal. When this new spinal endoscopy technique was started in early 2000, the author intentionally

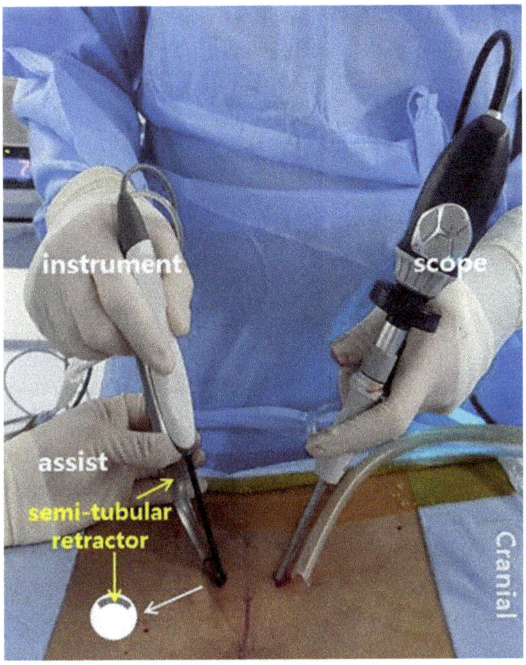

Fig. 2.7 UBE is unilateral biportal endoscopy. The nondominant hand of the surgeon holds the endoscope and the other hand handles the instruments. The assistant places a specially designed semi-tubular retractor in the working portal. The small portion of the circle in the working portal is covered by the retractor and the other portion is free. Then, UBE adopts a semi-tubular system

called "unilateral biportal endoscopy (UBE)" to differentiate it from the "bilateral biportal approach" in PELD.

The benefit of the unilateral approach is that the surgeon uses the same surgical route as in open surgery and the benefit of biportal endoscopy is that the endoscope of the endoscopic portal and the instruments of the working portal move independently. The functionality of the independent movement of the devices in each portal enables the surgeons to eliminate visual and motion limitations.

2. Fluid-medium surgery

UBE uses irrigating saline, whereas open surgery does not use any medium. While performing UBE, the working space becomes filled with irrigating saline and that is why it is called fluid-medium surgery. Continuous saline output is critically important, and the controlled management of the saline output influences the hydrostatic pressure in the working space, which enables the surgeons to have a clear view of the surgical field, facilitating safer surgery. For details, please refer to the "UBE is fluid-medium surgery, not air-based" section.

3. Triangulation

The lens of the endoscope is located in the front-most position of the endoscope. In the beginning stage of UBE surgery, it is not easy to place the instruments under endoscopic view due to many reasons. A triangular formation should be made by positioning the endoscope and surgical instruments very close together at the tips of the devices. True triangulation means locating the ends of the instruments just in front of the lens of the endoscope (Fig. 2.2a). If the endoscope and instruments are crossing each other in the shaft, each interferes with the other's movement. This situation is called 'early triangulation' and repositioning should be performed under c-arm radiography. Also, if the endoscope cannot be made to face the instruments at the tip, it will not be possible to find the instrument in the endoscopic view. This is called "open triangulation" and this should also be repositioned under c-arm radiography.

4. Semi-tubular system at the working portal

Although open surgery has no visual or motion limitations because the surgical field is a sufficient size, it has the disadvantage that it could be destructive surgery. To overcome this handicap, many trials of minimally invasive surgical approaches have taken place. The first and typical concept is the tubular system. Microendoscopic discectomy (MED) and PELD are representative examples of the effort to overcome the destructive aspect of open surgery [12].

UBE adopts a semi-tubular system. A semi-tubular retractor is tugged into the working portal by a surgical assistant to help the surgeon place and remove instruments while maintaining the smooth outflow of saline and tugging away neural system or soft tissue in the working space for a clear view. A small portion of the circle in the working portal is covered by the retractor and it functions just like in the tubular system. The other portion of the working space is exposed without any covering by a rigid tubular-like device. Thus, the free movement of instruments is secured as in open surgery. This is called a semi-tubular system.

The semi-tubular retractor has additional benefits from the unique features of the design. It has a groove in the shaft, so it guarantees better output flow, enables a working space by retracting the upper small muscle of the multifidus, performs the role of an instrument guide, and retracts nerve root if needed.

5. Generally, One-hand surgery

In open surgery, especially while doing some sensitive surgical actions in a risky anatomical space, the non-dominant hand supports the main acting hand for safe performance. But, in UBE, the non-dominant hand holds the endoscope, and the dominant hand operates the surgical instruments. Accordingly, the dominant hand should function without any support from the non-dominant hand. That is why this is called one-hand surgery.

No matter what, safe surgery is most important. To compensate for the lack of a backup hand, we need instrument modifications such as blunt-edge instruments and varied-angled freer. The corresponding changes should be made in surgical skills like the splitting and elevating technique while eliminating the ligament flavum and securing enough surgical space followed by gentle motions for safe surgery at the sensitive cord level.

6. Lens inside the body

The lens of the endoscope is put inside the patient's body, so it is easy to determine the pathologic region directly. This is not possible in microscopic surgery. The contralateral side of the spinal canal, foraminal area, the L5-S1 extra-foraminal area, and the ventral side of the thoracic dura are not exceptions.

Irrigating saline is continually in-flowed through the tip of the sheath of the endoscope and the flow pressure somewhat controls hemorrhage and washes away the hematoma for a clear surgical field.

7. A movable, not fixed lens

Because the non-dominant hand holds the endoscope, the surgeon might experience a trembling endoscopic view. This can be prevented somewhat by placing the arm close to the body. In surgery performed under triangulation formation, the endoscope and the instruments work independently very adjacent to each other, and the wide vision is an advantage, but there is a high risk of causing damage to the endoscope lens by speeding drill burrs and energy from the RF wand. To prevent this, a consistent distance between the endoscope and the instruments should be maintained. Keep in mind that a small movement of the tip of the endoscope results in very different surgical vision.

8. Instrument and endoscope to be handled with pivot movement

In open surgery, the surgical field is open, so when moving the instruments, horizontal movement should be considered. But in UBE, pivot movements should be made, using the two portals as the central pivot point. For example, if you plan to move the tip of the instruments forward, then you should move the tip of the other instruments, which are outside of the patient's body, backward. It takes some time to become accustomed to this during the learning curve period.

References

1. Spaner SJ, Warnock GL. A brief history of endoscopy, laparoscopy, and laparoscopic surgery. J Laparoendosc Adv Surg Tech A. 1997;7(6):369–73.
2. Jackson RW. A history of arthroscopy. Arthroscopy. 2010;26(1):91–103.

3. Telfeian AE, Veeravagu A, Oyelese AA, Gokaslan ZL. A brief history of endoscopic spine surgery. Neurosurg Focus. 2016;40(2):E2.
4. Mayer HM. A history of endoscopic lumbar spine surgery: what have we learnt? Biomed Res Int. 2019;2019:4583943.
5. Arangio G, Kostelnik KE. Intraarticular pressures in a gravity-fed arthroscopy fluid delivery system. Arthroscopy. 1992;8(3):341–4.
6. Lin CY, Chang CC, Tseng C, Chen YJ, Tsai CH, Lo YS, et al. Seizure after percutaneous endoscopic surgery-incidence, risk factors, prevention, and management. World Neurosurg. 2020;138:411–7.
7. Tabandeh H. Intraocular hemorrhages associated with endoscopic spinal surgery. Am J Ophthalmol. 2000;129(5):688–90.
8. Ahrens P, Mueller D, Siebenlist S, Lenich A, Stoeckle U, Sandmann GH. The influence of radio frequency ablation on intra-articular fluid temperature in the ankle joint - a cadaver study. BMC Musculoskelet Disord. 2018;19(1):413.
9. Podhajsky RJ, Sekiguchi Y, Kikuchi S, Myers RR. The histologic effects of pulsed and continuous radiofrequency lesions at 42 degrees C to rat dorsal root ganglion and sciatic nerve. Spine (Phila Pa 1976). 2005;30(9):1008–13.
10. Leach EH, Peters RA, Rossiter RJ. Experimental thermal burns, especially the moderate temperature burn. Q J Exp Physiol Cogn Med Sci. 1943;32(1):67–86.
11. Kambin P, O'Brien E, Zhou L, Schaffer JL. Arthroscopic microdiscectomy and selective fragmentectomy. Clin Orthop Relat Res. 1998;347:150–67.
12. Clark AJ, Safaee MM, Khan NR, Brown MT, Foley KT. Tubular microdiscectomy: techniques, complication avoidance, and review of the literature. Neurosurg Focus. 2017;43(2):E7.

3 Instruments and Settings of Unilateral Biportal Spinal Endoscopic Surgery

Young Ha Woo, Su Ki Jeon, and Seung Deok Sun

3.1 Introduction

3.1.1 Anesthesia and Position

1. Anesthesia

- Epidural anesthesia is performed on patients at a level 1 or 2 above the index level.
- In the case of epidural anesthesia, sedation is performed with midazolam or propofol to minimize the impact on the surgical procedure (Fig. 3.1).
- Sometimes, if anesthesia is not possible due to the narrow interlaminar space, anesthesia is also performed at the index level.
- In the case of cervical and thoracic lesions, general anesthesia is applied in advance of the surgery.

2. Position

- The patient is positioned prone on a Wilson frame comfortably placed on a standard operating room table (Fig. 3.2).
- A waterproof surgical drape is applied due to continuous saline irrigation. If a waterproof surgical drape cannot be used, use a surgi-drape on a general surgical drape (Fig. 3.3).
- The surgeon and scrub nurse are positioned on the side of the lesion, the radiologist operates the C-arm on the opposite side of the surgeon, and the surgical assistant nurse assists in the operation process on the other side of the surgeon. The anesthesiologist monitors the patient on the patient's head (Fig. 3.4).
- Camera, shaver and radiofrequency (RF) system: In the Unilateral Biportal Endoscopy (UBE) camera system, the camera monitor is located at the top, and at the bottom, there is a console to connect to 4 k equipment. Underneath, it has a console to connect shaver, equipment to control water pressure, drill console for the endoscope, and a console to connect to radiofrequency (RF) equipment (Fig. 3.5).

Supplementary Information The online version contains supplementary material available at [https://doi.org/10.1007/978-981-16-8201-8_3].

Y. H. Woo
Department of Orthopaedic Surgery, Busan Keun Hospital, Busan, South Korea
e-mail: microsun@dreamwiz.com

S. K. Jeon
Department of Neurospine Surgery, Daejeon Woori Hospital, Daejeon, South Korea

S. D. Sun (✉)
Department of Orthopaedic Surgery, Sun's Orthopedic Clinic, Seoul, South Korea

D. H. Heo et al. (eds.), *Unilateral Biportal Endoscopic Spine Surgery*,
https://doi.org/10.1007/978-981-16-8201-8_3

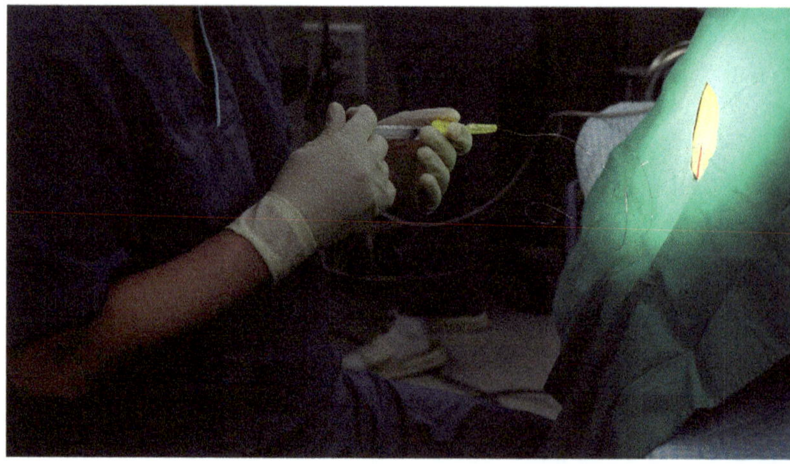

Fig. 3.1 Anesthesiologist performs epidural anesthesia

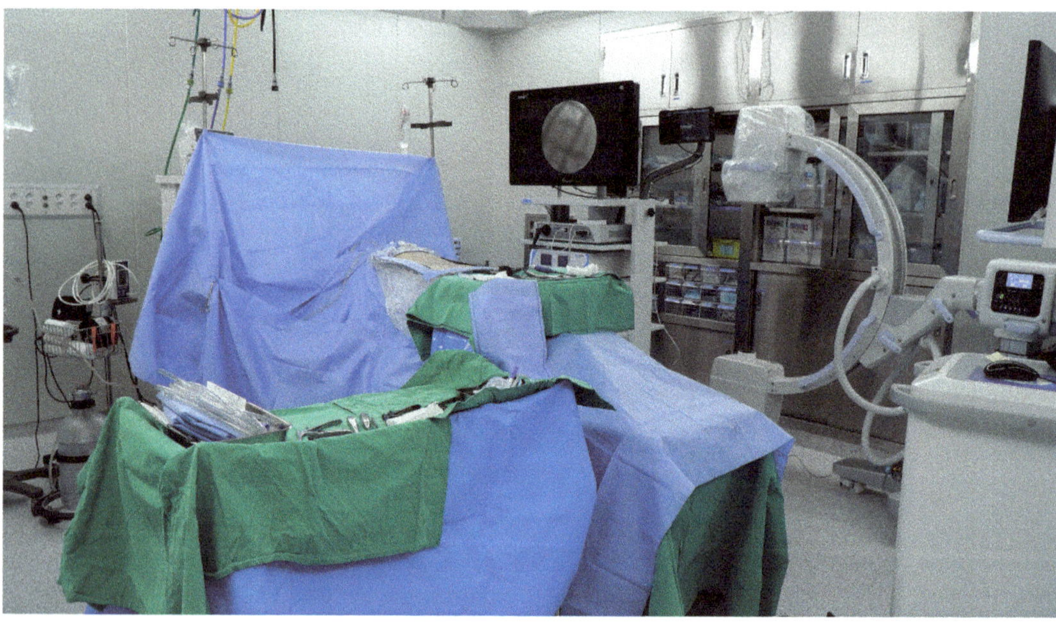

Fig. 3.2 Patient positioning and operating room setup

3.1.2 UBE Instrument Settings

- Scope: Use a zero-degree endoscope that can be used on the spine (Fig. 3.6). Additionally, depending on the operator's preference, a 30-degree scope is also used. The 30-degree scope is useful for decompression of the intervertebral foramen.
- Kerrison punch and pituitary forceps: Instruments used in conventional spine surgery can be used together. Angled instruments can be used freely. It has the advantage of being able to be used with rotatory Kerrison punch and curved Kerrison punch in UBE (Fig. 3.7a). Pituitary forceps also consist of holding straight and holding at an angle (Fig. 3.7b).
- Diamond drills: We use an endoscope drill that can be used underwater. It uses a diamond burr and has a variety of sizes from 2, 3, 4, to 5 mm (Fig. 3.8).
- Straight and angled curettes, probe: Curette is a device used to drop the yellow ligament, and a probe is used to drop the middle part of the

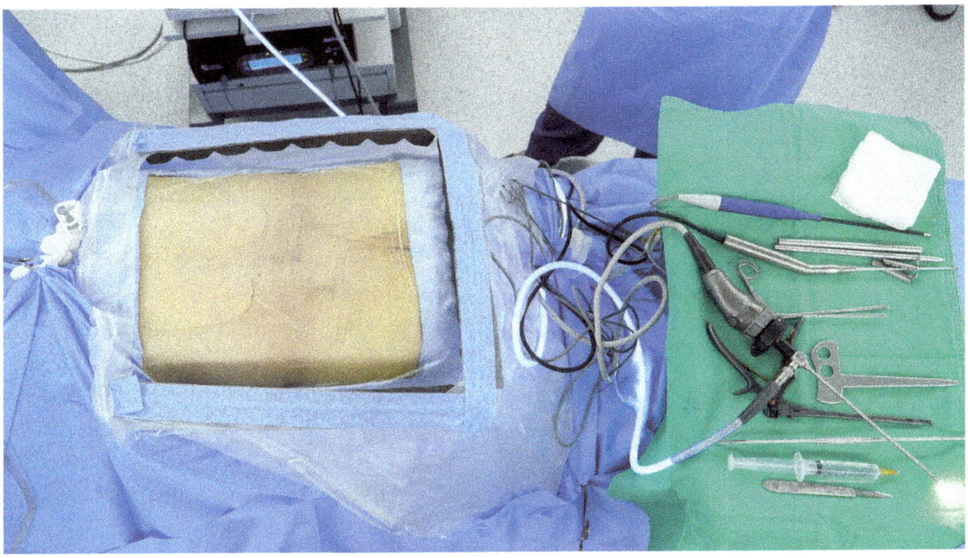

Fig. 3.3 Waterproof surgical drape for left-sided L4-5 approach

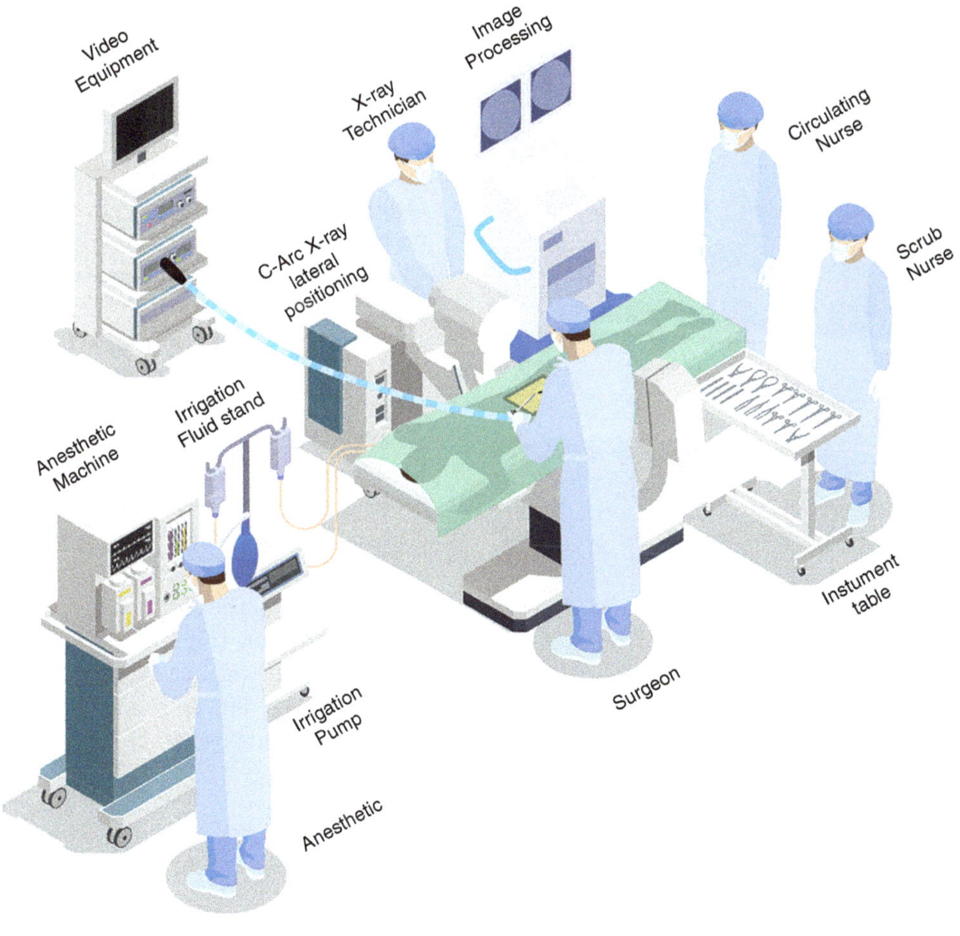

Fig. 3.4 Standard operating room setup

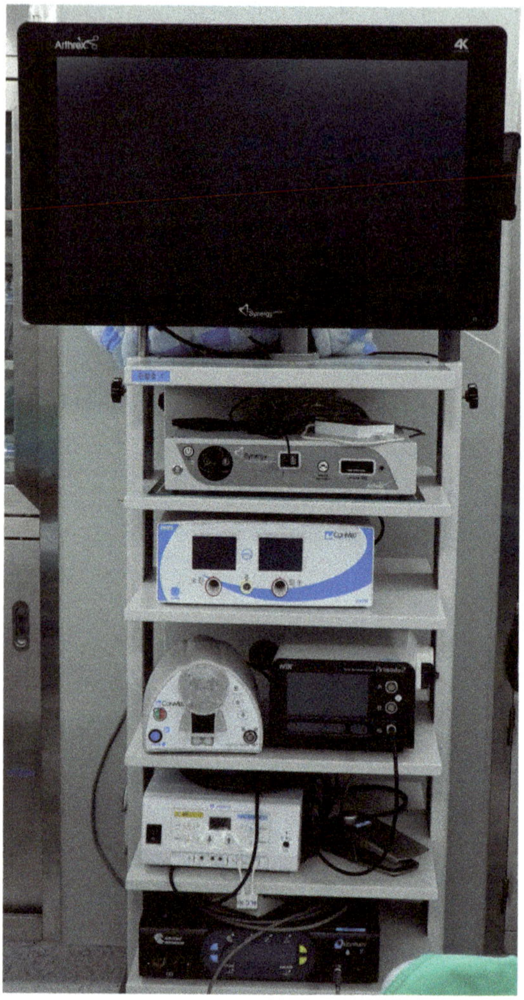

Fig. 3.5 Camera, shaver, and RF system

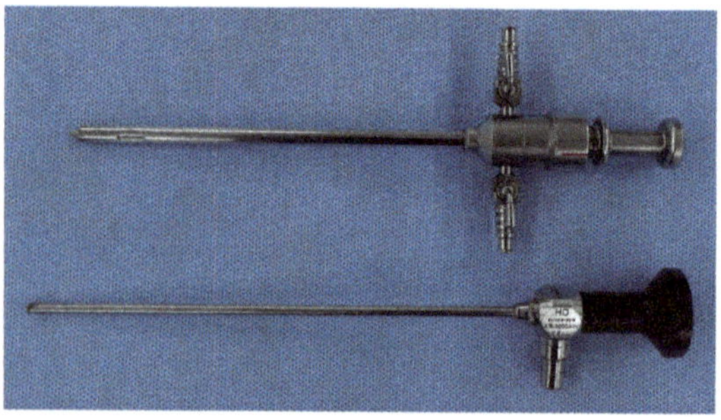

Fig. 3.6 It consists of a 0-degree endoscope scope and endoscope sheath

yellow ligament or to find hidden disc pieces (Fig. 3.9).

- T-shape handle: The T-shape handle is a device to secure a space for water to fill between the lamina and muscles. It is a device that works to slightly detach the muscle from the lamina (Fig. 3.10).
- Working sheath, scope retractor: It is the working sheath that assists with the endoscopy and water drainage. The scope retractor is inspired by the instrument of the uniportal endoscope, which allows the nerve to be retracted without the help of an assistant (Fig. 3.11).
- Serial dilators: It is a device to sequentially secure intramuscular space before inserting the working sheath, and insert it sequentially after using the T-shape handle (Fig. 3.12).
- Root retractors: The instrument used in general spinal surgery has been altered for use in endoscopy, with a slightly higher length and a variable size. Specially, there is a retrator that can be safely inserted when inserting a cage in fusion and is designed to be used in disc surgery as well(Fig. 3.13).
- Double-ended instruments: This instrument makes it easy to use in endoscopy by lengthening instruments used in general spinal surgery (Fig. 3.14).
- Shaver, bone chip cannular, and impactor: This is a device that organizes the disk before inserting the cage and a device that sets artificial bones before inserting the cage (Fig. 3.15).
- RF probe: A RF probe is composed of 90 degrees, 30 degrees, and ball type. The 90 degrees probe is the first to be used and is used to create space when doing UBE for the first time (Fig. 3.16). The 30-degree probe is useful for disk ablation (Fig. 3.17). The ball-type probe is useful when cauterizing small blood vessels around the disk and blood vessels mixed around adipose tissue (Fig. 3.18).

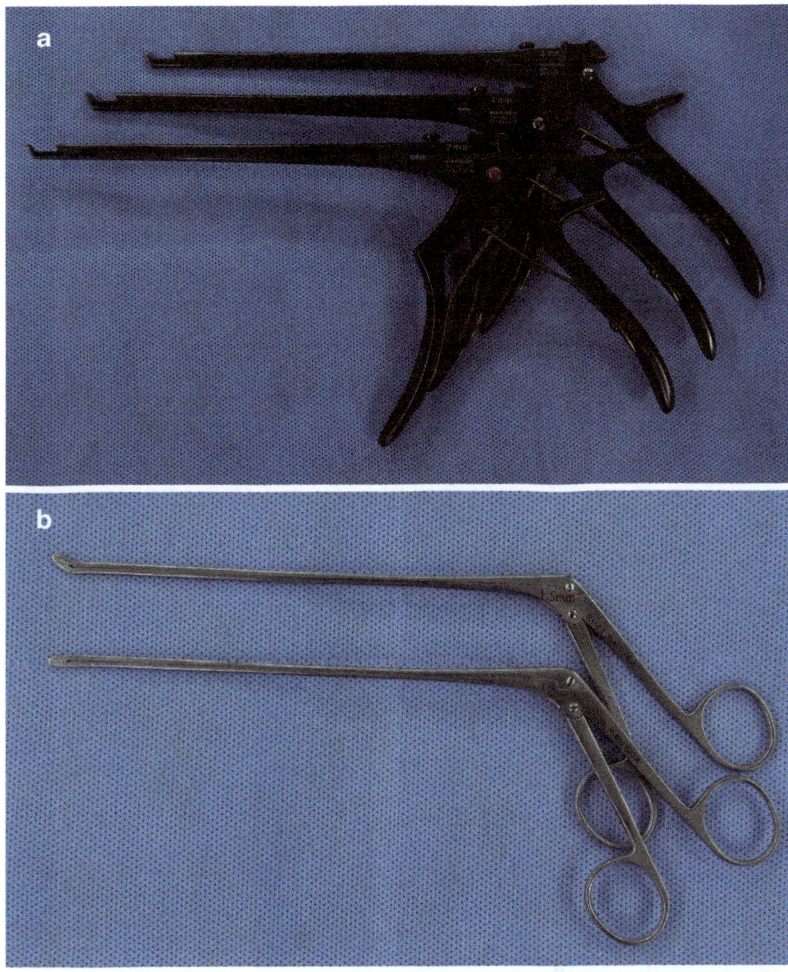

Fig. 3.7 (**a**) Straighted Kerrison punch. (**b**) Straighted and angled Pituitary Forceps

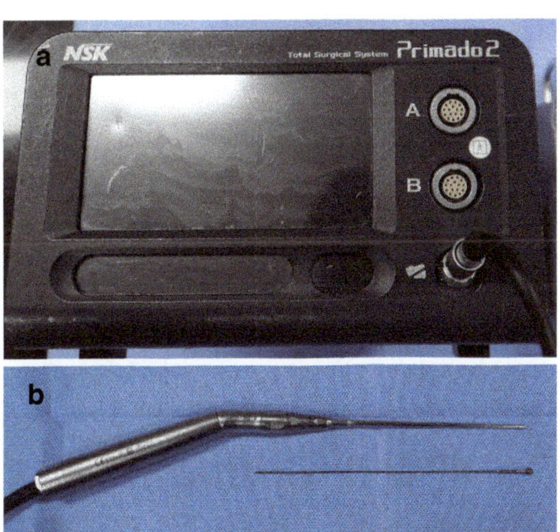

Fig. 3.8 (**a**) Waterproof endoscopic Diamond drill set-up box (**b**) handpiece and diamond drill

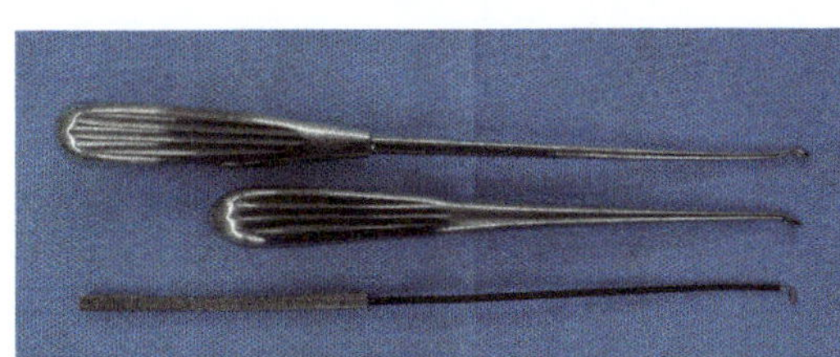

Fig. 3.9 Straight and angled curettes, probe

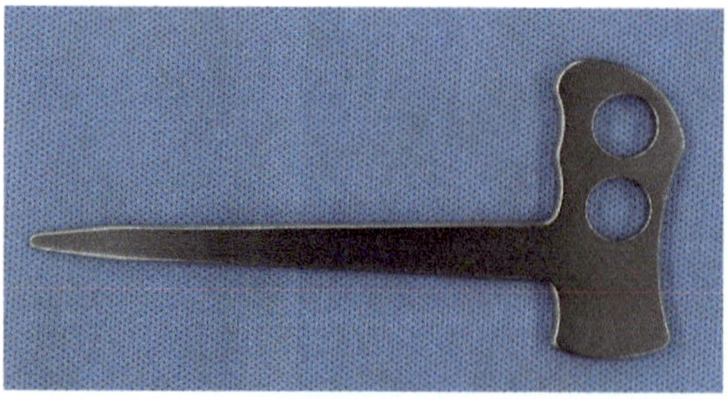

Fig. 3.10 T-shape handle

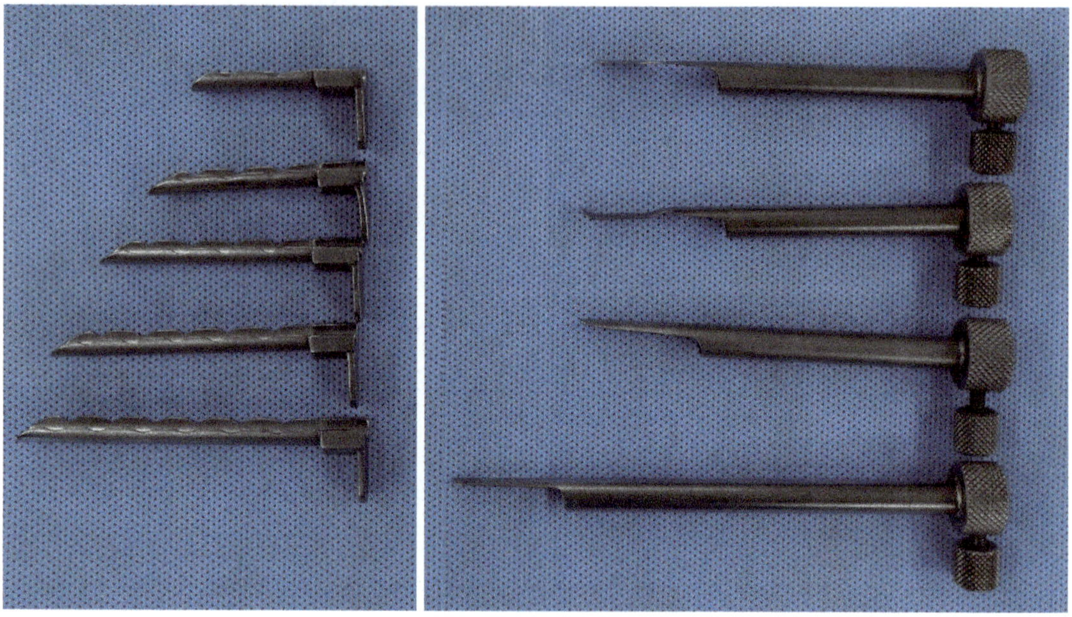

Fig. 3.11 Working sheaths (left) and scope retractors (right)

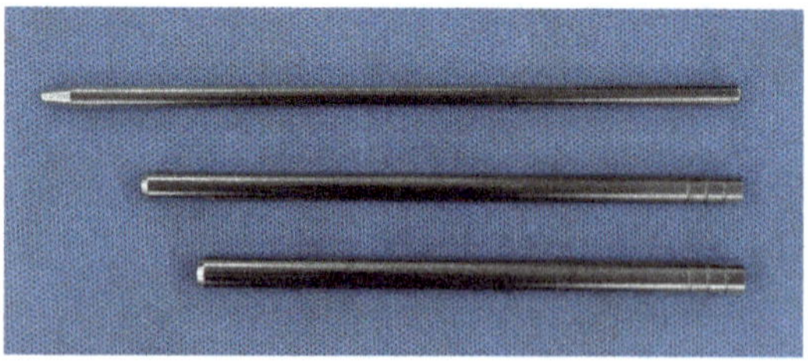

Fig. 3.12 Serial dilators

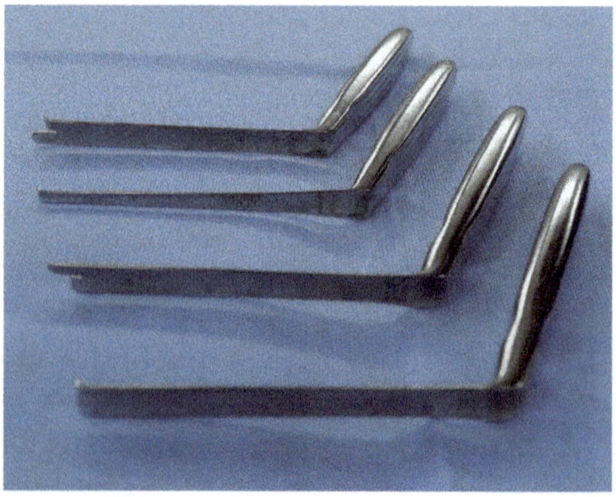

Fig. 3.13 Nerve root retractors

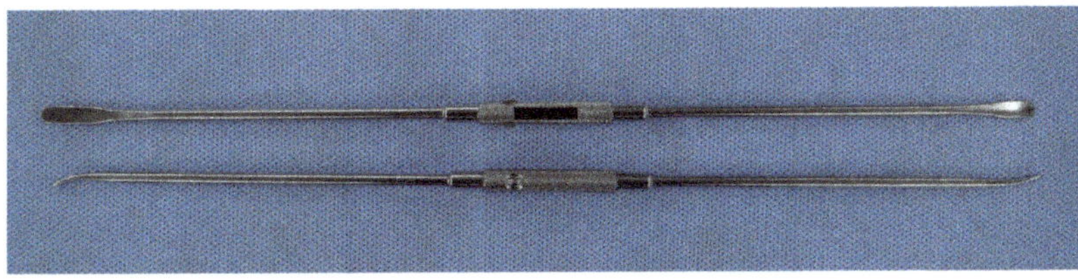

Fig. 3.14 Double-ended instruments

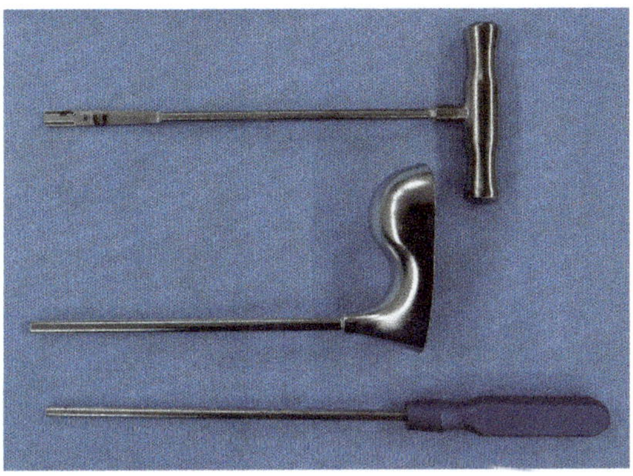

Fig. 3.15 Shaver, bone chip cannular, and bone chip impactor

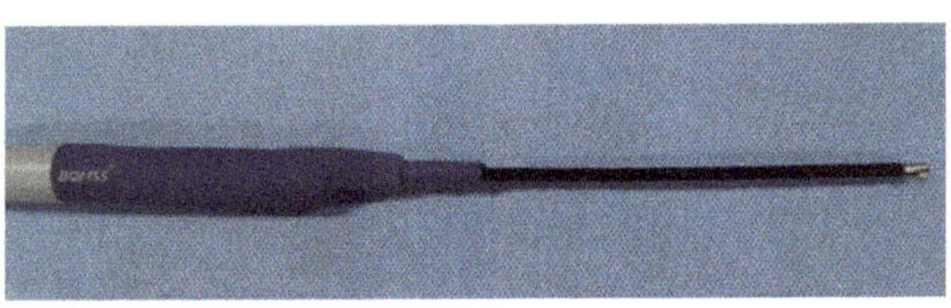

Fig. 3.16 90 degree RF probe

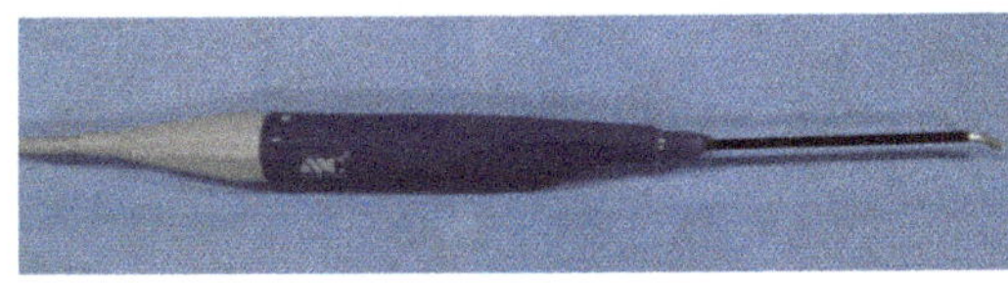

Fig. 3.17 30 degree RF probe

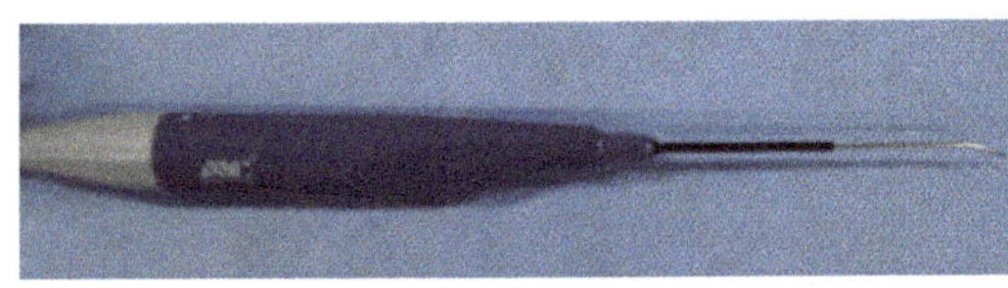

Fig. 3.18 Ball-type RF probe

3.1.3 Startup Process After Initial Setting

This is the scene that begins early after the UBE system is in place. If you check the location, create a working portal and a viewing portal, and see water entering and exiting, you are ready for surgery (Video 3.1).

Part II

Lumbar Disc Herniation

Unilateral Biportal Endoscopy for Herniated Lumbar Disc

4

Seung Kook Kim, Seong Yi, and Jeong Yoon Park

4.1 Introduction

Herniated lumbar disc (HLD) is a common cause of back and leg pain. The initial treatment for HLD is conservative and includes analgesics, physiotherapy, and epidural steroid injections. However, upon failure of conservative treatment, especially when neurological deficits are present with matched radiologic findings, discectomy can be considered [1]. Since 1970, microscopic laminectomy and disc removal have been the gold standard for HLD; however, over the last few years, the progress of endoscopic techniques with the development of new endoscopic instruments and video equipment has led to similar or superior outcomes to microscopic discectomy [2, 3].

Recently, unilateral biportal endoscopic (UBE) spine surgery has been introduced for various spinal diseases [4]. Unlike one-portal endoscopy, biportal endoscopic spinal surgery has a long and wide field of view and the axes and portals for the endoscope and surgical instruments are separated. Therefore, the instruments can be used over a relatively long distance and wide field of view, and this unique feature of the biportal endoscopy facilitates anatomical orientation and handling of instruments. In biportal endoscopic spine surgery, the endoscope and instrument angles are independent and separated, so that the instrument angle does not interfere with vision. In addition, conventional surgical instruments, such as drills and punches, can be used through a working portal. The ability to use conventional instruments has the advantage that the initial setting cost is lower than that in percutaneous one-portal endoscopic spine surgery. One of the main differences between biportal and one-portal endoscopic spine surgery is that various general surgical instruments can be used during the biportal procedure because of the independent working portal. Furthermore, UBE has advantages over the conventional approach in muscle preservation and bone manipulation [5]. To increase the understanding of the procedure, we describe the details below.

Supplementary Information The online version contains supplementary material available at [https://doi.org/10.1007/978-981-16-8201-8_4].

S. K. Kim
Himchan Spine and Joint Centre, University Hospital Sharjah, Sharjah, United Arab Emirates

S. Yi
Department of Neurosurgery, Severance Hospital, Yonsei University College of Medicine, Seoul, South Korea

J. Y. Park (✉)
Department of Neurosurgery, The Spine and Spinal Cord Institute, Gangnam Severance Hospital, Yonsei University College of Medicine, Seoul, South Korea
e-mail: spinepjy@yuhs.ac

D. H. Heo et al. (eds.), *Unilateral Biportal Endoscopic Spine Surgery*,
https://doi.org/10.1007/978-981-16-8201-8_4

4.2 Indications and Contraindications

The indications of UBE for HLD are very similar to those of microscopic lumbar discectomy. All types of lumbar disc herniation including protrusion, extrusion, sequestration, and central, paracentral, foraminal, and extraforaminal disc herniations can be removed and decompressed with UBE. Recurrent and calcified disc herniation and cauda equina syndrome are also included in UBE indications [6, 7]. HLD with stenosis was previously considered a contraindication for endoscopic discectomy, but biportal endoscopic surgery can effectively achieve central decompression followed by additional discectomy, thus adding this diagnosis to the indications for biportal endoscopic discectomy [8].

4.3 Special Instruments

The surgical instruments are the same as in standard UBE stenosis decompression surgery. A standard conventional laminectomy set (pituitary forceps, punches, drill, hook, etc.), zero-degree endoscopy, radiofrequency device, and 3000 cc normal saline for continuous irrigation are essential. Additional angle endoscopic views such as 12° and 30° are helpful when a wider field of view is needed. Continuous saline flow is essential, and serial dilators (Fig. 4.1a), various working sheath (Fig. 4.1b), and scope retractor (Fig. 4.1c) are necessary for unimpeded saline flow. Because nerve protection is more important than simple decompression scope retractors (Fig. 4.1c) or assistant retractors (Fig. 4.1d) should be prepared. Various types of radiofrequency (RF) coagulators (Fig. 4.1e) for bleeding control, dissectors (Fig. 4.1f) for adhesiolysis, and variously angled osteotomes/chisels are necessary. A high-speed drill exclusively for endoscopy is helpful, but a conventional drill (such as Midas Rex®) is sufficient.

4.4 Anesthesia and Positioning of the Patient

Epidural, spinal, or general anesthesia can be selected depending on institutional policy and patient condition. The patient can be positioned either on the spine table or Wilson frame, while the C-arm is placed in the anteroposterior (AP) direction for level checking (Fig. 4.2a). A surgical drape is placed in a water-tight fashion and widely, at least 10 cm, apart from the incision site. Recently, a special drape for UBE has been developed and is convenient to use (Fig. 4.2b and c).

4.5 Surgical Steps

4.5.1 Skin Mark and Incision

The surgical level and landmarks are determined during fluoroscopy in the AP direction. The lateral direction can help in the final conformation and in lumbarization or sacralization cases. Generally, the instrumental portal is made on the disc level first, and then the scope portal is made 2.0–3.0 cm apart from the instrumental portal. However, in cases of obese patients, presence of high-level disc, or hyperlordosis this distance may need to be modified. The endoscopic portal is located 2.0–3.0 cm cranially for a left-sided approach and caudally for a right-sided approach (Fig. 4.3a and b), in the case of a right-handed surgeon. For sufficient internal discectomy, unlike simple ruptured particle removal, the instrumental portal should be decided carefully depending on the disc space angle. Preoperative radiologic images should be evaluated to determine this angle (Fig. 4.3a, b). Therefore, the instrumental portal is determined first and the scope portal is determined later. The two portals should be at least 2.0–3.0 cm apart to prevent interruption (Fig. 4.3c, d). Transverse or horizontal incisions are possible, and in the case of longitudinal incision, it is advantageous for

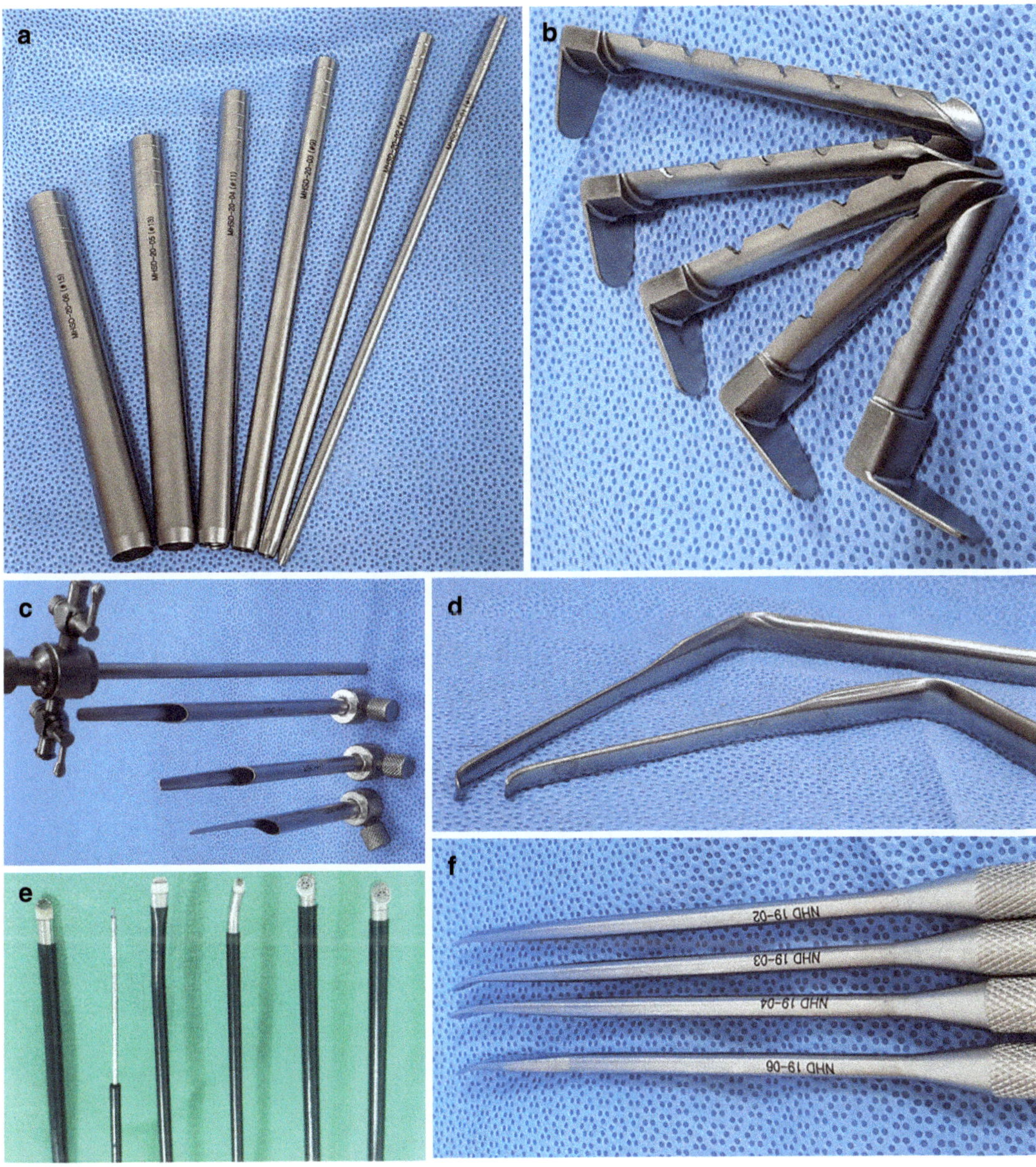

Fig. 4.1 Special instruments for unilateral biportal endoscopic discectomy. Serial dilators (**a**), working cannula for continuous irrigation (**b**), and scope retractors (**c**), assistant retractors (**d**), radiofrequency coagulators (**e**), and dissectors (**f**)

contralateral decompression to be made on the medial pedicle line.

4.5.2 Creation of Two Portals

Portal size should be at least 0.7 cm in diameter for unimpeded saline flow. Transverse incision facilitates saline flow more than horizontal incision due to fascia and muscle fiber dissection. Adequate muscle dissection with a serial dilator or dissector is necessary for this purpose. A 3000 cc saline bag placed 100 cm above the operation area (100 cm H_20 injection pressure) or an automatic injector could be used. Water pressure should be maintained below 23 mmHg dur-

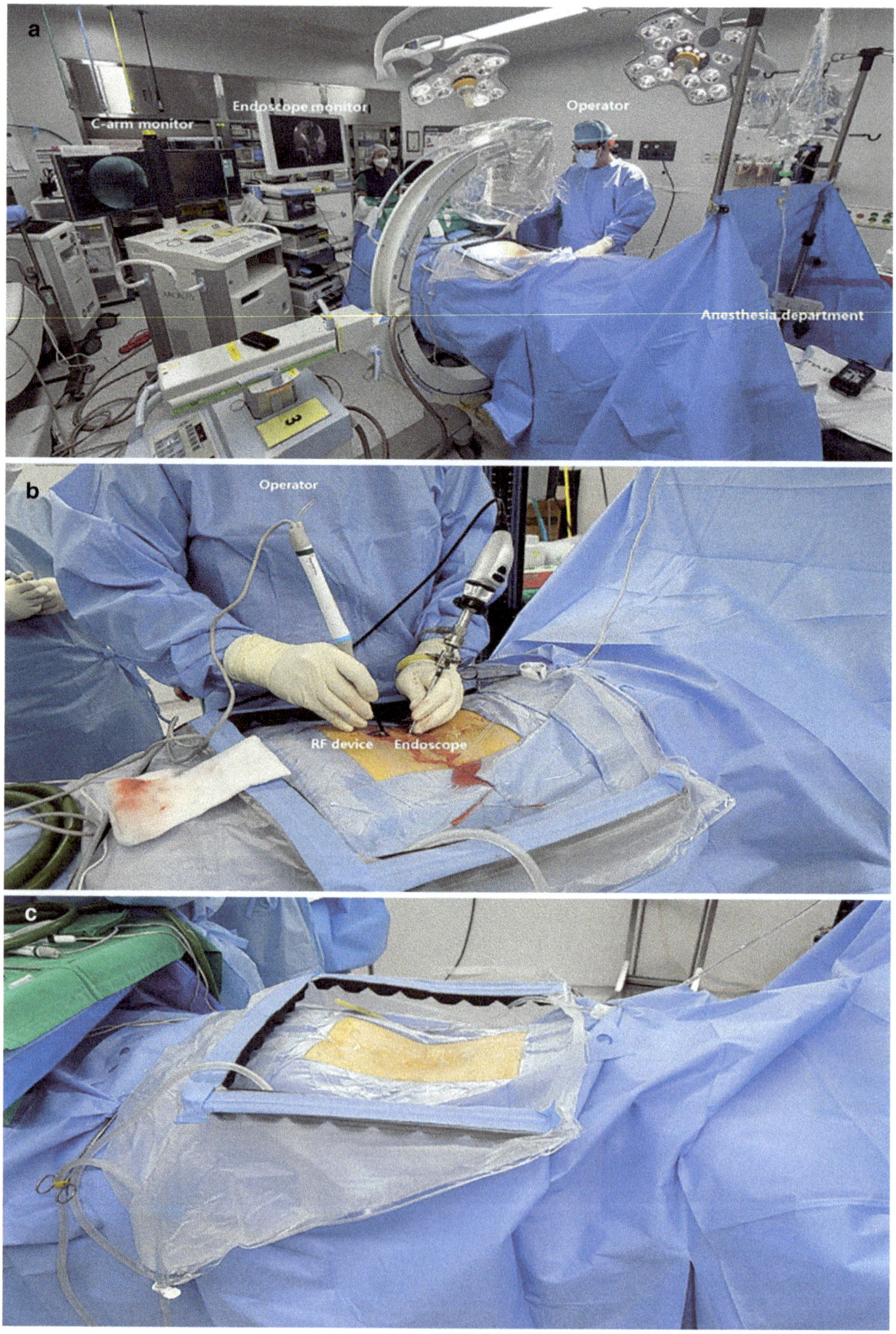

Fig. 4.2 Operation room arrangement and surgical drape (**a**). Detailed view of operation site (**b**). Water-tight surgical drape (**c**)

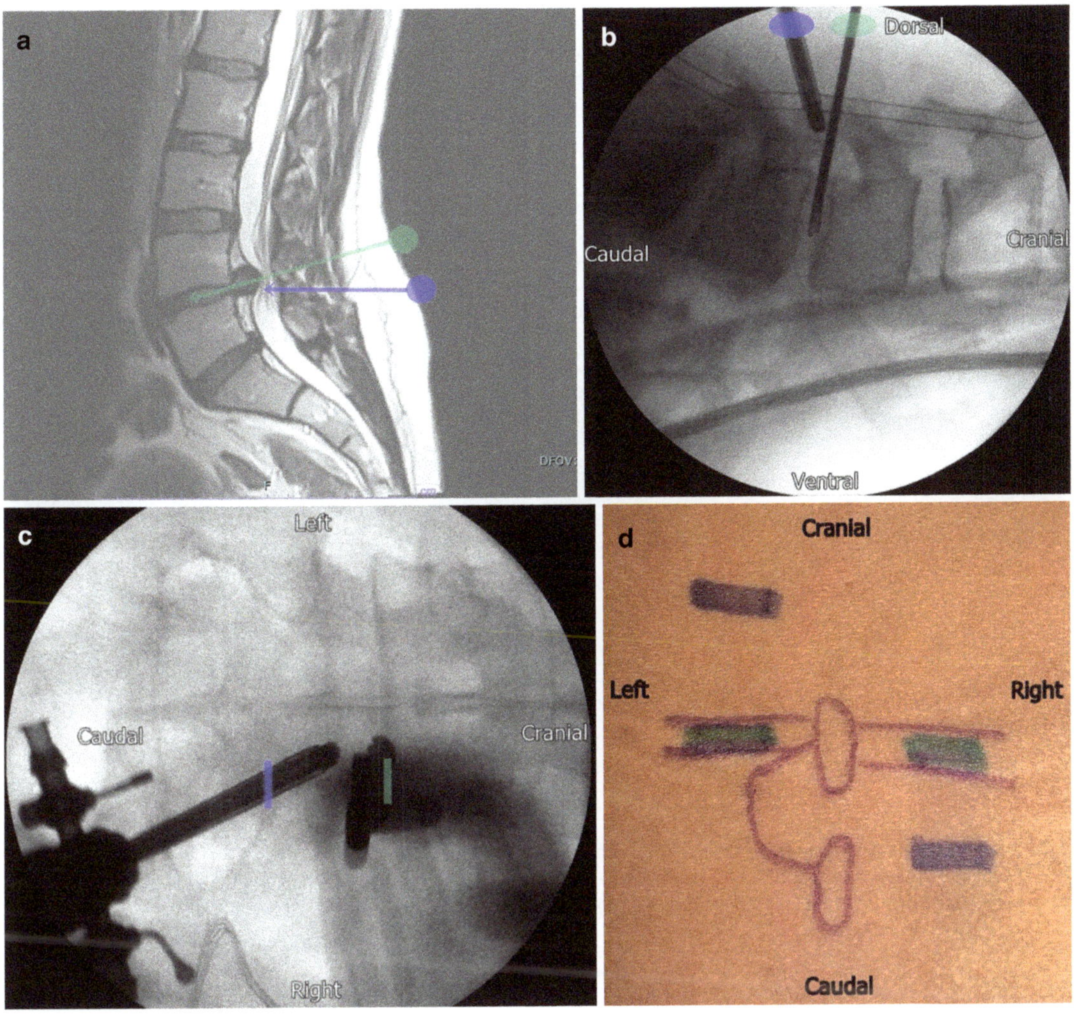

Fig. 4.3 Decision of incision site. Preoperative T2 weighted magnetic resonance (MR) sagittal imaging is important. For a right-sided approach, instrumental portal (green) and scope portal (blue) are decided from preoperative MR sagittal image (**a**). The same portals are confirmed by intraoperative fluoroscopic lateral (**b**) and anteroposterior image (**c**). Skin marks for left and right-sided approach. Instrumental portal (green) and scope portal (blue) should be different according to the approach side (**d**)

ing the procedure [9]. If blurred vision in the absence of bleeding or water retention are noted due to water retention, portal dilatation and fascia dissection should be repeated. Obese and young male patients with large muscle mass need more careful portal preparations or maintenance of working sheaths or cannulas (Fig. 4.1b) for unimpeded saline flow during the procedure (Video 4.1).

4.5.3 Working Space Preparation

Using a muscle detacher, muscle detachment should be performed on the lower border of the upper lamina and upper border of the lower lamina (Fig. 4.4a). For working space preparation, coagulation of muscle with a radiofrequency (RF) coagulator and soft tissue removal with a muscle shaver is helpful. The first step after the

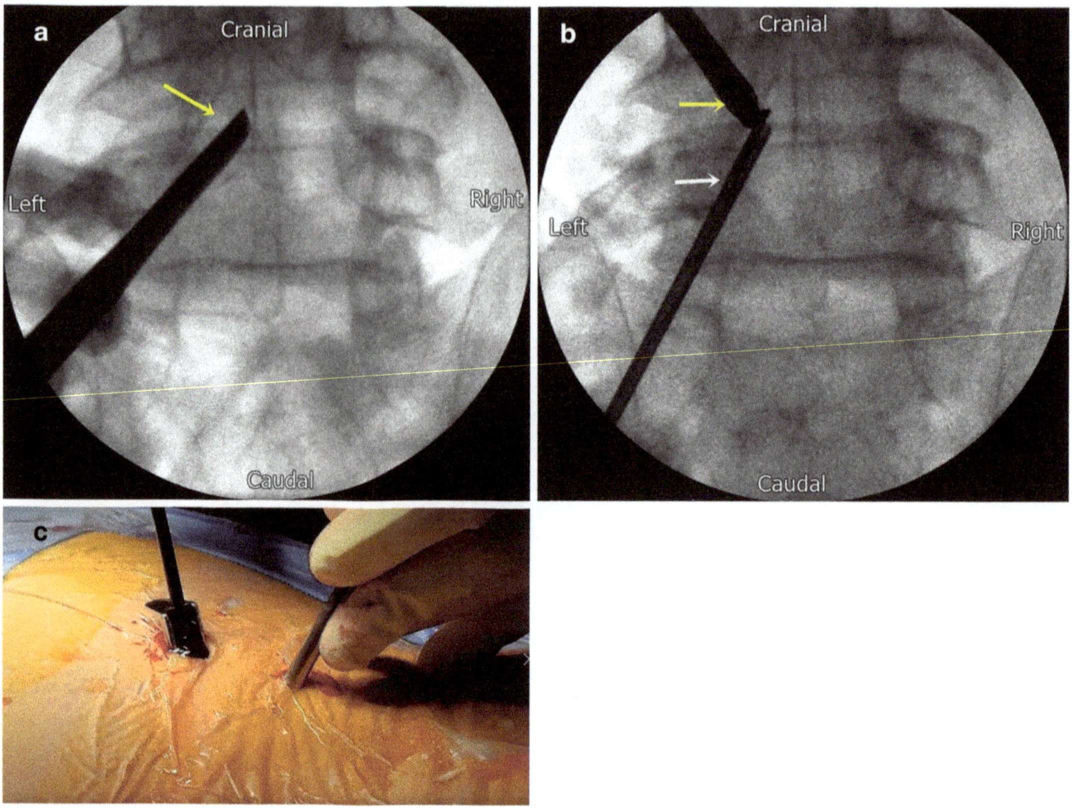

Fig. 4.4 Working space preparation. Muscle detachment on lower end of upper lamina (yellow arrow, left-sided approach) (**a**). Instrumental portal (white arrow) and scope portal (yellow arrow) are identified over lamina (**b**). Intraoperative field image of adequate saline flow (**c**). Single-wing type working cannula was used

creation of the portal involves coagulating the soft tissues around both the scope and instrument portals as needed and locating the tip of the RF coagulator on endoscopic vision or under fluoroscopy (Fig. 4.4b). Using a Kerrison punch or pituitary forceps, the outer layer of the ligamentum flavum and bulky soft tissues are removed for identification of landmarks for laminectomy. Adequate saline flow should be ensured before starting the laminectomy (Fig. 4.4c). Th3e importance of continuous and adequate saline flow during UBE cannot be overemphasized.

4.5.4 Laminectomy and Flavectomy (Video 4.2)

An illustrative case with a left-sided approach at L4/5 is demonstrated in its entirety in Video 4.2. Partial hemi-laminectomy starts with an automated drill or osteotome until a point slightly medially to the midline and by the upper free margin of the ligamentum flavum cranially. After the L4 lower laminar border is confirmed, laminectomy starts from the lower margin with the drill (Fig. 4.5a). L4 partial laminectomy continues until the upper free margin of the ligamentum flavum is exposed (Fig. 4.5b). The ligamentum flavum lower free margin is then detached from the L5 upper laminar border (Fig. 4.5c) and is removed using pituitary forceps, and the lateral margin of the dural sac and nerve root are confirmed (Fig. 4.5d). To avoid excessive traction of the nerve, sufficient ligamentum flavum removal and partial removal of the superior articular process are necessary. Dissection begins from the origin of the traversing root and proceeds between the nerve and discussing dissectors (Fig. 4.5e).

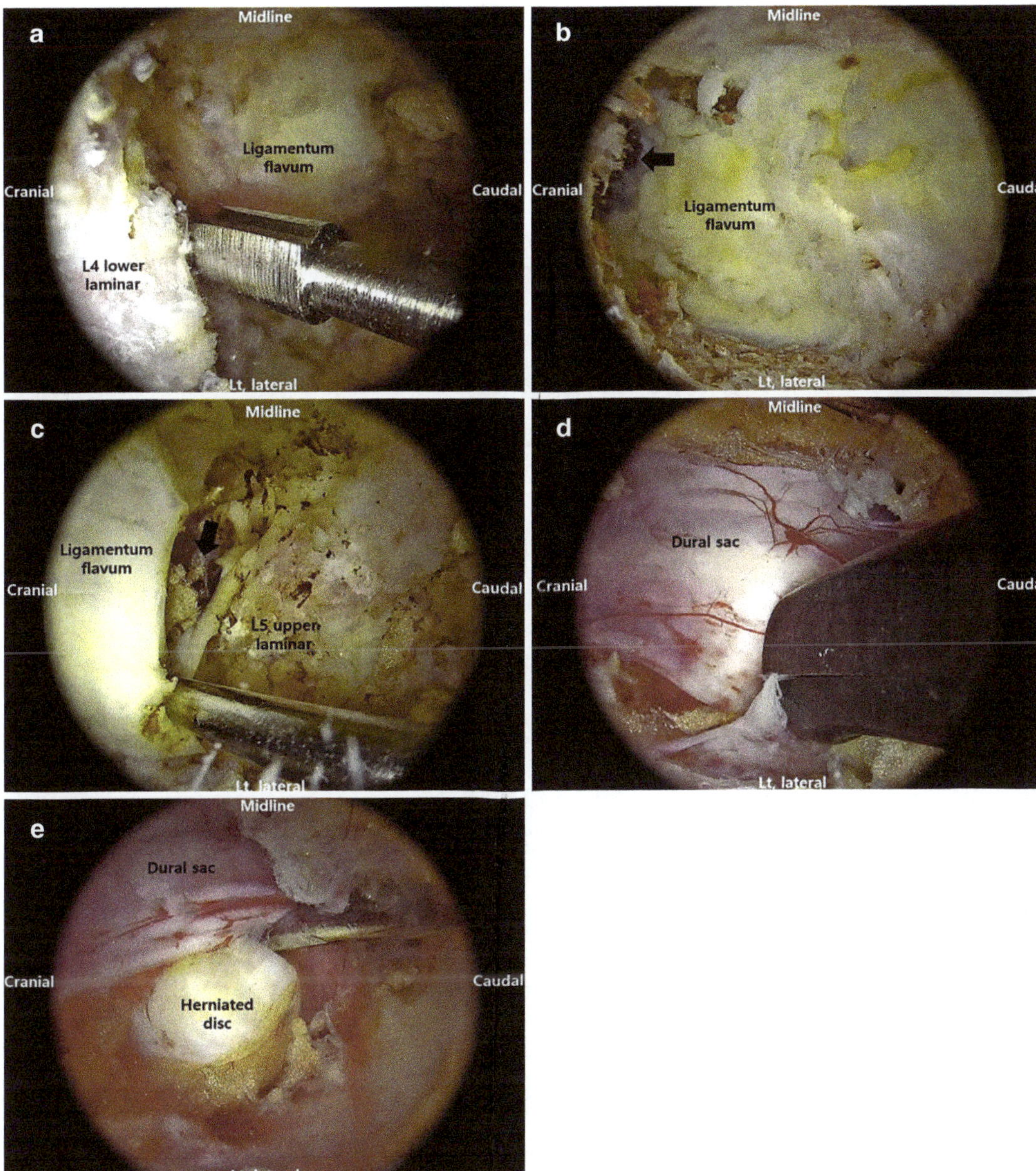

Fig. 4.5 Laminectomy and flavectomy at L4/5 from a left-sided approach. After the L4 lower laminar border is confirmed, laminectomy is started from the L4 laminar lower margin with drill (**a**). L4 partial laminectomy is performed until the ligamentum flavum upper free margin (black arrow) is exposed (**b**). The ligamentum flavum lower free margin (black arrow) is detached from the L5 upper laminar border (**c**). The ligamentum flavum is removed and the dural sac and root lateral margin are confirmed (**d**). Starting from the origin of the traversing root, dissection proceeds between the nerve and disc with the use of dissectors (**e**). The full procedure can be viewed in Video 4.2

4.5.5 Discectomy (Video 4.2)

The disc space is located medially to the superior articular process. After locating the herniated disc (Fig. 4.5e), the ruptured disc particle is removed (Fig. 4.6a). Additional discectomy is performed using pituitary forceps ensuring root protection with a root retractor (Fig. 4.6b). Bleeding control and annuloplasty can be achieved with RF coagulators, whereas annulotomy can be performed with an Indian knife. Removal of the ruptured disc with forceps with concomitant nerve protection is important. Scope retractors and assistant retractors are also helpful for nerve protection. With a scope retractor more efficient nerve protection can be expected compared to assistant retractors. Intermittent root traction and release are important to prevent nerve traction injuries. There are four corridors for discectomy: ipsilateral shoulder (Fig. 4.6c),

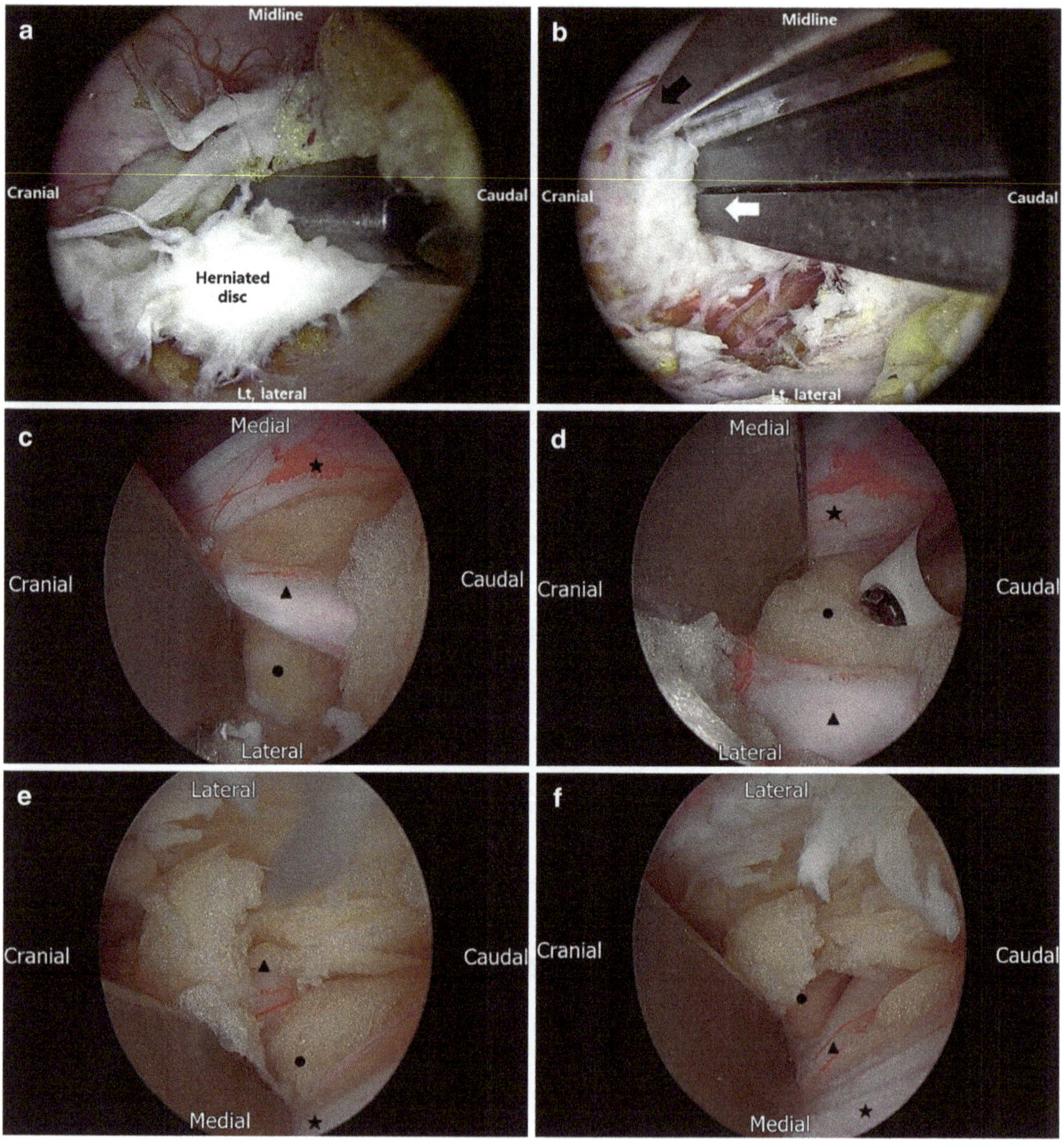

Fig. 4.6 Discectomy at L4/5 from a left-sided approach. The herniated and ruptured disc is located and removed (**a**). Additional discectomy is done with pituitary forceps (white arrow), after ensuring root protection with root retractor (black arrow) (**b**). There are four corridors for discectomy, ipsilateral shoulder (**c**), ipsilateral axillary (**d**), contralateral axillary (**e**) and contralateral shoulder (**f**) (triangle: nerve root, dot: disc, star: thecal sac). Depending on location and characteristics of disc, the appropriate approach should be chosen to reduce chances of nerve traction injury. After complete discectomy, the surgeon must confirm complete neural structure decompression (**g**). In this case, an incidental dural tear (black arrow) was discovered (**g**) and addressed with direct dural repair (**h**). The full procedure can be viewed in Video 4.2

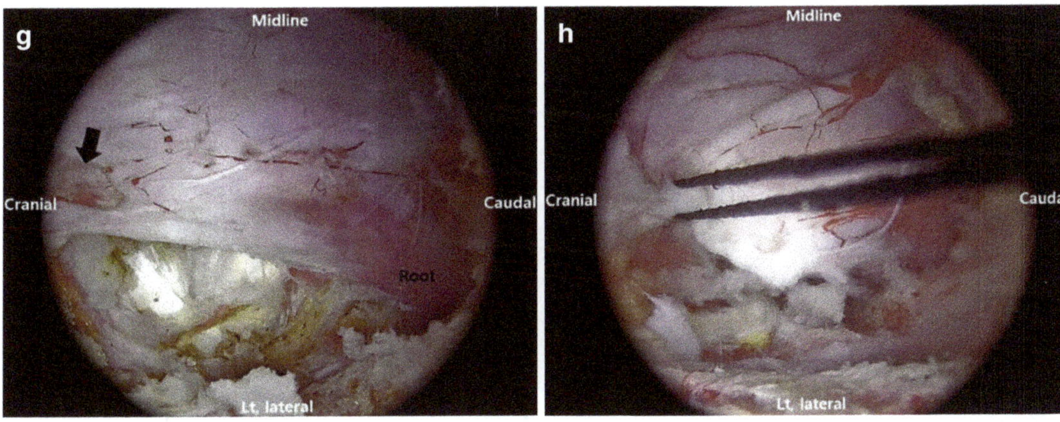

Fig. 4.6 (continued)

ipsilateral axillary (Fig. 4.6d), contralateral axillary (Fig. 4.6e), and contralateral shoulder (Fig. 4.6f). Depending on the location and characteristics of the disc, an appropriate approach for reducing root traction injury should be chosen. Soft disc material can be removed with pituitary forceps, whereas calcified disc particles can be detached with Kerrison punches or osteotomes. Regarding internal disc decompression, which, if performed, is associated with less risk of recurrence, it can be accomplished by the use of pituitary forceps or RF ablation to remove the internal nucleus. After sufficient decompression, annuloplasty with an RF coagulator can be performed. After complete discectomy, the surgeon must confirm complete neural structure decompression (Fig. 4.6g). In the presented case, an incidental dural tear (Fig. 4.6g, black arrow) was discovered which was addressed with direct dural repair (Fig. 4.6h).

4.5.6 Drainage and Closure

Surgical drain insertion is optional in unilateral laminectomy and discectomy procedures. To skip drain insertion, meticulous bleeding control is mandatory. Repetitive skin compression around the portal can decrease soft tissue water retention before suturing. A 50 cc or 100 cc drain can be inserted under endoscopic guidance or blindly through the instrumental or endoscopic portal over the laminar or dural sac (Fig. 4.7a). The skin is sutured with nylon 3:0 at both portals and a tagging drainage tube is left in the portal site (Fig. 4.7b). We recommend the insertion of a drain line through the instrumental rather than the endoscopic portal because it is the instrumental portal patency that maintains unimpeded saline flow during the entire procedure.

4.6 Illustrated Cases

4.6.1 Case 1 (Left Side Axillar Approach, Video 4.3)

A 37-year-old woman was seen for a 1-year history of back and right leg radiating pain. The straight leg raise test (SLRT) was 30 °. Magnetic resonance imaging (MRI) showed severe disc herniation and left inferior migration at the L5/S1 level (Fig. 4.8). For a left-sided approach, the instrumental portal was placed on the disc space level, and the scope portal was placed 3 cm above. Laminectomy and flavectomy were performed in the same manner as described above. The entire discectomy procedure is presented in Video 4.3. After ligamentum flavum removal, the migrated disc material was located in the axillary space. The large migrated disc was removed, followed by a thorough exploration of the shoulder space and additional internal discectomy. The discectomy was performed with pituitary forceps, whereas an RF coagulator was used for concurrent annuloplasty. A drain was inserted, and the skin was sutured with 3-0 nylon. Immediately postoperatively the leg radiating pain improved while the back pain at the operation site resolved on postoperative day 3.

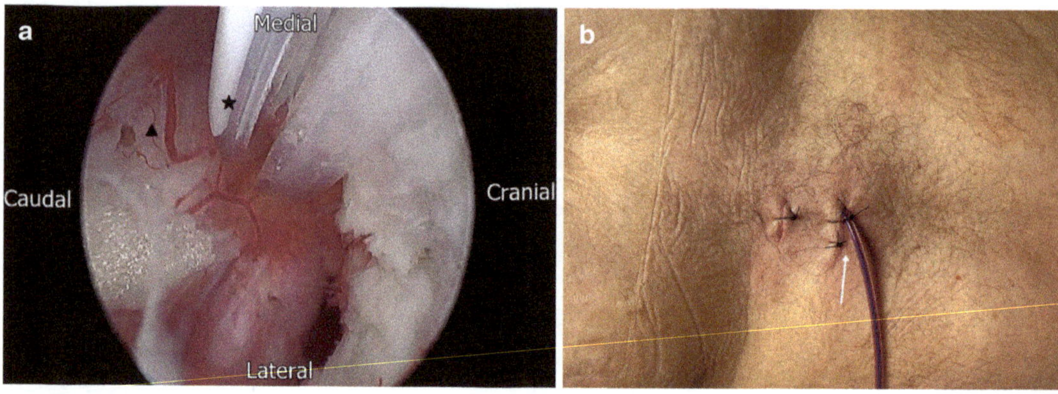

Fig. 4.7 Drain insertion under endoscopic guidance (star: hemovac, triangle: thecal sac) (**a**). Skin suture and drain tagging (white arrow) (**b**)

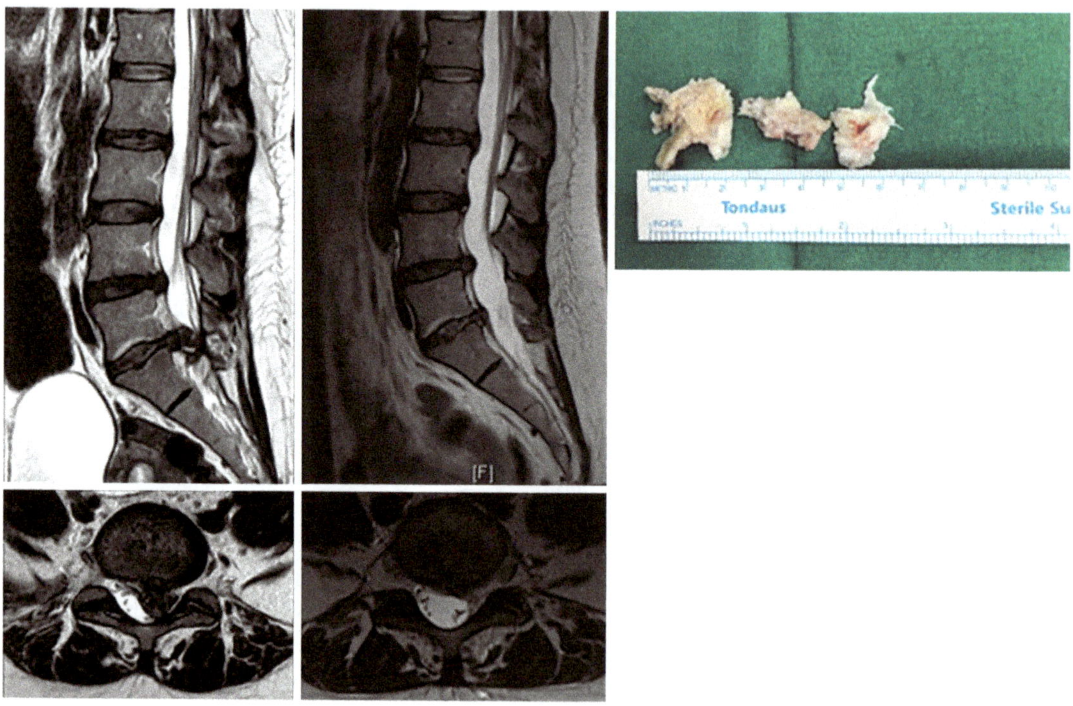

Fig. 4.8 Case 1. MRI showed severe disc herniation and inferior migration at the L5/S1 level on the left. From the left: preoperative, postoperative MRI and removed disc particles

4.6.2 Case 2 (Left-sided Shoulder Approach, Video 4.4)

A 43-year-old female presented to the outpatient clinic with left buttock pain for 6 months. Visual analogue scale (VAS) score was 3 for the back and 9 for buttock to leg. Mild weakness of the left ankle was noted. The SLRT was positive at 30 °. MRI showed a superiorly migrated large disc at L5/S1 level on the left (Fig. 4.9). For a left-sided approach, the instrumental portal was placed on the disc space level, and the scope portal was placed 3 cm above. Laminectomy and flavectomy were performed in the same manner as described above. The entire discectomy procedure is described in Video 4.4. First, the lower margin of

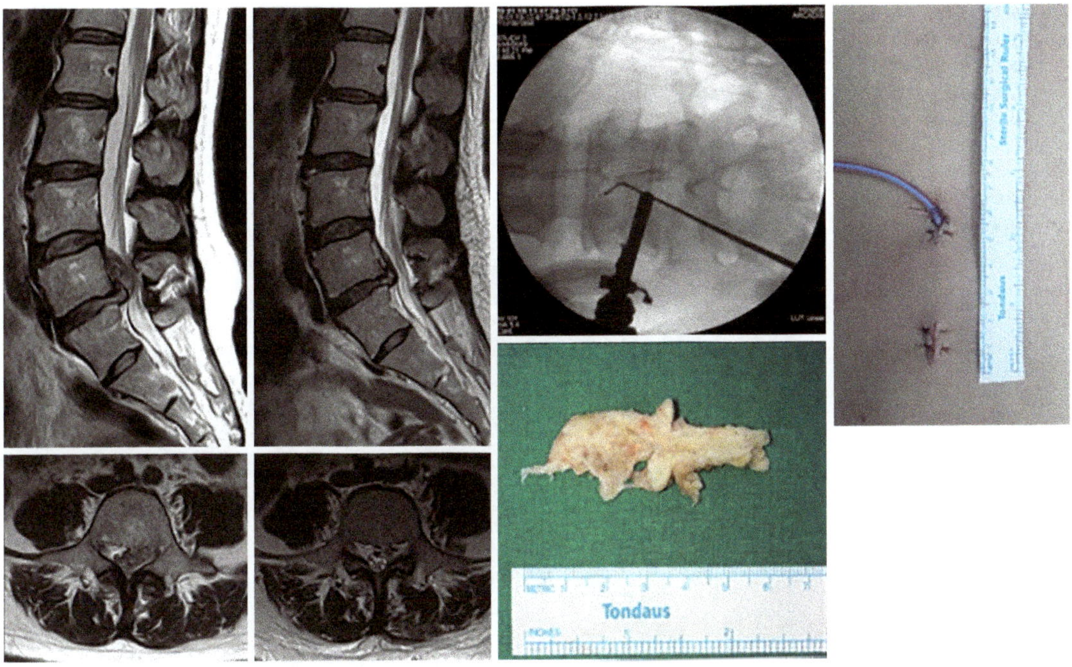

Fig. 4.9 Case 2. MRI showed large superior migrated disc at the L5/S1 level on the left. From left: preoperative, postoperative MRI, X-ray image during operation, removed disc particles, and final wound

the L5 lamina was identified using an RF coagulator. After sufficient L5 laminar drilling, the upper free margin of the ligamentum flavum was exposed and the S1 laminar upper margin was identified. Using Kerrison punches, the S1 upper lamina was partially removed to confirm the lower free margin of the ligmentum flavum. After careful dissection with a blunt hook, the ligamentum flavum was removed and the large superior migrated disc was located and removed (Fig. 4.9). A blunt hook was used to explore disc remnants superiorly (Fig. 4.9). After confirming complete removal of the migrated disc, a 100 cc drainage bag was inserted and the skin was sutured. On a postoperative day 1 VAS scores were 4 for the back and 3 for the leg, and after POD 7 VAS decreased to 1 for both the back and leg.

4.6.3 Case 3 (Left-sided Contralateral Approach to Right Foramen, Video 4.5)

A 71-year-old female with right buttock and leg pain for 6 months presented to the outpatient clinic. The VAS score was 7 for buttock to leg. Mild weakness was observed in the right knee, and the SLRT was positive at 30°. Conservative treatment, including physiotherapy and medication, was not helpful. MRI showed foraminal disc herniation at the L 2/3 level on the right (Fig. 4.10). Laminectomy was performed in the same manner as described above. For the contralateral approach, additional midline laminectomy was performed over the ligamentum flavum midline slit with an osteotome and punch. The entire discectomy procedure is described in Video 4.5. After sufficient L2 laminar removal to the contralateral foramen, the ligamentum flavum was removed to the level of L2/3 right foramen, and the contralateral foramen was explored to find the ruptured disc. After careful dissection with a hook, the superiorly migrated disc was found and removed. With a blunt hook, the superior foraminal space was explored to find any disc remnants. After confirming complete removal of the migrated disc, a 100-cc drain was inserted and the skin was sutured. The patient was discharged 3 days later, and on postoperative day 3, the VAS score was 2 for the leg.

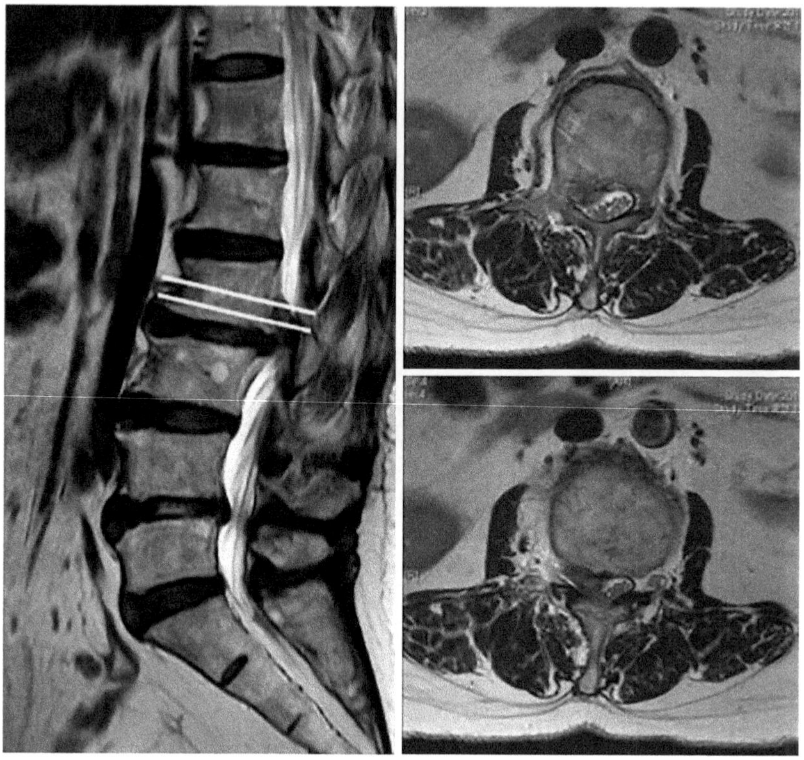

Fig. 4.10 Case #3. MRI showed foraminal disc herniation at the L2/3 level on the right. From left: preoperative sagittal, lower pedicle level, and lower endplate level axial MRI image (white line)

4.7 Complications and Their Management

4.7.1 Bleeding

Bone bleeding can be controlled using bone wax or an RF coagulator. A small tip RF coagulator (Fig. 4.1e) is helpful for controlling small vessel bleeding. In the case of diffuse spontaneous bleeding without major visible bleeding vessels a hemostatic matrix (Floseal®) is useful. Influent saline can be falsely perceived as operation site bleeding. Before attempting to control bleeding, the saline flow should also be checked. It has been reported that the use of an infusion pump may increase the risk of epidural hematoma because high water pressure may hide bleeding during surgery.

4.7.2 Traction Injury and Dural Tear

Excessive traction and aggressive adhesiolysis can cause dysesthesia and paresthesia after surgery. Regarding the choice of retractor, we recommend a scope retractor (Fig. 4.1c). Between the scope retractor and assistant retractor, the scope retractor can avoid excessive retraction because the operator can feel the resistance of the nerve. However, even with the use of a scope retractor, intermittent release of retractor tension should be applied to prevent nerve traction injury. During laminectomy, the ligamentum flavum should not be removed too early. The ligamentum flavum is an important protector against the sharp side of the instrument during laminectomy. If the epidural space is already exposed, the ligamentum flavum should be removed from above the epidural fat, as hidden neural structures may be located under the fat. After ligamentum flavum removal, the use of the RF coagulator on coagulation mode only, or on ablation mode with low power (20 w) is recommended as high power energy can induce nerve injury or dural tears. If a dural tear has already occurred, the water pressure should be decreased and the size of the dural tear determined. Depending on the size of the injury, we chose observation, fibrin sealant patch, non-penetrating clip, or endoscopic suture (Fig. 4.6h, Video 4.1).

4.7.3 Learning Curve and Important Points

UBE discectomy requires nerve protection and skillful disc removal, which are important steps in the preparation of interbody fusion surgery. Simple lumbar stenosis decompression without discectomy with working space preparation, laminectomy, safe ligamentum flavum removal, and exposure of the nerve root should be repeated before starting discectomy. In the early stages of the learning curve, identifying important anatomical landmarks (origin of traversing nerve root and medial wall of pedicle) before discectomy and using discrimination dye (Indigo carmine) could be helpful.

4.7.4 Surgical Tips and Pitfalls

Currently, one prospective [8] and three retrospective studies [3, 5, 10] have reported on UBE discectomy. These studies showed that UBE had similar, but not superior, results to other discectomy techniques. Advantages were less postoperative back pain and shorter hospital stay, and possible disadvantages were persistent back pain, dural tear, and incomplete disc decompression [11]. To overcome these possible disadvantages we offer the following surgical tips.

Blurred vision due to excessive saline flow and lack of experience with the endoscopic procedure can result in incomplete surgery and increased perioperative risks. Sufficient muscle detachment, portal widening with serial dilation, soft tissue reduction with muscle shaver, and careful bleeding control with an RF device are the first and most important steps for all kinds of UBE procedures. The importance of continuous and unimpeded saline flow during UBE cannot be overemphasized, and the above steps can help to ensure this. Compared to microscopic procedures and percutaneous one-portal endoscopic discectomy, UBE allows various working distances and viewing angles; therefore, surgeons should be familiar with the control of the endoscope. For example, most of the scope has two controllers: focus control and magnification control. Both should be properly adjusted during the entire procedure.

Incomplete discectomy and dural tear can occur due to insufficient laminectomy and incorrect use of instruments. In cases of soft disc herniation without degeneration, target-oriented small laminectomy and ligamentum flavum splitting techniques are helpful. However, with calcified and degenerated migrated discs enough bone should be removed, the ligamentum flavum should be resected in its entirety, and all anatomical landmarks should be identified carefully. Kerrison punches, osteotomes, and various scope retractors can decrease the risk of incomplete discectomy. If a dural tear occurs unexpectedly a sufficient effort should be made to achieve enough decompression and ligamentum flavum removal followed by disc removal as planned, before the dural injury is managed. Unlike open surgery, endoscopic spine surgery usually does not result in cerebrospinal fluid leakage because of strong muscle barriers. UBE discectomy is a safe and effective surgery with many benefits. As more UBE-specific instruments are developed, and UBE surgical skills improve we expect to see better outcomes for the proper indications.

Acknowledgments Instruments are designed by "MD & company" (Seoul, Korea) without any commercial relationships.

References

1. Awad JN, Moskovich R. Lumbar disc herniations: surgical versus nonsurgical treatment. Clin Orthop Relat Res. 2006;443:183–97.
2. Gibson JNA, Subramanian AS, Scott CEH. A randomised controlled trial of transforaminal endoscopic discectomy vs microdiscectomy. Eur Spine J. 2017;26(3):847–56.
3. Barber SM, Nakhla J, Konakondla S, Fridley JS, Oyelese AA, Gokaslan ZL, et al. Outcomes of endoscopic discectomy compared with open microdiscectomy and tubular microdiscectomy for lumbar disc herniations: a meta-analysis. J Neurosurg Spine. 2019;31:1–14.

4. Kambin P, Nass. Arthroscopic microdiscectomy. Spine J. 2003;3(3 Suppl):60S–4S.
5. Heo DH, Lee DC, Park CK. Comparative analysis of three types of minimally invasive decompressive surgery for lumbar central stenosis: biportal endoscopy, uniportal endoscopy, and microsurgery. Neurosurg Focus. 2019;46(5):E9.
6. Kang T, Park SY, Park GW, Lee SH, Park JH, Suh SW. Biportal endoscopic discectomy for high-grade migrated lumbar disc herniation. J Neurosurg Spine. 2020;33:1–6.
7. Choi DJ, Jung JT, Lee SJ, Kim YS, Jang HJ, Yoo B. Biportal endoscopic spinal surgery for recurrent lumbar disc herniations. Clin Orthop Surg. 2016;8(3):325–9.
8. Choi DJ, Choi CM, Jung JT, Lee SJ, Kim YS. Learning curve associated with complications in biportal endoscopic spinal surgery: challenges and strategies. Asian Spine J. 2016;10(4):624–9.
9. Hong YH, Kim SK, Hwang J, Eum JH, Heo DH, Suh DW, et al. Water dynamics in unilateral biportal endoscopic spine surgery and its related factors: an in vivo proportional regression and proficiency-matched study. World Neurosurg. 2021;149:e836–e43.
10. Choi KC, Shim HK, Hwang JS, Shin SH, Lee DC, Jung HH, et al. Comparison of surgical invasiveness between microdiscectomy and 3 different endoscopic discectomy techniques for lumbar disc herniation. World Neurosurg. 2018;116:e750–e8.
11. Kim W, Kim SK, Kang SS, Park HJ, Han S, Lee SC. Pooled analysis of unsuccessful percutaneous biportal endoscopic surgery outcomes from a multi-institutional retrospective cohort of 797 cases. Acta Neurochir. 2020;162(2):279–87.

5 Foraminal and Extraforaminal HNP (Paraspinal Approach)

Ho Jin Lee, Ju Eun Kim, and Dae Jung Choi

5.1 Introduction

Lumbar foraminal or extraforaminal disc herniation (FDH) accounts for 7–12% of all lumbar disc herniations [1, 2]. FDH compresses the nerve root in the intervertebral foramen and affects its extraforaminal course. Patients with FDH manifest radicular pain that can be more severe than in other types of lumbar herniation, such as relatively mild low back pain. This notable feature is caused by direct irritation and compression of the nerve root and its dorsal root ganglion, which is more sensitive to pain in a narrow intervertebral foramen [3].

For surgical treatment, a midline or paramedian approach with partial or total laminectomy is usually applied to obtain access to the lesion. Although many spine surgeons are familiar with this approach, it can lead to spinal instability and often requires additional fixation, even in a minimally invasive manner. The posterolateral approach, such as Watkins' method or Wiltse's paraspinal sacrospinalis-splitting approach, minimizes spinal instability [4, 5]. However, a large portion of the isthmus must be removed to decompress the root, resulting in fracture.

The paraspinal approach using unilateral biportal endoscopy (UBE) has been introduced, with favorable clinical outcomes [6, 7]. This method has many advantages and overcomes the drawbacks of the earlier open, microendoscopic, and endoscopic procedures, including easy access to L5–S1 lesions, independent movement of the working channel, minimal chance of facet instability, high-quality imaging, and no requirement for specialized endoscopic instruments [6].

5.2 Indications and Contraindications

- Indications
  - Foraminal lumbar disc herniation
  - Extraforaminal lumbar disc herniation
  - Recurrent foraminal or extraforaminal lumbar disc herniation
- Relative contraindications
  - FDH with degenerative spondylolisthesis
- Contraindications

No author has any relevant financial relationship to disclose.
None of the content of this paper has been presented previously.

Supplementary Information The online version contains supplementary material available at [https://doi.org/10.1007/978-981-16-8201-8_5].

H. J. Lee
Department of Orthopaedic Surgery, Chungnam National University College of Medicine, Daejeon, South Korea

J. E. Kim (✉) · D. J. Choi
Department of Orthopaedic Surgery, Himnaera Hospital, Busan, South Korea

D. H. Heo et al. (eds.), *Unilateral Biportal Endoscopic Spine Surgery*, https://doi.org/10.1007/978-981-16-8201-8_5

– FDH with segmental instability
– FDH with lytic spondylolisthesis
– Coexisting pathological conditions
  Spine infection
  Spine tumor

5.3 Special Instruments

Angled instruments are useful to access foraminal structures (Fig. 5.1). We used an angled curette to detach the ligamentum flavum from the deep portion of the foramen around the medial part of the facet joint. An upward-curved pituitary rongeur is necessary to remove the detached tissues from the operative field around the canal. The upward-curved Kerrison punch and burr effectively cut and enlarge the foraminal canal located under the pedicle.

5.4 Anesthesia and Positioning

The surgical procedure was performed under general or epidural anesthesia. The patient was placed prone with the abdomen free from pressure on a radiolucent frame, with the hip and knee joints flexed to open the foraminal space.

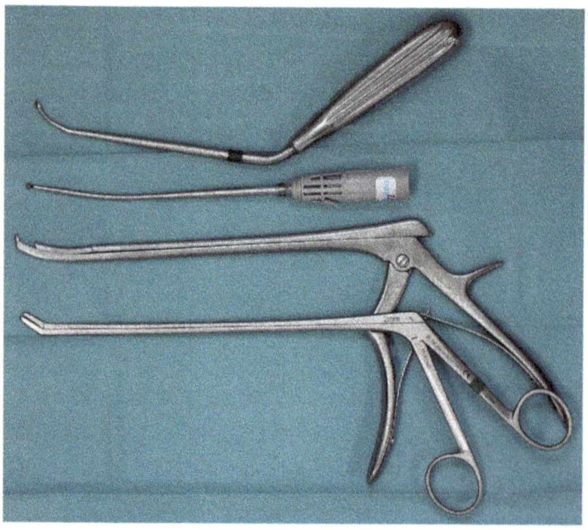

Fig. 5.1 Useful UBE instruments for foraminal discectomy. Top to bottom: angled curette, upward-curved burr, upward-curved Kerrison punch, and upward-curved pituitary rongeur

5.5 Surgical Steps

1. **Placement of the two portals**

Under C-arm fluoroscopic imaging, the upper and lower pedicles, and their transverse processes, were marked on the skin at the surgical level. The C-arm intensifier was set parallel to the upper endplate of the proximal vertebral body at the operative level. Portal incisions were made 2–3 cm lateral to the lateral border of each pedicle on the midline of the transverse process (Fig. 5.2). Different portal placements were used when the L5–S1 level was treated due to the iliac crest. The left portal was the same as described for the left L5–S1, but the right portal was moved to a point 1 cm medial from the conventional right portal. Both portals were changed to a point 1 cm proximal from the original portals for the right L5–S1.

2. **Constructing the surgical field**

This step exposes the lateral edge of the isthmus, the superior articular process (SAP) of the facet joint, and the transverse process surrounding the exit of the foramen. The guide pin should be

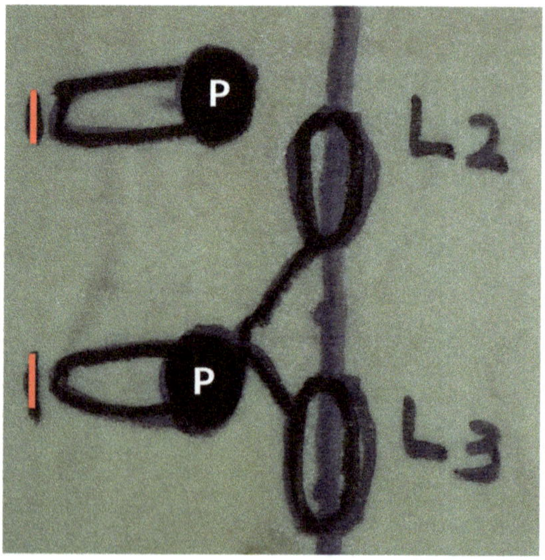

Fig. 5.2 Placement of the portals. One-centimeter vertical incisions were made 2–3 cm lateral to the lateral margin of the pedicle line, on the midline of each of the two transverse processes. "P" indicates the location of the pedicle and the red lines represent the actual incisions

inserted into the isthmus under the C-arm intensifier before beginners start this step; the guide pin was introduced through the right skin incision (the working portal for the endoscope), which allows the surgeon to obtain access to the exit of the foramen (Fig. 5.3). Using a narrow Cobb elevator, the soft tissues were gently detached from the lateral edge of the isthmus, SAP, and transverse process of the targeted foramen surrounding the fixed guide pin. A 0° scope was initially inserted through the viewing portal after inserting the cannula. A saline irrigation pump was connected to the endoscope, set to a pressure of 23–30 mmHg during the procedure, and controlled within this range depending on the surgical view. A continuous flow of saline solution was critical to control minor bleeding and maintain clarity of the surgical field. After separating the soft tissue, a shaver and radiofrequency probe were used to manage the remnant tissues and bleeding (Video 5.1). Construction of the surgical field was finished following complete exposure of the lateral edge of the isthmus, SAP, and transverse process (Video 5.1, Fig. 5.4).

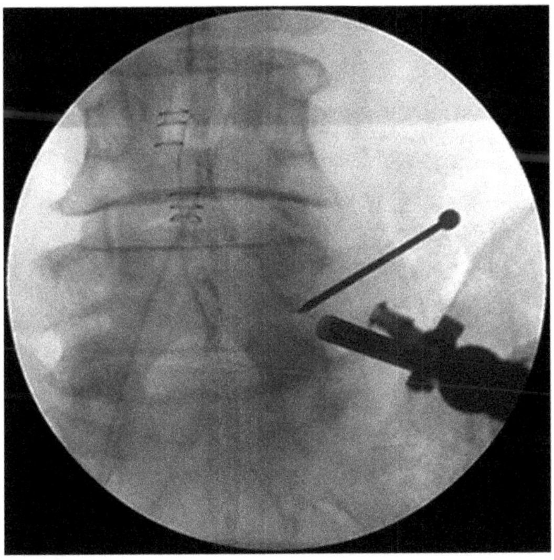

Fig. 5.3 Anteroposterior C-arm fluoroscopic image showing a guide pin inserted into the lateral edge of the isthmus, which allows access to the exit of the foramen

3. **Foraminoplasty and nerve root exposure**

Care should be taken to meticulously expose the compressed exiting nerve roots, which are vulnerable to damage. This foraminoplasty procedure is helpful to decompress the nerves and remove the surrounding tissues, including the ligamentum flavum, without injuring the nerve before the discectomy. The lateral edge of the isthmus and tip of the SAP are the key structures and were peeled off with the burr and Kerrison punch. The burr was used to enlarge the roof of the foramen by thinning out the lateral edge of the isthmus and tip of the SAP, followed by the Kerrison punch (Video 5.2). After the foraminoplasty, the ligamentum flavum was detached and removed from the undersurface of the isthmus and the SAP using an angled curette, upward-curved Kerrison punch, and upward-curved pituitary rongeur (Fig. 5.1, Video 5.2). The exiting nerve root was exposed after flavectomy, and the decompression procedure was performed around the nerve using the Kerrison punch, curettes, and a burr.

4. **Discectomy**

After exposing the nerve root with appropriate decompression, the herniated disc compressing the nerve was confirmed. Discectomy was performed with the pituitary rongeur, probe, and curette (Video 5.3).

5. **Closure**

After adequate hemostasis with a radiofrequency probe, a suction drain was inserted through the instrument portal (working portal). The endoscope and instruments were extracted. Any remaining saline was discharged by manual squeezing around the portals. The skin was repaired with a skin stapler after a 1-point subcutaneous suture with absorbable material.

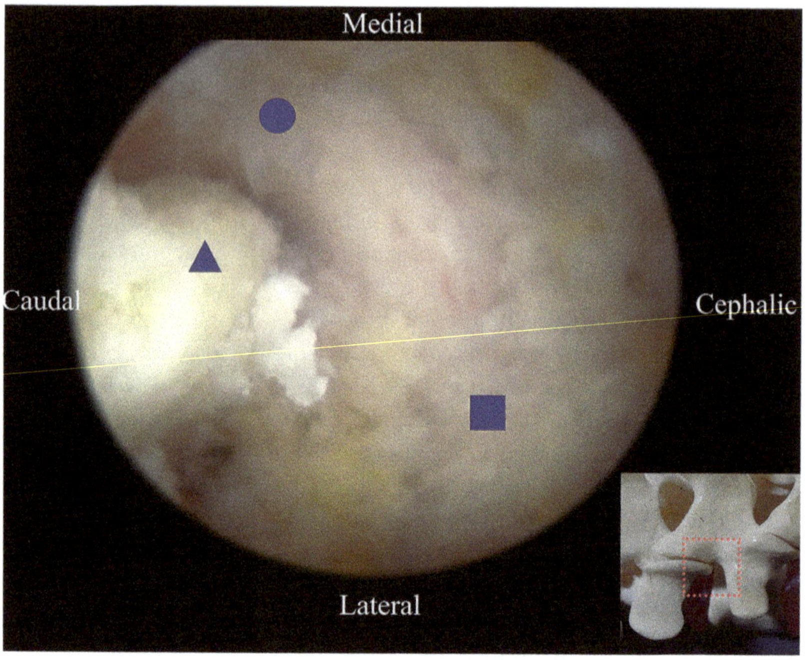

Fig. 5.4 Endoscopic image showing the construction of the surgical field before foraminal discectomy via UBE. The triangle indicates the tip of the superior articular process, and the circle represents the lateral edge of the isthmus, and the square represents the transverse process

5.6 Illustrated Cases

1. Case 1: A 55-year-old female suffered from severe radiating pain in the left anterior thigh with intermittent neurological claudication.

Preoperative magnetic resonance imaging (MRI) showed left FDH at L2–3 (Fig. 5.5). We performed the endoscopic discectomy using the UBE paraspinal approach (Fig. 5.6). The symptoms improved significantly immediately after the operation.

2. Case 2: A 66-year-old male suffered from severe radiating pain in the left posterior calf with intermittent neurological claudication.

Preoperative MRI images revealed left FDH at L5–S1 (Fig. 5.7). We performed the endoscopic discectomy using the UBE paraspinal approach (Fig. 5.8). The symptoms improved significantly immediately after the operation.

5.7 Management of Complications

The complications of this foraminal discectomy using the UBE paraspinal approach were usually minor.

1. Dural tear: A small-sized tear (<1 mm) was treated by covering it with a collagen patch. Non-penetrating vascular clipping was another treatment option for more significant-sized tears.
2. Abdominal discomfort with distension: This complication can result from the collection of retroperitoneal fluid after the UBE paraspinal approach. The majority of cases resolved spontaneously without any additional treatment. We recommend controlling the saline irrigation pressure within 30 mmHg during surgery to prevent saline from leaking into the retroperitoneal space.

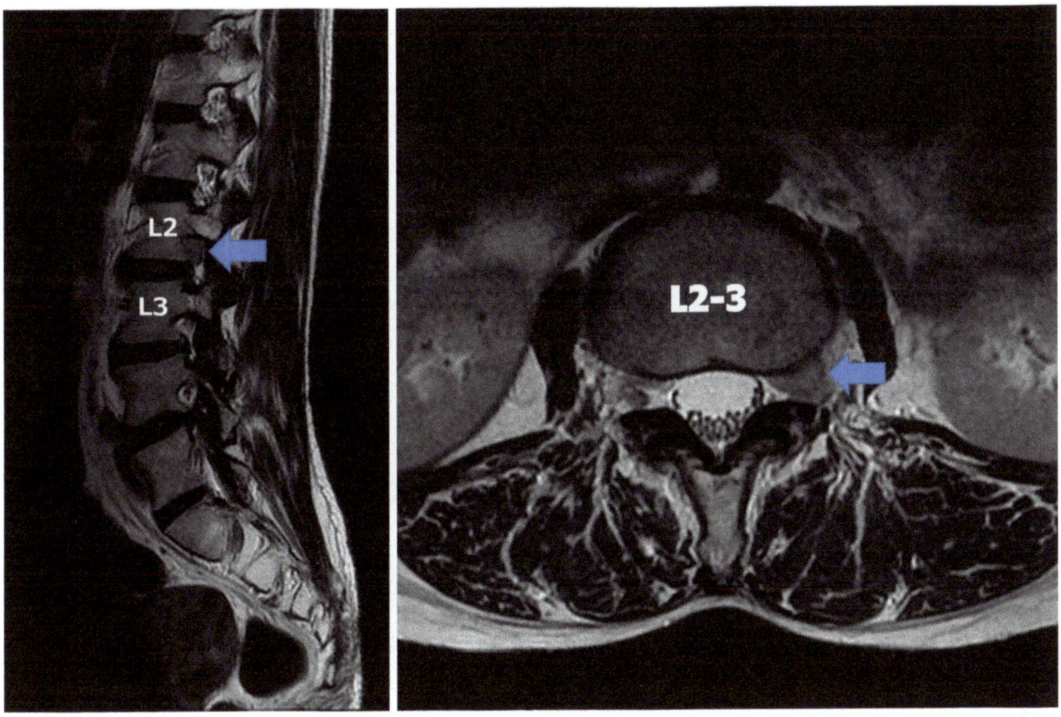

Fig. 5.5 Preoperative magnetic resonance image of Case 1 showing left foraminal disc herniation at L2–3. *Blue arrow* indicates the foraminal herniated disc

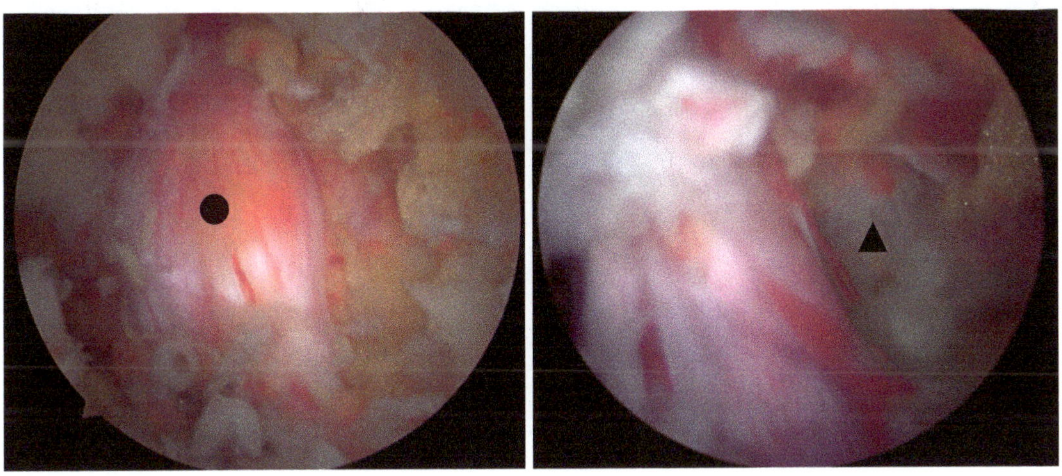

Fig. 5.6 Endoscopic image showing the dorsal root ganglion of the L2 nerve root compressed by the herniated disc (Left), and the herniated disc located under the axillary portion of the L2 nerve root (Right). The circle indicates the dorsal root ganglion, and the triangle indicates the herniated disc

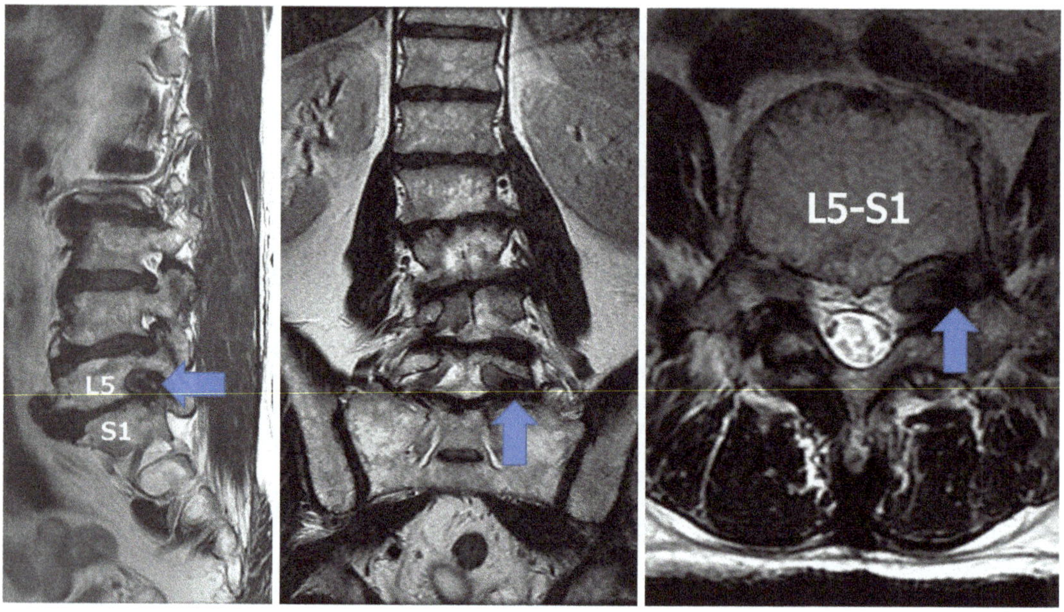

Fig. 5.7 Preoperative magnetic resonance image of Case 2 showing left foraminal disc herniation at L5–S1. The blue arrow indicates the foraminal herniated disc

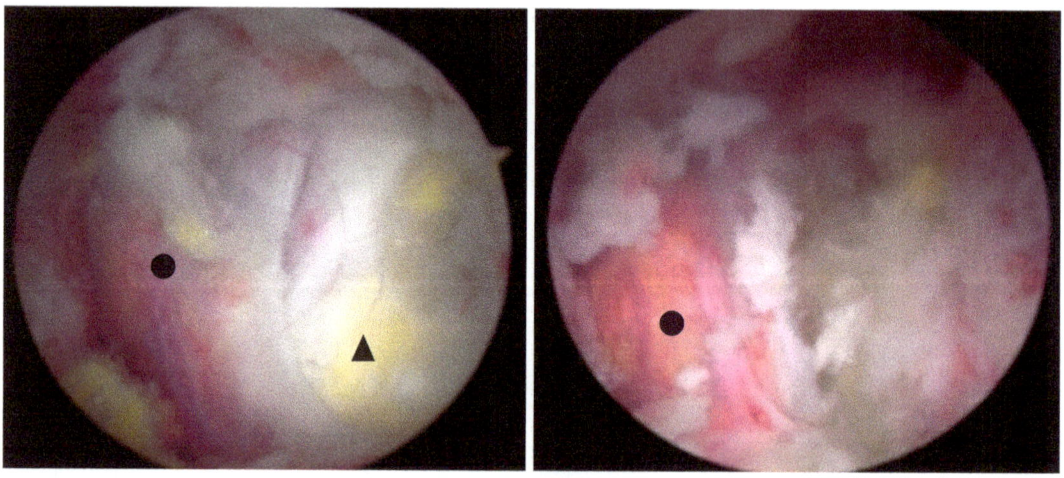

Fig. 5.8 Endoscopic image showing the L5 nerve root compressed by the herniated disc (Left) and the nerve root after the discectomy (Right). The circle indicates the L5 nerve root, and the triangle denotes the herniated disc

5.8 Surgical Tips and Pitfalls

Three factors need to be considered to perform an adequate discectomy. First, during construction of the surgical field, care should be taken not to injure the radicular artery around the SAP of the facet joint. Second, the tip of the SAP should be removed gradually during foraminoplasty. Instability after resecting the SAP may be a concern. The tip of the SAP is removed to allow an approach to the FDH, as described above. Because the foraminoplasty is limited to the tip of the SAP, it may not be lead to postoperative instability. However, more research is needed for confirmation. Third, when intra-foraminal lesions are treated, it is useful to use a specially designed angled curette, upward-curved Kerrison punch, and upward-curved pituitary rongeur.

References

1. Abdullah AF, Wolber PGH, Warfield JR, Gunadi IK. Surgical management of extreme lateral lumbar disc herniations: review of 138 cases. Neurosurgery. 1988;22(4):648–53.
2. Marquardt G, Bruder M, Theuss S, Setzer M, Seifert V. Ultra-long-term outcome of surgically treated far-lateral, extraforaminal lumbar disc herniations: a single-center series. Eur Spine J. 2012;21(4):660–5.
3. Epstein NE. Foraminal and far lateral lumbar disc herniations: surgical alternatives and outcome measures. Spinal Cord. 2002;40(10):491–500.
4. Watkins MB. Posterolateral fusion of the lumbar and lumbosacral spine. JBJS. 1953;35(4):1014–8.
5. Wiltse LL, Bateman JG, Hutchinson RH, Nelson WE. The paraspinal Sacrospinalis-splitting approach to the lumbar spine. JBJS. 1968;50(5):919–26.
6. Ahn J-S, Lee H-J, Choi D-J, Lee K-Y, Hwang S-J. Extraforaminal approach of biportal endoscopic spinal surgery: a new endoscopic technique for transforaminal decompression and discectomy. J Neurosurg Spine. 2018;28(5):492–8.
7. Choi D-J, Kim J-E, Jung J-T, Kim Y-S, Jang H-J, Yoo B, et al. Biportal endoscopic spine surgery for various foraminal lesions at the lumbosacral lesion. Asian Spine J. 2018;12(3):569–73.

Unilateral Biportal Endoscopy Via Contralateral Sublaminar Approach for Surgical Management of Lumbar Disc Herniation

6

Dong Hwa Heo, Cheol Woong Park, Seong Yi, and Hungtae Chung

6.1 Introduction

It may be difficult to treat upper lumbar disc herniation or migrated disc herniation via ipsilateral laminotomy [1]. Rarely, wide laminotomy with medial facetectomy is needed to remove migrated disc herniations. Especially, there may be a high possibility of injury to the isthmus and facet joint due to narrow laminar space in case of upper lumbar disc herniation [2, 3].

Contralateral sublaminar approach is a familiar strategy in endoscopic surgery for lumbar central or lateral recess stenosis. We have frequently performed decompression of contralateral traversing nerve root via removal of contralateral ligamentum flavum in cases of central or lateral recess stenosis during unilateral biportal endoscopy (UBE). Contralateral sublaminar discectomy is a modification of routine UBE contralateral decompressive procedures in central stenosis [3, 4]. Contralateral and exiting nerve roots can be accessed after midline laminotomy via contralateral approaches (Figs. 6.1a and b). Contralateral sublaminar lumbar discectomy has several advantages such as relatively small laminotomy, preservation of facet joint, and adequate demonstration of contralateral exiting or traversing nerve root [4]. Contralateral sublaminar approach might be appropriate for the treatment of foraminal disc herniation, migrated ruptured disc, and upper lumbar disc herniations [1, 3–5].

Supplementary Information The online version contains supplementary material available at [https://doi.org/10.1007/978-981-16-8201-8_6].

D. H. Heo
Neurosurgery, Endoscopic Spine Surgery Center, Seoul Bumin Hospital, Seoul, South Korea

C. W. Park (✉)
Neurosurgery, Spine Center, Daejeon Woori Hospital, Daejeon, South Korea

S. Yi
Neurosurgery, Severance Hospital, Yonsei University, Seoul, South Korea

H. Chung
Orthopedics, Endoscopic Spine Surgery Center, Seoul Bumin Hospital, Seoul, South Korea

6.2 Indications and Contraindications

Foraminal disc herniations, migrated disc herniation and upper lumbar disc herniations are the best indications for contralateral sublaminar approach in UBE. Both compression of exiting nerve root and traversing nerve root via concomitant central or lateral stenosis with disc herniation are other indications for this strategy, which

D. H. Heo et al. (eds.), *Unilateral Biportal Endoscopic Spine Surgery*,
https://doi.org/10.1007/978-981-16-8201-8_6

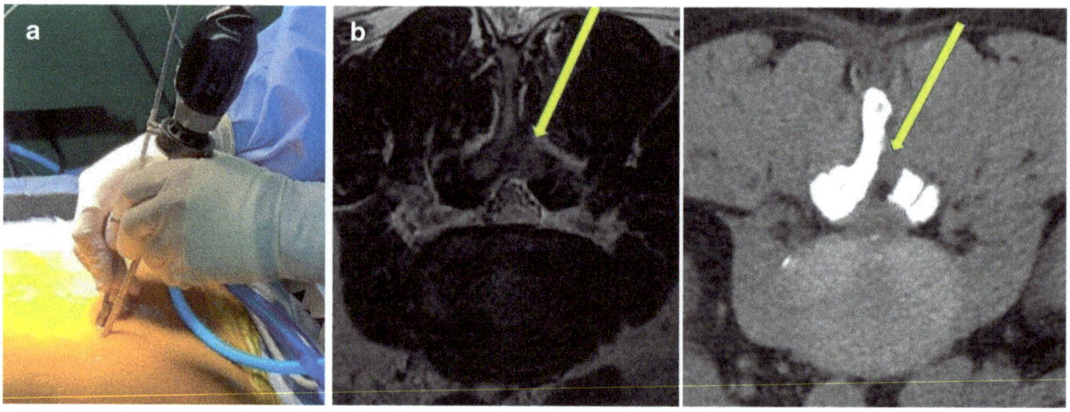

Fig. 6.1 The contralateral sublaminar approach in UBE is presented. Overview of UBE contralateral sublaminar approach (**a**). Midline laminotomy area in the contralateral sublaminar approach (**b**)

can be used to decompress exiting nerve root as well as traversing nerve root at the same time. Central disc herniation, calcified disc, and contained disc herniation are contraindications for contralateral sublaminar UBE.

- Indications: upper lumbar disc herniation, foraminal disc herniation, upward or downward migrated disc as well as compressive lesion of exiting nerve root and traversing nerve root
- Contraindications: contained disc herniation, central disc herniation, and calcified disc

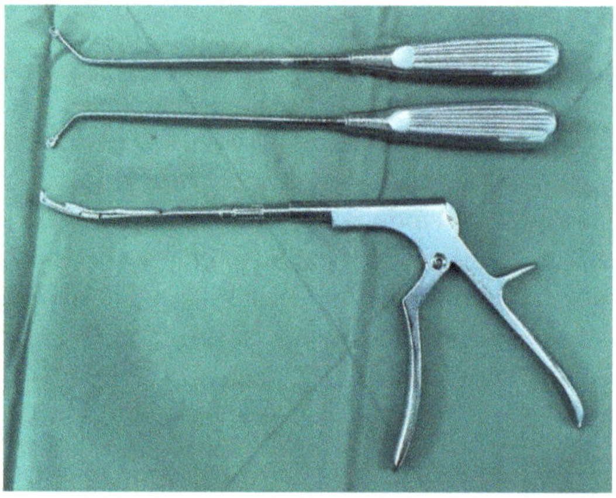

Fig. 6.2 Partially curved foraminal Kerrison punches and curved curettes used in contralateral sublaminar approach

6.3 Special Instruments

Partially curved foraminal Kerrison punches or rongeurs measuring 2–3 mm in diameter are highly useful in removing the foraminal ligament around the contralateral exiting nerve root (Fig. 6.2). Angled curettes are also useful to decompress an exiting nerve root. Kerrison 360° Rotating Rongeur is also very effective in resecting contralateral ligamentum flavum and foraminal ligament. Curve curettes are also used (Fig. 6.1). We prefer to use mini up-bite pituitary forceps when ruptured disc particles are removed in the contralateral foraminal area. Although a zero-degree endoscope was usually used in various UBE approaches, a 12° or 30° endoscope may facilitate the delineation of the contralateral foramen.

6.4 Anesthesia and Position

Both epidural anesthesia and general endotracheal anesthesia are used. Prone position is necessary for the contralateral approach. We prefer a prone position over Jackson table or Wilson flame to reduce abdominal pressure as well as epidural pressure.

6.5 Surgical Steps

6.5.1 Creation of Two Channels

The location of the two portals should be modified based on the targets (Fig. 6.3). For the decompression of a contralateral exiting nerve root and removal of up-migrated disc herniation or foraminal disc herniation, the two holes should be slightly lower than the routine two portals (Fig. 6.3a). In contrast, if the main target traverses the nerve root or down-migrated disc particles, the two channels should be slightly higher than the routine two portals (Fig. 6.3b). Modification of portal location may prevent excessive bone work.

6.5.2 Bone Work

Midline laminotomy was initiated at the junction of spinous process and lamina (Fig. 6.4a). In case of contralateral bony stenosis or osteophytes, we performed contralateral sublaminar bony decompression before disc removal (Fig. 6.4b).

If the right-sided ruptured disc particles are removed, a left-side laminotomy should be performed via two portals on the left side. Contralateral sides can be accessed through the small ipsilateral laminotomy area (Fig. 6.5).

Although the width of the laminotomy is small, the lower portion of the upper lamina must be removed sufficiently to expose the exiting nerve root. For the removal of down-migrated disc, we partially removed the superior articular process and the upper portion of the contralateral lower laminar area.

6.5.3 Removal of Ligamentum Flavum and Exposure of Nerve Root

Contralateral ligamentum flavum was partially removed to expose nerve root and ruptured disc particles (Fig. 6.6a). If patients exhibit central or lateral recess stenosis, we totally removed contralateral ligament flavum. It is necessary to remove the foraminal ligament to expose and decompress the contralateral exiting nerve root (Fig. 6.6b). The contralateral exiting nerve root is placed under the foraminal ligament (Fig. 6.6c).

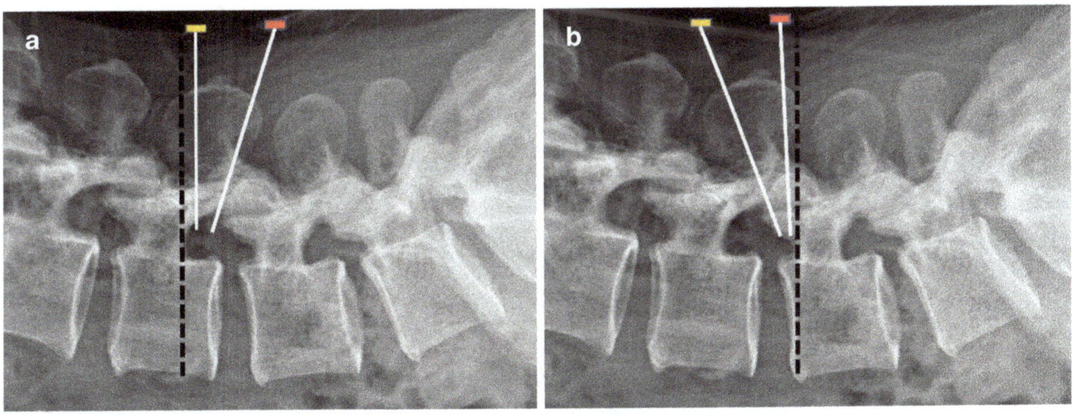

Fig. 6.3 Modification of the location of two portals in a case of left to right contralateral approach. If the main target is a contralateral exiting nerve root, endoscopic portal should be created below the lower margin of the upper pedicle (**a**). For the decompression of a contralateral traversing nerve root, the working portal should be created in the area superior to the upper margin of lower pedicle (**b**)

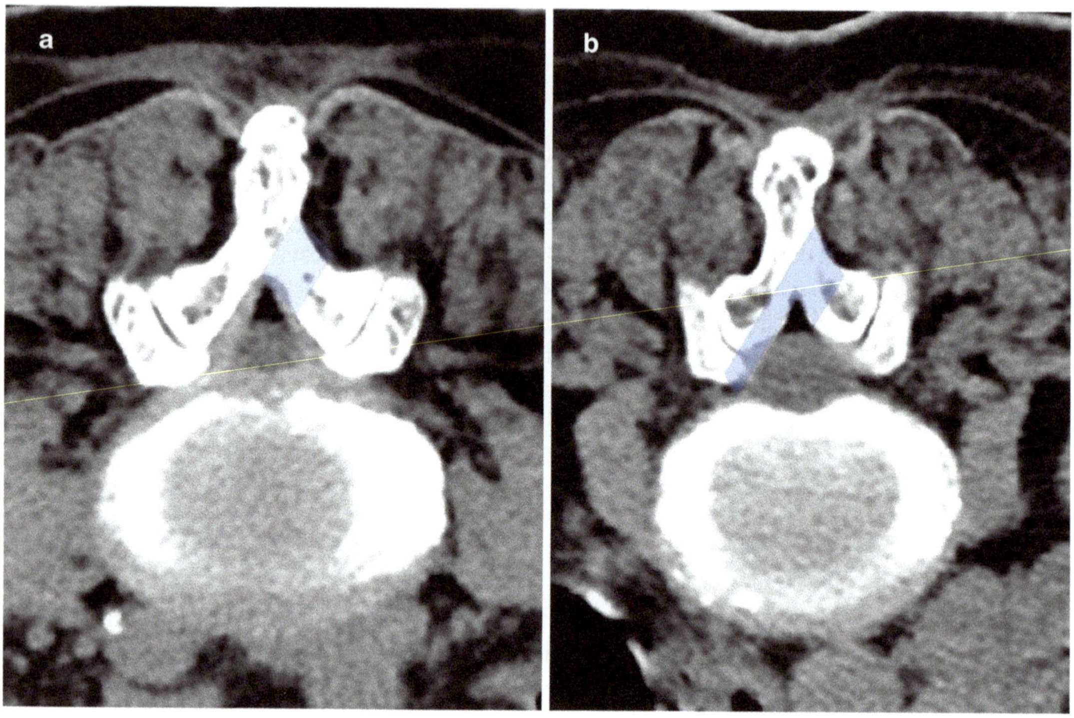

Fig. 6.4 The area of midline laminotomy in left-to-right approach (**a**). Central stenosis is an indication for contralateral sublaminar bony removal for easy access of contralateral foraminal area (**b**)

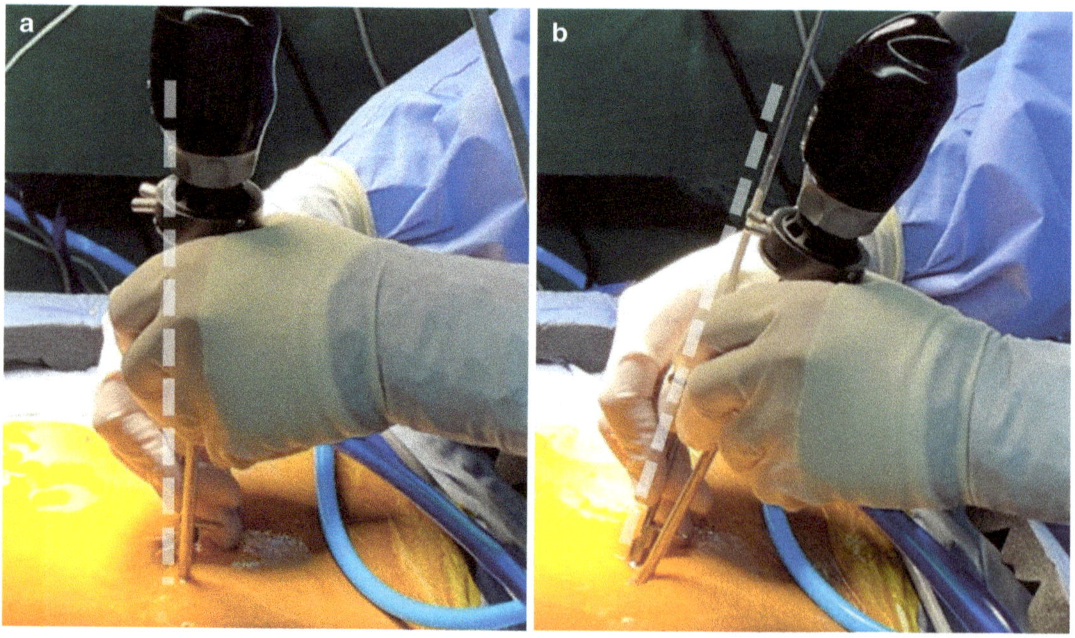

Fig. 6.5 Tilting of endoscope and spinal instruments. By tilting the two portals, the contralateral side can be easily accessed via small mid-line laminotomy area (**a**) before tilting, (**b**) after tilting of two portals

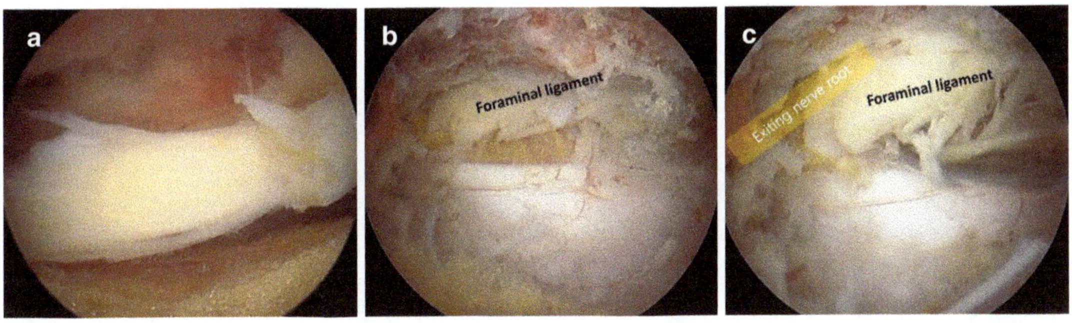

Fig. 6.6 Intraoperative endoscopic image of contralateral ligamentum flavum and foraminal ligament. Contralateral ligamentum flavum was removed to expose contralateral dura and traversing nerve root (**a**). Contralateral foraminal ligament should be removed to expose contralateral exiting nerve root (**b**). The exiting nerve root passes under foraminal ligament (**c**)

6.5.4 Removal of Ruptured Disc Particles

The ruptured disc particles were easily detected and exposed by retracting the dura medially (Figs. 6.5 and 6.6). Angled hoots enabled the removal of disc particles. We removed disc particles using small pituitary forceps or angled up-bite pituitary.

6.5.5 Bleeding Control

A small-diameter RF probe is recommended and extreme care is required when using RF around the root.

Bleeding around nerve roots or pedicles can be controlled with an RF probe. Packing with pieces of Gelfoam or tachosil is also very useful for hemostasis. An epidural drainage catheter is placed after surgery. This catheter is usually removed the second day after surgery.

@Brief Summary of Surgical Steps

1. Creation of modified two portals
2. Ipsilateral midline laminotomy
3. Removal of contralateral ligamentum flavum
4. Exposure of dura and nerve roots
5. Disc particle rupture after slight retraction of dura
6. Bleeding control
7. Epidural catheter insertion
8. Wound closure

6.6 Illustrated Cases

6.6.1 Case 1: Foraminal Up-migrated Disc (Fig. 6.7 and Video 6.1)

A 41-year-old female patient presented with complaints of left leg pain and L3 dermatome refractory to conservative management. Preoperative MRI revealed a foraminal up-migrated disc at L3–4 Lt (Fig. 6.7). The left-sided L3 nerve root was compressed by foraminal ruptured disc particles. We performed disc particle removal via UBE contralateral sublaminar approach from right to left side (Fig. 6.7). Foraminal ruptured disc particles were completely removed after surgery. Postoperative MRI revealed total removal of ruptured disc particles and adequate decompression of left L3 exiting nerve root (Fig. 6.7, red arrow). The patient's pain was significantly alleviated postoperatively.

6.6.2 Case 2: Upper Lumbar Disc Herniation, Down Migration (Fig. 6.8 and Video 6.2)

A 65-year-old female patient presented with left leg pain. Preoperative MRI showed left-sided ruptured disc herniation at L2–3 and migration to L3 level (Fig. 6.8). Ruptured disc particles were removed via the right-sided UBE contralateral sublaminar approach of L2–3 (Fig. 6.8). Surgery

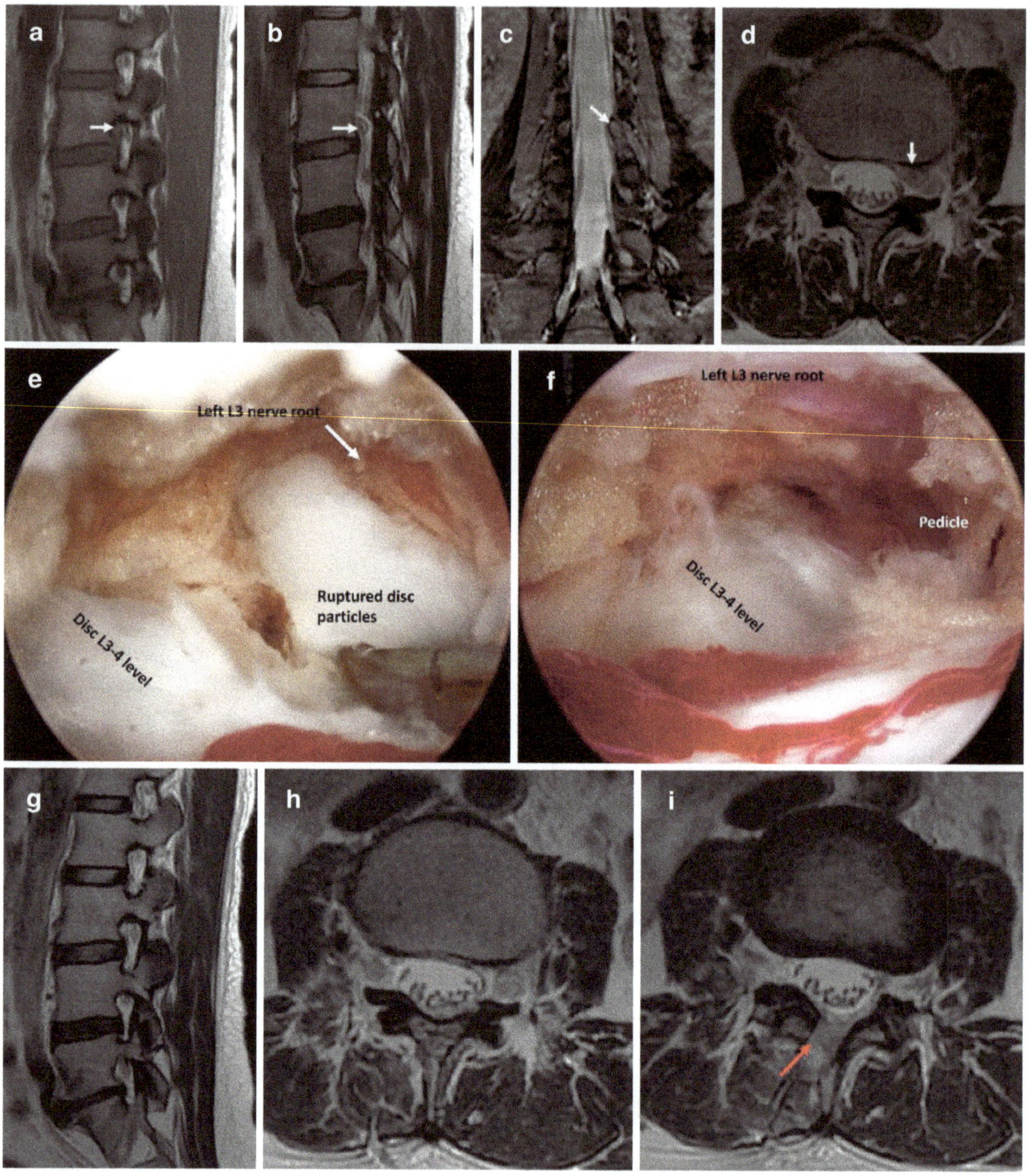

Fig. 6.7 Preoperative MRI reveals foraminal ruptured disc herniation at left L3–4 (White arrow, **a**: T1 sagittal, **b**: T2 sagittal, **c**: MR myelogram, and **d**: T2 axial). The patient underwent UBE surgery via contralateral sublaminar approach (**e** and **f**). Foraminal ruptured disc particles compressed left L3 exiting nerve root (**e**). The left L3 exiting nerve root was completely decompressed after removal of disc particles (**f**). Postoperative MRI shows complete removal of ruptured disc herniation (**g, h**, and **i**) and small and narrow area of laminotomy [1]

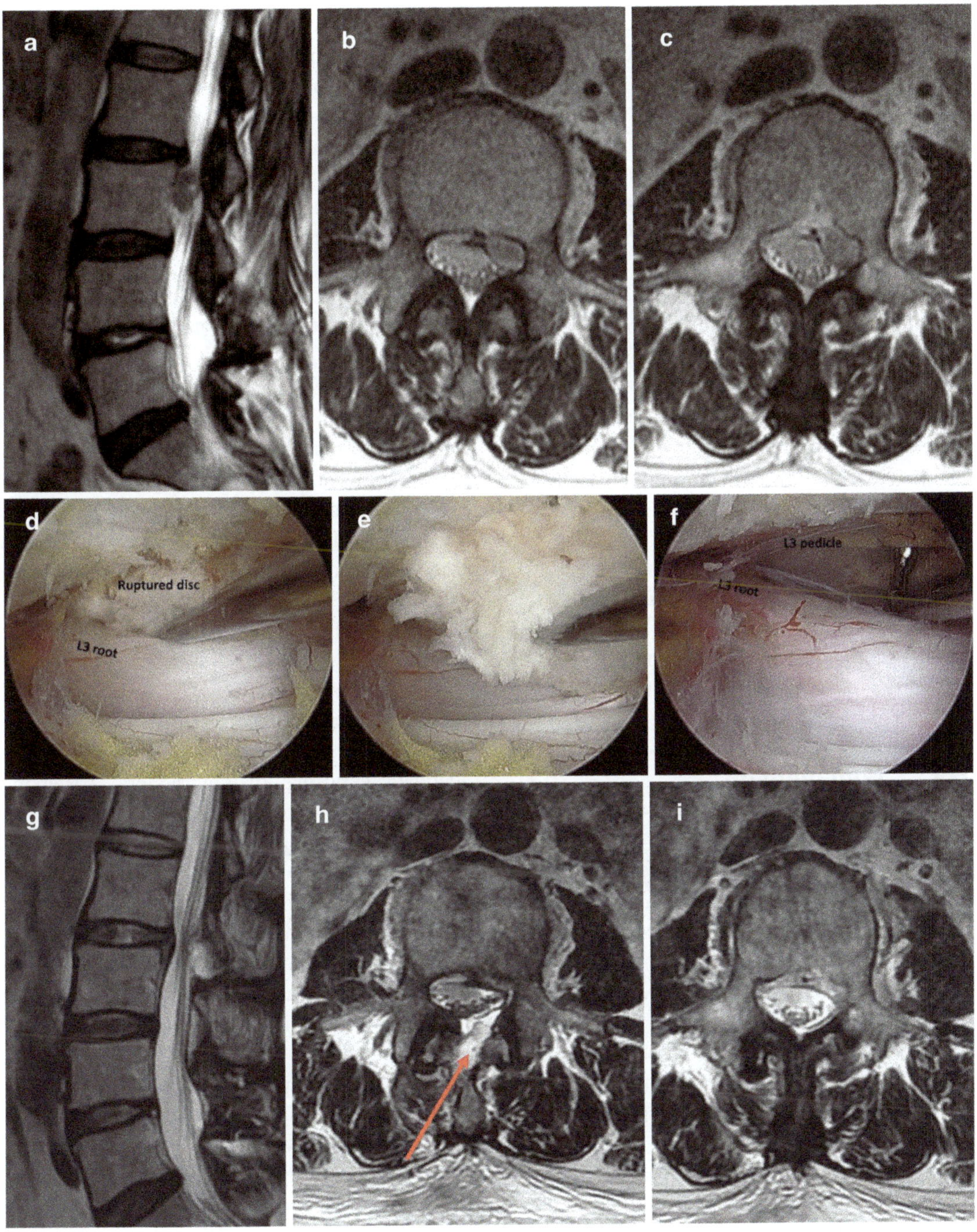

Fig. 6.8 Preoperative MRI shows left disc herniation with down migration at L2–3 (**a, b**, and **c**). We performed right-sided UBE contralateral sublaminar approach for removal of ruptured disc (**d, e** and **f**). The ruptured disc particles were detected under left L3 traversing nerve root (**d** and **e**). Following the removal of disc particles, the medial wall of left pedicle was clearly seen (**f**). Postoperative MRI revealed complete removal of ruptured disc particles (**g, h**, and **i**). Small laminotomy area was detected after UBE contralateral approach (**h**)

completely eliminated ruptured disc particles and resolved the patient's pain completely.

6.6.3 Case 3. Dual Roots Decompression. Foraminal HNP with Lateral Recess Stenosis (Fig. 6.9 and Video 6.3)

A 75-year-old female patient routinely complained of intermittent claudication of right leg and received treatment for spinal stenosis for a long time. The patient recently presented with radiating pain involving the right lower extremity, which had suddenly worsened. Preoperative lumbar MR images showed right foraminal ruptured disc herniation with central stenosis at L3–4 (Fig. 6.9). We performed left-to-right UBE contralateral sublaminar intervention for ruptured disc removal at L3 and decompression of L4 nerve (Fig. 6.9). Postoperative MR images showed total removal of ruptured foraminal disc and decompression of lateral recess of right L4–5 (Fig. 6.9).

6.7 Management of Complications

1. Recurrent disc herniation: The possibility of recurrent disc herniation remains. The contralateral approach entailed only sequestrectomy or removal of ruptured disc particles. This approach cannot be used to perform internal decompression or intradiscal discectomy. If patients manifest concomitant central disc herniation or contained disc herniation, ipsilateral laminotomy and discectomy were more appropriate.
2. Incomplete removal of ruptured disc particles: Rarely, the ruptured disc particle is fragmented into multiple pieces, warranting careful exploration around the nerve root for any residual disc fragments or remnants using a hook or dissectors. Intraoperative C arm fluoroscopy monitoring strongly facilitated optimal decompression (Fig. 6.10).
3. Postoperative epidural hematoma: Epidural bleeding usually occurs after the removal of ruptured disc particles. Epidural bleeding should be completely controlled using RF coagulation and packing of Gelfoam pieces.

6.8 Surgical Tips and Pitfalls

Adequate upper laminotomy is required over the exposed proximal portion of ligamentum flavum for the decompression of exiting nerve root via removal of up-migrated foraminal herniated disc. In case of concomitant foraminal stenosis, contralateral sublaminar bony decompression and complete removal of foraminal ligament are indicated. Angled up-bite pituitary forceps facilitate the removal of up-migrated disc or foraminal disc herniation.

In cases of down-migrated disc herniation, partial removal of upper area of lower laminae and superior articular process is necessary for adequate exposure of contralateral traversing nerve root and ruptured disc particle.

Surgical landmarks of contralateral exiting nerve root include tip of the superior articular process and foraminal ligament. If the foraminal ruptured disc particles are removed, the exiting nerve root can be detected easily without locating surgical landmarks. However, surgical landmarks may be important if patients manifest foraminal or central stenosis.

Bleeding generally occurs around the contralateral foramen and medial border pedicle following total removal of ruptured disc particles. Epidural vein is the main bleeding focus after discectomy and can be easily controlled via RF (small diameter steering RF tip) coagulation or Gelfoam packing. Floseal application is another option available for hemostasis.

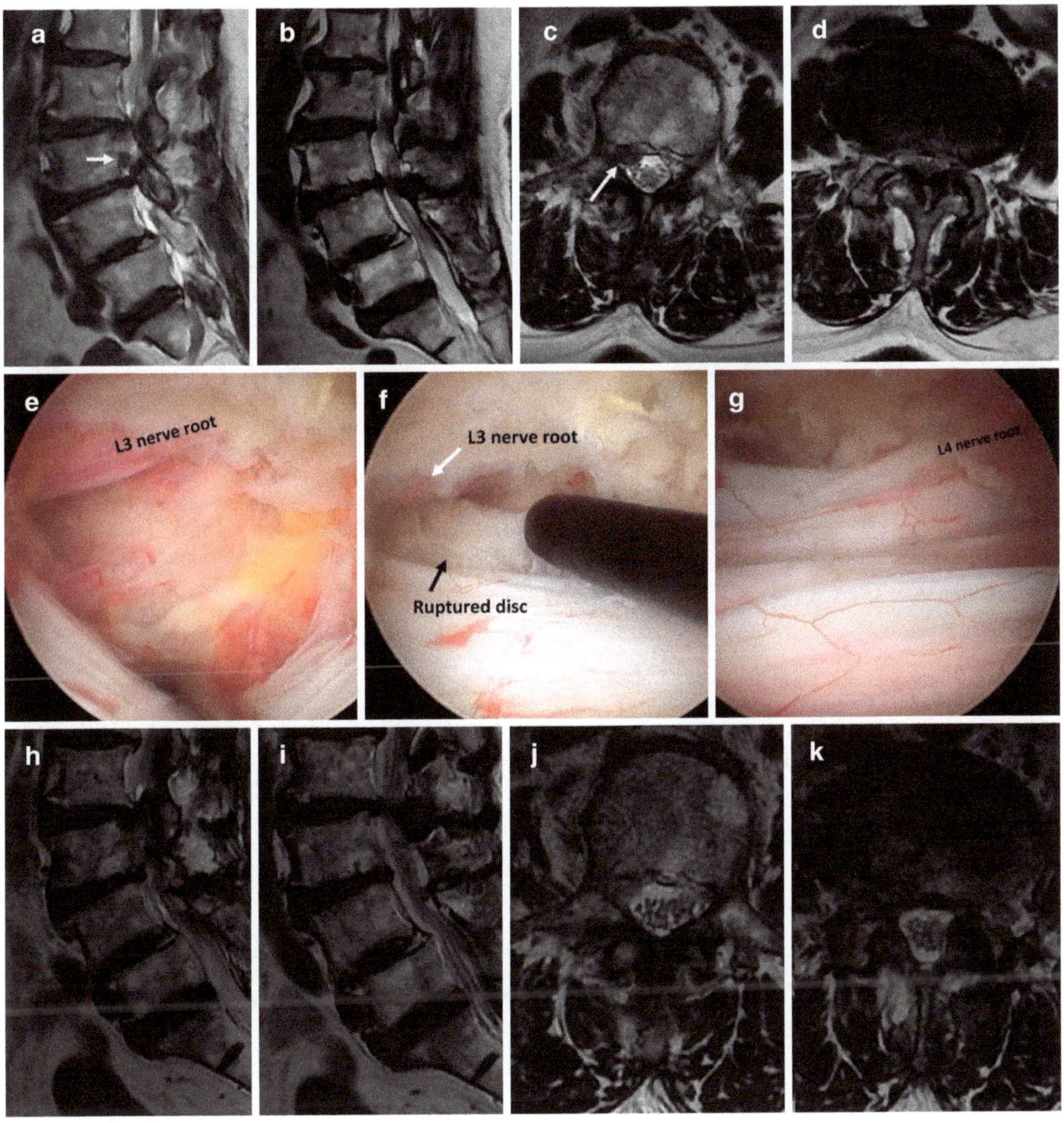

Fig. 6.9 A 75-year-old female patient suffered from radiating pain and claudication of right leg. Preoperative MR images revealed a right foraminal ruptured disc and lateral recess stenosis at L3–4. (Sagittal: **a** and **b**, axial: **c** and **d**). This patient was surgically treated via UBE using the left-sided contralateral sublaminar approach (**e**, **f** and **g**). After disc particles removal through contralateral sublaminar approach (**f**), L3 and L4 nerve roots were completely decompresse (**e** and **g**). Postoperative MR images depicted complete removal of ruptured disc particles and decompression of right lateral recess at L3–4 (**h**, **i**, **j** and **k**). UBE surgery resulted in significant alleviation of pain

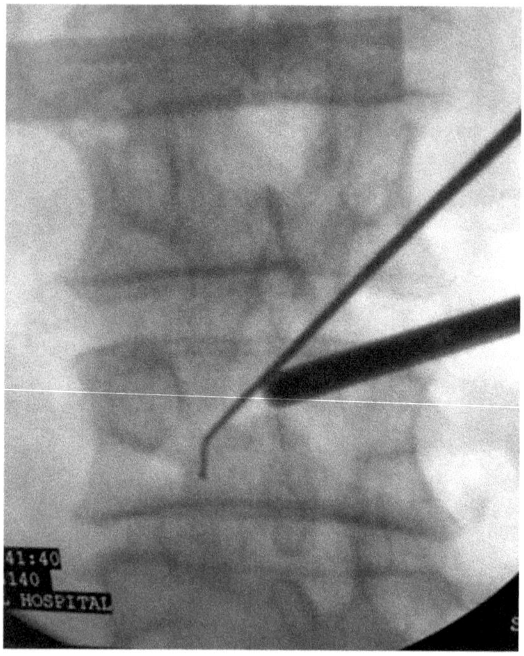

Fig. 6.10 Intraoperative C arm image highlighting UBE contralateral sublaminar approach. The degree of decompression of contralateral traversing nerve root was evaluated via real-time C-arm imaging

References

1. Akbary K, Kim JS, Park CW, Jun SG, Hwang JH. Biportal endoscopic decompression of exiting and traversing nerve roots through a single interlaminar window using a contralateral approach: technical feasibilities and morphometric changes of the lumbar canal and foramen. World Neurosurg. 2018;117:153–61.
2. Hwang JH, Park WM, Park CW. Contralateral interlaminar keyhole percutaneous endoscopic lumbar surgery in patients with unilateral radiculopathy. World Neurosurg. 2017;101:33–41.
3. Heo DH, Kim JS, Park CW, Quillo-Olvera J, Park CK. Contralateral sublaminar endoscopic approach for removal of lumbar Juxtafacet cysts using percutaneous biportal endoscopic surgery: technical report and preliminary results. World Neurosurg. 2019;122:474–9.
4. Park JH, Jang JW, Park WM, Park CW. Contralateral keyhole biportal endoscopic surgery for ruptured lumbar herniated disc: a technical feasibility and early clinical outcomes. Neurospine. 2020;17(Suppl 1):S110–s9.
5. Heo DH, Lee N, Park CW, Kim HS, Chung HJ. Endoscopic unilateral laminotomy with bilateral discectomy using biportal endoscopic approach: technical report and preliminary clinical results. World Neurosurg. 2020;137:31–7.

Unilateral Biportal Endoscopy for Revision Lumbar Discectomy

7

Min Seok Kang, Hyun Jin Park, and Dae Jung Choi

7.1 Introduction

Lumbar discectomy is a successful treatment for symptomatic lumbar disc herniation, but at least 8-years of follow-ups have reported an incidence of recurrent lumbar disc herniation of 38%, total reoperation rate of 15%, and a reoperation rate for recurrent lumbar disc herniation of 9.1% [1]. In particular, recurrent lumbar disc herniation, which is defined as the presence of herniated disc material at the same level as previously operated upon in patients who experienced a pain-free phase for more than 6 months, is known most common cause of surgical failure of lumbar discectomy.

Despite the relatively high incidence and reoperation rates, it is still controversial whether the optimal treatment for recurrent lumbar disc herniation is revision lumbar discectomy or instrumented fusion. In particular, given the disruption of anatomic planes and formation of peridural fibrotic tissue following lumbar discectomy, revision surgery can be a more technically complicated operation. The midline approach for the conventional revision lumbar discectomy is performed through a surgical corridor that requires traversing potentially confusing scar tissue, often requiring more surgical dissection and bony resection than the first-time operation [2]. This can be a potential risk of incidental durotomy or postoperative segmental instability. The incidence of incidental durotomy was reported at 3.5% for primary lumbar discectomy and 13.2% for revision lumbar discectomy [3]. In addition, concern over repeat recurrent lumbar disc herniation may lead surgeons to advocate posterior instrumented fusion surgery even in the absence of instability [4]. Revision lumbar discectomy was known to lead good probability for improvement, although not as good as for primary lumbar discectomy, and patients undergoing revision surgery were less satisfied [5, 6].

Although controversial, the minimally invasive approach can lead to significant improvement of back pain and reduce the complications rates compared with the open microscopic approach [7]. In this respect, full-endoscopic spine surgery may be a good alternative to revision lumbar discectomy [8–10]. However, unilateral biportal endoscopy can be a better alternative to revision lumbar discectomy in that both hands

Supplementary Information The online version contains supplementary material available at [https://doi.org/10.1007/978-981-16-8201-8_7].

M. S. Kang
Department of Orthopedic Surgery, Endoscopic Spine Surgery Center, Seoul Bumin Hospital, Seoul, South Korea

H. J. Park (✉)
Department of Orthopedic Surgery, Kangnam Sacred Heart Hospital, Hallym University College of Medicine, Seoul, South Korea

D. J. Choi
Department of Orthopedic Surgery, Spine Center, Himnaera Hospital, Busan, South Korea

D. H. Heo et al. (eds.), *Unilateral Biportal Endoscopic Spine Surgery*,
https://doi.org/10.1007/978-981-16-8201-8_7

can be used independently compared to percutaneous uni-portal full-endoscopic surgery. In the text below, the surgical procedure for recurrent lumbar disc herniation using unilateral biportal endoscopy will be described in detail.

7.2 Indications and Contraindications

The surgical indications were as follows: (1) Patients who previously received a lumbar laminotomy (or partial hemilaminectomy) and discectomy due to symptomatic lumbar disc herniation, (2) had leg pain of lumbosacral radiculopathy after being pain free for at least 6 months, (3) a herniated disc materials located at the same area as the previous surgery, as confirmed through magnetic resonance imaging, and (4) did not respond to conservative treatments. However, if the radicular pain remains after first-time surgery, or if the radicular pain has recurred after a brief improvement, it may also require a repeat lumbar discectomy when a residual or local recurrence of disc herniated is confirmed.

In fact, there are no specific contraindications. However, the Modic change in vertebral endplates (level 2), severe disc degeneration (Pfirrmann grade III), and increasing segmental sagittal rotations are the confounding factors that may affect the prognosis of lumbar discectomy, so sufficient information must be provided to the patient before surgery [11].

7.3 Anesthesia and Position

Once general endotracheal or epidural anesthesia is performed and appropriate IV access is obtained, the patient was placed in the prone position on the operating table over a radiolucent Wilson frame in a kneeling position. The patient was then prepped and water-proof draped in a sterile fashion. This is the same as lumbar discectomy or decompressive laminectomy using unilateral biportal endoscopy.

7.4 Surgical Steps

Under C-arm fluoroscopy, the target level was confirmed and identified on the patient's skin above the margin of the spinous process, lamina, facet joints, and intervertebral disc spaces. At the point where the line of the medial border of preserved facet articular processes and the line of the intervertebral disc space meet, two 0.7-cm skin incisions are made at the point of 1-cm top and bottom. (Fig. 7.1).

After sufficient incise to the lumbar fascia, the muscle detacher is used for subperiosteal dissection, which peels the multifidus muscles above the vertebral lamina and facet joint, facilitating the identification of medial border of facet articular process, laminar border, isthmus, multifidus muscles, and peridural fibrotic tissue. (Fig. 7.2a) (Video 7.1) If the anatomical landmarks are unclear by overgrowing scar tissue, the outer cortex of the vertebral lamina and facet articular processes is decorticated using a small-head diamond drill until boundaries of the vertebral lamina, the facet articular process, and scar tissue are identified. (Video 7.2) And then, with a small-head curved curette, chisel, or a diamond drill, the caudal border of the superior lamina and the medial border of the facet articular processes are undercut until a portion of healthy dura of traversing nerve root is exposed sublaminar. (Fig. 7.2b, c).

The exposure of the lateral margin of traversing nerve root is followed by a careful mobilization of the nerve root to the medial side. (Fig. 7.2d) If adhesion exists between the nerve root and the outer annulus of intervertebral disc, it is advisable to leave the nerve root in place and open the scar tissue by releasing it repeatedly lateral to the nerve root to get a safe access to the recurrent disc materials using a blunt dissector or small nerve hook. If the sequestrated nucleus pulposus is identified during this process, nucleus sequestrectomy is performed. Then, limited lumbar discectomy was performed meticulously (Fig. 7.2e, f) (Video 7.3). Complete neural decompression was confirmed by dural pulsation restoration. Bleeding control was achieved using

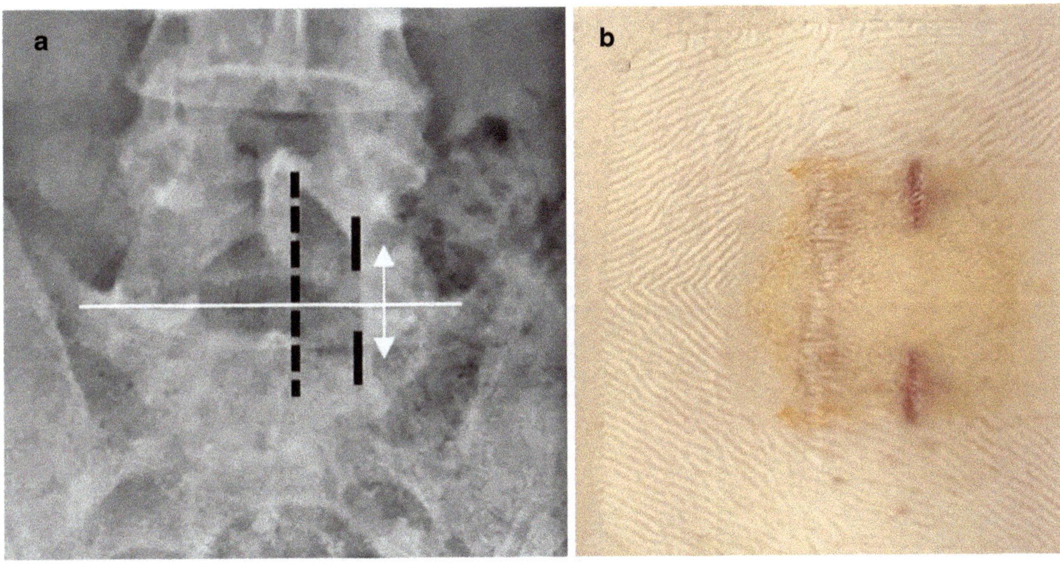

Fig. 7.1 Location of surgical portals. (**a**) Under C-arm fluoroscopy, the margin of the spinous process, lamina, facet articular processes, and intervertebral disc spaces was identified. At the point where the line of the medial border of preserved facet articular processes and the line of the intervertebral disc space meet, two 0.7-cm skin incisions are made at the point of 1-cm top and bottom. (**b**) Two weeks after surgery, wound photographs

the bipolar radiofrequency probe and bone wax, and a surgical drain was placed prior to skin closure.

7.5 Illustrated Cases

(1) **Case 1:** A 42-year-old male patient complained of severe right leg pain from a month ago. He underwent lumbar discectomy L5-S1 right side 15 months ago and has been doing well for three months after surgery. Preoperative plain radiographs showed right laminotomy status of L5-S1. And preoperative magnetic resonance imaging study showed recurrent herniated disc material at the same level as previously operated upon at right subarticular area of L5-S1. Lastly, he was undergone revision lumbar discectomy using unilateral biportal endoscopy. We obtained anatomical landmark without touching peridural fibrotic scar tissue as much as possible, and we could easily separate scar tissue from medial margin of facet articular process using curette or dissector and so on, and identify and remove the recurrent disc materials. (Fig. 7.3). After operation, preoperative symptoms were significantly improved postoperative 2 days.

(2) **Case 2:** A 57-year-old female patient who underwent lumbar discectomy L5-S1 left side 2 years ago, visited our clinic for a relapse of the left leg radicular pain 2 months ago. Left laminotomy status was observed and recurrent lumbar disc herniation from central to left subarticular area was observed in MR imaging. (Fig. 7.4) The revision lumbar discectomy using unilateral biportal endoscopy can be found in Video 7.4. The disc herniation was well removed after surgery, and a little additional laminotomy was required. (Fig. 7.4)

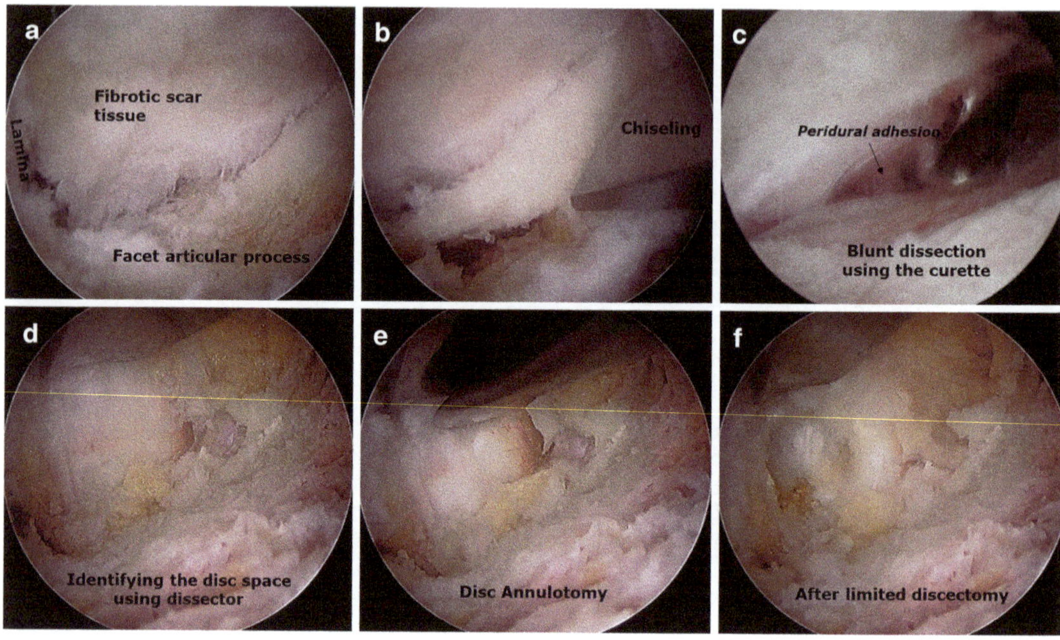

Fig. 7.2 Surgical steps of revision lumbar discectomy using unilateral biportal endoscopy. (**a**) Endoscopic visualization of the medial border of facet articular process, laminar border, and peridural fibrotic tissue was obtained. If the anatomical landmarks are unclear by overgrowing scar tissue, the outer cortex of the vertebral lamina and facet articular processes is decorticated using a small-head diamond drill until boundaries of the vertebral lamina, the facet articular process, and scar tissue are identified. (**b**) Additional laminotomy was performed using a chisel to identify traversing nerve root. (**c**) If extended laminotomy was performed in the first-time lumbar discectomy, blunt dissection can be performed directly on a layer of scar tissue, which is left on the dura of nerve root, at the medial border of the facet articular process using a curette. (**d**) The exposure of the lateral margin of traversing nerve root is followed by a careful mobilization of the nerve root to the medial side. (**e**) If the sequestrated disc material is identified, performed disc sequestrectomy, then annulotomy was performed for disc fragmentectomy and limited discectomy. (**f**) Limited discectomy was performed

7.6 Complications and Its Management

In the biportal endoscopic revisional lumbar discectomy, there are no major complications. Most have reported minor complications such as incidental durotomy, nerve root irritation, postoperative dysesthesia, and postoperative epidural hematomas, these complications usually improve after conservative managements including oral medication and physical therapy. If durotomy is recognized during surgery, direct repair with application of TachoSil (Absorbable fibrin sealant patch) and nonpenetrating clips can be expected a good outcome.

7.7 Surgical Tips and Pitfall

In the first-time lumbar discectomy, laminotomy (or partial hemilaminectomy) and partial flavectomy were performed, and the inevitable formation of peridural fibrotic tissue in this area after surgery, which can cause technical challenges when performing repeated discectomy. In particular, revision lumbar discectomy requires more paravertebral muscle dissection than the first-time surgery to secure anatomical landmarks and may cause iatrogenic spondylolysis or segmental instability following additional laminotomy. If necessary, a computerized tomography scan gives detailed information about the extension of

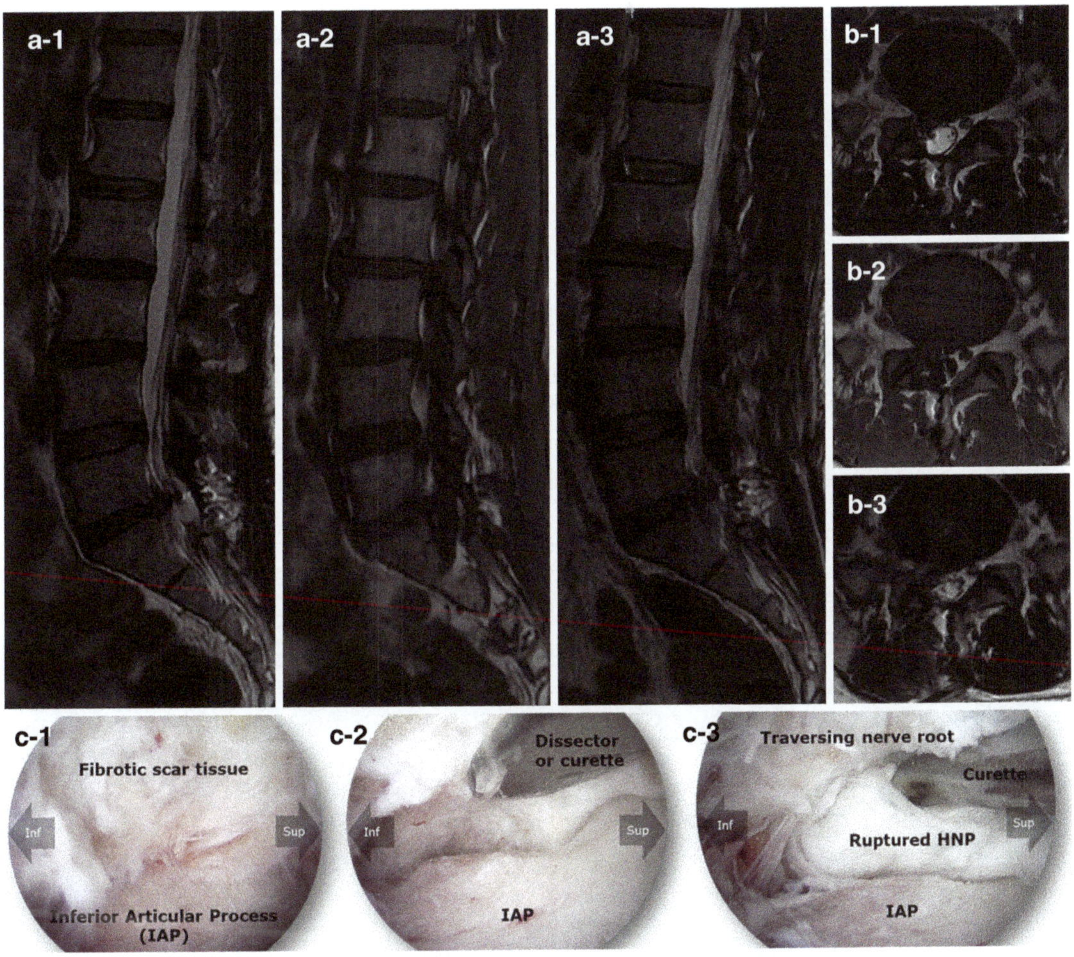

Fig. 7.3 Case presentation of a 42-year-old male patient. (**a**) Sagittal image of magnetic resonance imaging study. (**a-1**) Preoperative T2 weighted image. (**a-2**) Preoperative T1 weighted image. (**a-3**) Postoperative T2 weighted image. (**b**) Axial image of magnetic resonance imaging study. (**b-1**) Preoperative T2 weighted image. (**b-2**) Preoperative T1 weighted image. (**b-3**) Postoperative T2 weighted image. (**c**) Operative findings. (**c-1**) Easy access to the operation field without touching a fibrotic scar tissue. (**c-2**) Easy detachment a fibrotic scar tissue from the bony lamina. (**c-3**) Easy isolation of sequestration disc

the previous laminotomy, hemilaminectomy, facetectomy status, and presence of posterior limbus or ossification in the annulus.

In order to successfully remove recurrent disc materials using biportal endoscopic technique, the authors suggest approaching the space between facet articular processes and traversing nerve root where is relatively less adhesion, without touching the scar tissue as possible. In particular, making skin incisions on the outside rather than the previous incision is important because an endoscope and surgical instruments can safely land just above the preserved vertebral lamina and facet joints, and may prevent the risk of loss of orientation by peridural scar tissue. In addition, arthroscopic tissue shaver releases a normal muscle tissue more easily than fibrotic scar tissue, and the use of coagulation mode in the bipolar radiofrequency ablator allows for adequate tissue and vascular cauterization without lateral tissue damage than the use of electrocautery.

After endoscopic visualization of anatomical landmarks, it is simple and effective to separate

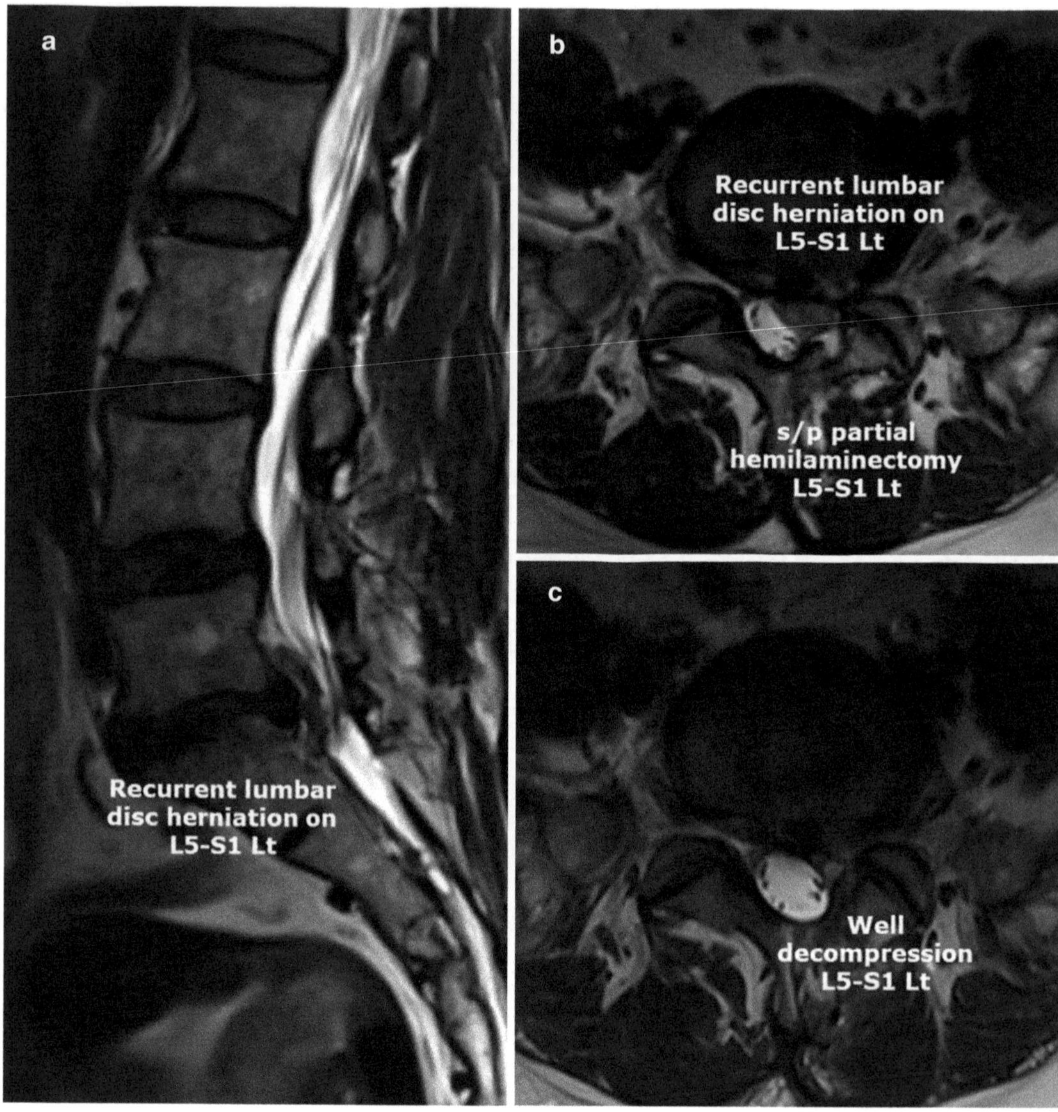

Fig. 7.4 Case presentation of a 57-year-old female patient. (**a**) Preoperative magnetic resonance T2-weighted lateral image. (**b**) Preoperative magnetic resonance T2-weighted axial image. (**c**) Postoperative magnetic resonance T2-weighted axial image

the scar tissue containing the transversing nerve root from the medial boundary of the facet articular processes and to repeatedly mobilization the traversing nerve root in the medially direction. In particular, even if significant peridural fibrotic scar tissue formation, a layer of scar tissue is left on the dura of nerve root can rather prevent incidental dural tear.

Posterior ring apophysis separation, other called posterior limbus, with lumbar disc herniation is probably more common than is generally recognized. And it is known that a posterior limbus is not associated with recurrent disc herniation or a fair outcome. However, in patients with large disc re-herniation through annular defect following fist-time lumbar discectomy, posterior limbus existed at the site where the annular defect occurred, and a disc fragmentectomy may be limited by posterior limbus. In these conditions, large annular incision may be considered inevitable, but UBE uses a bipolar radiofrequency ablator to identify and remove posterior limbus fragments without large annular incisions only limited circular annuloplasty [10].

References

1. Leven D, Passias PG, Errico TJ, Lafage V, Bianco K, Lee A, et al. Risk factors for reoperation in patients treated surgically for intervertebral disc herniation: a subanalysis of eight-year SPORT data. J Bone Joint Surg Am. 2015;97(16):1316–25.
2. Felbaum DR, Stewart JJ, Distaso C, Sandhu FA. Complication rate in minimally invasive revision lumbar discectomy: a case series and technical note. Clin Spine Surg. 2018;31(5):E266–e9.
3. Tafazal SI, Sell PJ. Incidental durotomy in lumbar spine surgery: incidence and management. Eur Spine J. 2005;14(3):287–90.
4. Guan J, Ravindra VM, Schmidt MH, Dailey AT, Hood RS, Bisson EF. Comparing clinical outcomes of repeat discectomy versus fusion for recurrent disc herniation utilizing the N(2)QOD. J Neurosurg Spine. 2017;26(1):39–44.
5. Fritzell P, Knutsson B, Sanden B, Strömqvist B, Hägg O. Recurrent versus primary lumbar disc herniation surgery: patient-reported outcomes in the Swedish spine register Swespine. Clin Orthop Relat Res. 2015;473(6):1978–84.
6. Nolte MT, Basques BA, Louie PK, Khan JM, Varthi A, Paul J, et al. Patients undergoing revision microdiskectomy for recurrent lumbar disk herniation experience worse clinical outcomes and more revision surgeries compared with patients undergoing a primary microdiskectomy. J Am Acad Orthop Surg. 2019;27(17):e796–803.
7. Dower A, Chatterji R, Swart A, Winder MJ. Surgical management of recurrent lumbar disc herniation and the role of fusion. J Clin Neurosci. 2016;23:44–50.
8. Shin KH, Chang HG, Rhee NK, Lim KS. Revisional percutaneous full endoscopic disc surgery for recurrent herniation of previous open lumbar discectomy. Asian Spine J. 2011;5(1):1–9.
9. Choi DJ, Jung JT, Lee SJ, Kim YS, Jang HJ, Yoo B. Biportal endoscopic spinal surgery for recurrent lumbar disc herniations. Clin Orthop Surg. 2016;8(3):325–9.
10. Kang MS, Hwang JH, Choi DJ, Chung HJ, Lee JH, Kim HN, et al. Clinical outcome of biportal endoscopic revisional lumbar discectomy for recurrent lumbar disc herniation. J Orthop Surg Res. 2020;15(1):557.
11. Brooks M, Dower A, Abdul Jalil MF, Kohan S. Radiological predictors of recurrent lumbar disc herniation: a systematic review and meta-analysis. Journal of neurosurgery. Spine. 2020;34:1–11.

Part III

Lumbar Stenosis

Lumbar Stenosis: Central and Lateral Recess Stenosis

8

Jae Won Jang, Chung Kee Chough, Dong Geun Lee, and Choon Keun Park

8.1 Introduction

Lumbar central and lateral recess stenosis is one of the most common causes of leg radiating pain, buttock pain, and neurogenic leg claudication. Treatment options for lumbar central and lateral recess stenosis have two main categories: conservative management and surgical interventions. The main surgical option for lumbar central and lateral recess stenosis is decompressive laminectomy. Open subtotal decompressive laminectomy can provide broad decompression of the central spinal canal and lateral recess and it had been widely used by spine surgeons [1]. However, it is associated with extensive injuries of normal spinal structures such as bone, facet joints, paraspinal muscles, and ligaments [2].

Interlaminar approach to decompress the central spinal canal and lateral recess using microscopy was introduced in 1978 [3]. This method had been considered the gold standard approach for lumbar stenosis for a long time. It can minimize damages to normal spinal bone and collateral paraspinal soft tissues compared to previous conventional total or subtotal laminectomy. Successful adoption of microscopic spinal surgery through lumbar interlaminar approach makes it possible to safely perform complete nerve root decompression while reducing iatrogenic injury of the spinal column and paraspinal soft tissues. Microscopic unilateral laminectomy for bilateral decompression (ULBD) is introduced as a less invasive technique that is performed through mini-open or tubular approaches of lumbar central and lateral recess stenosis [4]. However, it also has several drawbacks, including paraspinal muscle injury, violation of facet joint, and technical difficulty for contralateral decompression.

Endoscopic spine surgery has been the hot issue of spine surgery in the last two decades with the concerns about reducing normal structure damage during surgery. Uniportal endoscopic spine surgery is theoretically true and full endoscopic surgery, but endoscopic handling and restricted available instruments are not familiar to most spine surgeons [5]. Therefore, a well-known limitation of uniportal endoscopic surgery is its stiff learning curve [6]. Unilateral biportal endoscopy (UBE) for spine surgery has been recently used for various spinal diseases from lumbar disease to cervical and thoracic lesions [7–10]. UBE surgery can offer a relatively early adaptation of surgical technique for beginners of endoscopic

Supplementary Information The online version contains supplementary material available at [https://doi.org/10.1007/978-981-16-8201-8_8].

J. W. Jang · D. G. Lee · C. K. Park
Department of Neurosurgery, Suwon Leon Wiltse Memorial Hospital, Suwon, Republic of Korea

C. K. Chough (✉)
Department of Neurosurgery, Yeouido St. Mary's Hospital, The Catholic University of Korea, Seoul, Republic of Korea

D. H. Heo et al. (eds.), *Unilateral Biportal Endoscopic Spine Surgery*,
https://doi.org/10.1007/978-981-16-8201-8_8

surgery. It may have an advantage in overcoming the steep learning curve of endoscopic spine surgery. The decompression for lumbar central and lateral recess stenosis can be easily performed with a clear magnified surgical view from the ipsilateral side to the contralateral side via a UBE surgery [8, 11, 12]. UBE for lumbar decompression may provide better clinical outcomes including less muscle damage, less use of postoperative opioids, and shorter hospital stay compared to microscopic decompression [13–16].

In this chapter, the authors introduce the current step-by-step technique of ULBD using UBE, and also discuss the surgical pitfalls of this technique.

8.2 Indications & Contraindications

Indications and contraindications of a UBE surgery are very similar to those of a microscopic lumbar canal decompression for central and lateral recess stenosis.

8.2.1 Indications

- Unilateral lumbar lateral recess stenosis
- Bilateral lumbar lateral recess stenosis
- Central lumbar canal stenosis
- Lumbar canal stenosis caused by justa-facet cysts
- Lumbar canal stenosis caused by Grade I spondylolisthesis
- Lumbar canal stenosis caused by epidural abscess

8.2.2 Relative Contraindications

- Lumbar canal stenosis caused by Grade II spondylolisthesis
- Postoperative lumbar canal re-stenosis

8.2.3 Contraindications

- Lumbar canal stenosis caused by high-grade spondylolisthesis
- Tumorous conditions
- Lumbar canal stenosis caused by uncontrolled spinal infections

8.3 Surgical Instruments

Special tool kits including serial dilators and muscle dissector for making working and endoscopic portals are required (Fig. 8.1a). Radiofrequency (RF) and shaver are used for bleeding control and soft-tissue dissection. A semi-circular tube can be used in the working portal to maintain fluent fluid flow (Fig. 8.1b). To reduce the possibility of nerve injury from RF, RF tips with various angles (0 degree, 45 degrees, and 90 degrees) can be used. Endoscopic drill and general spinal instruments such as Kerrison punches, disc forceps, curettes, root retractor, nerve freer, and endoscopic hook are needed for decompression of spinal canal (Fig. 8.1c). Small straight or curved osteotomes are also needed, especially for decompression of lateral recess (Fig. 8.1d).

8.4 Anesthesia & Positions

Epidural or general anesthesia can be utilized to perform UBE surgery. Initially, general anesthesia is recommended for beginners because full muscle relaxation under general anesthesia helps maintain fluid passage through the working portal to make a clean operation field by fluent washing out of blood and bone dust. Epidural anesthesia is recommended for experts of UBE surgery with the use of sedative drugs. After epidural or general anesthesia, the patient is placed in the prone-flexed position over the radiolucent spine frame.

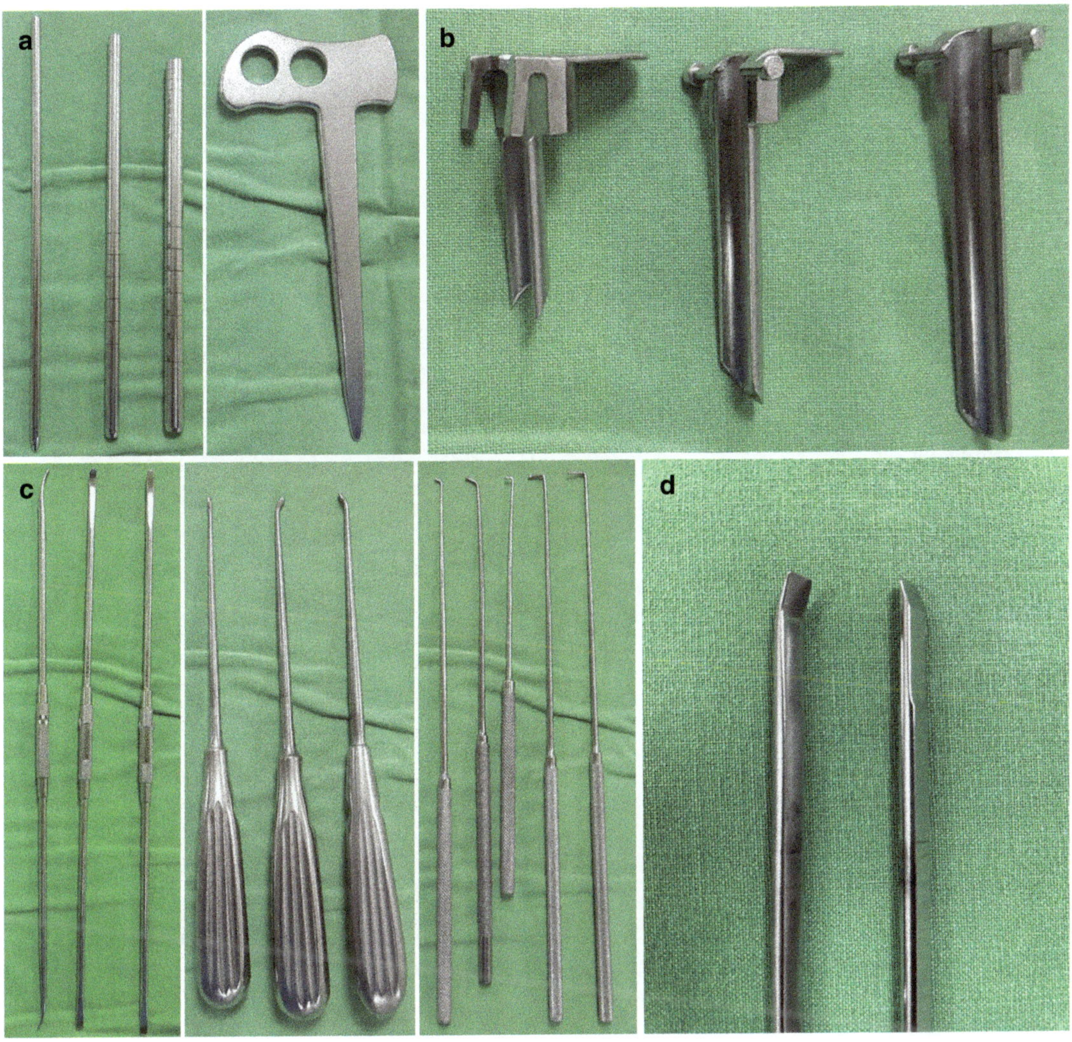

Fig. 8.1 General instruments for unilateral biportal endoscopic (UBE) spine surgery. (**a**) Serial dilators and muscle dissector for making working and endoscopic portals. (**b**) Semi-circular tube for maintenance of fluent saline outflow. (**c**) Soft tissue and nerve freer, curettes, and endoscopic hooks. (**d**) Straight and curved osteotomes

8.5 Surgical Steps

8.5.1 Skin Entry Points and Making Two Holes (Working and Endoscopic Port)

The target level for surgical decompression was localized by fluoroscopy. A waterproof surgical drape was applied through a sterile process. A drainage system of irrigation fluid should also be set up. The medial pedicular line of the pathologic target level is drawn under a true anteroposterior fluoroscopic view. Two vertical or transverse skin incisions are made on junctional points between the drawn medial pedicular line and the distal transverse pedicle line of the upper and lower vertebra of pathologic level on true lateral fluoroscopic lateral view (Fig. 8.2a, b).

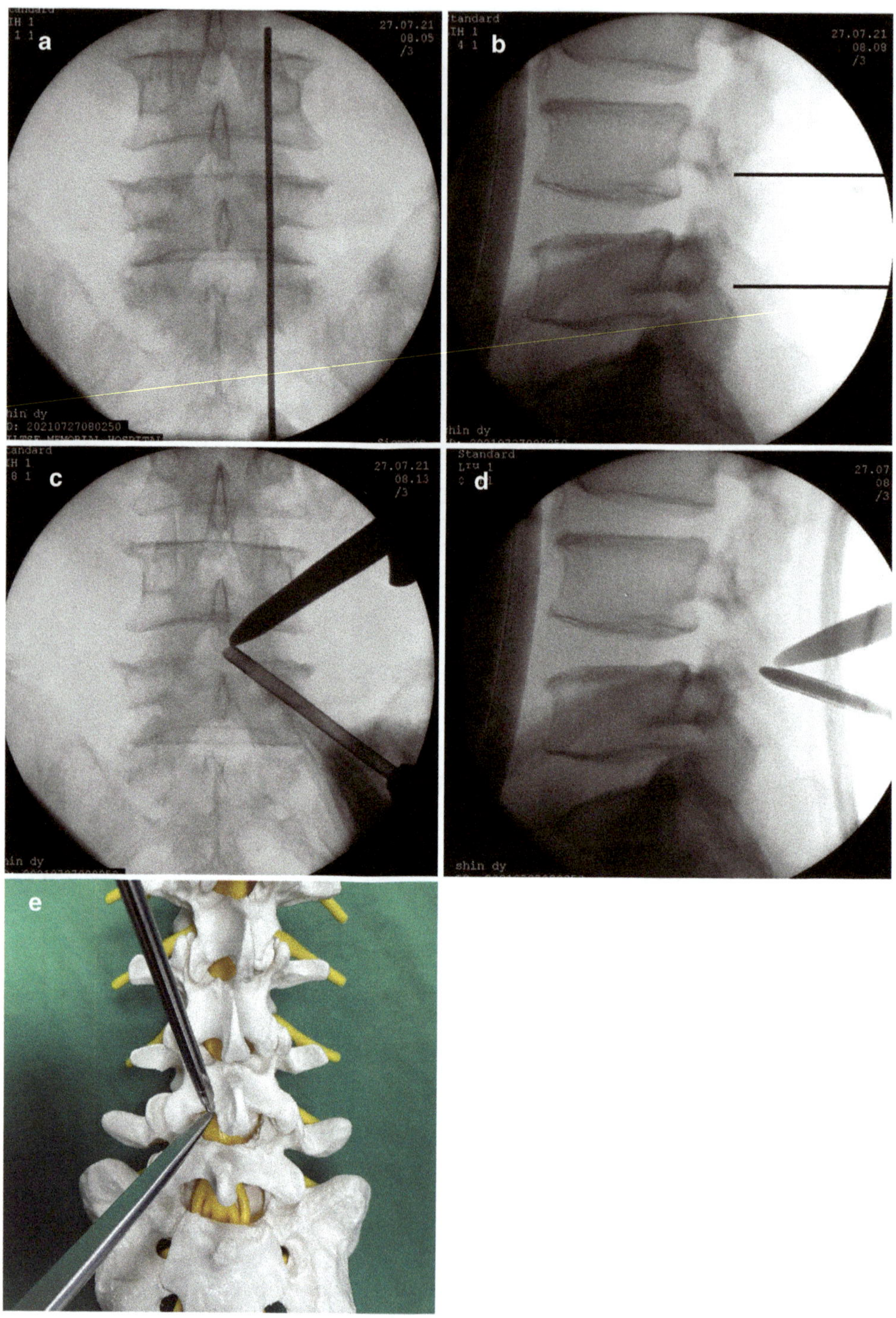

Fig. 8.2 Entry points for working and endoscopic portals and making holes. (**a**) Skin incision sites are made around the pedicle area. The medial pedicular line of approach site was firstly checked in the true anteroposterior radiograph. (**b**) Two skin incisions were made around the lower margin of the proximal and distal pedicle of lesion level on the medial pedicular line in the true lateral radiograph. (**c** and **d**) After serial dilation, the surgeon can fight instruments with triangular formation through each port on spino-laminar junction, initial target area of operation. (**e**) Meeting points endoscopy and surgical instruments in spino-laminar junction on artificial lumbar spine model

About 6–7 mm incision is needed for insertion of a spinal endoscope. About 9–10 mm incision is generally needed to maintain fluent outflow of irrigation saline and freely pass of general spinal instruments. The distance between the endoscopic portal and the working portal is generally about 2–3 cm. Deep fascial incision is also required to maintain fluent outflow. If outflow is not maintained fluently, cruciate deep fascial incision may be required, especially during a contralateral decompression. After incision of skin and deep fascia, working space can be made by serial dilation and blunt dissection using special serial dilator systems (Video 8.1). The initial docking point of endoscopy and the serial dilator is the spino-laminar junction of the pathologic level (Fig. 8.2c–e). The fatty space is generally located between the multifidus and lamina on the spino-laminar junction. The surgeon can make a working space non-traumatically. Continuous fluent irrigation should be also maintained to have a clean operative surgical view. A water pressure pump can be applied to maintain fluent saline outflow, but the authors prefer natural drainage of irrigation fluid by adjusting saline bag height.

8.5.2 Soft-tissue Dissections

A free-fat space between the spino-laminar junction and the multifidus is usually seen in computed tomography (CT) or magnetic resonance imaging (MRI) scan. The space is expanded with insertion of the endoscope and initiation of saline irrigation. The surgeon can easily find the spino-laminar junction of target level. Soft tissues around the spino-laminar junction and the interlaminar space can be dissected and removed using RF ablation, Kerrison punch, and disc forceps. Ligamentum flavum of the interlaminar space at the target level should be exposed clearly. Soft-tissue dissection should be minimized as much as possible to preserve paraspinal soft tissues.

8.5.3 Ipsilateral Laminotomy and Decompression

Ipsilateral laminectomy is performed on the spino-laminar junction of the target level using endoscopic drills or small osteotomes. Central fissure of ligamentum flavum can be identified after expansion of laminotomy from the spino-laminar junction to the centro-cranial part of the spinous base. After confirmation of central fissure of ligamentum flavum, laminotomy should be done under a clean magnified endoscopic view until the medial part of superior articular process is exposed. The proximal origin of the ligamentum flavum is V-shaped. It is attached superior-laterally up to intervertebral foramen. Therefore, lateral laminotomy should be done more cranially from central fissure of ligamentum flavum until the edge of ligamentum flavum is freely detached. However, proximal edge of ligamentum flavum can be detached using curved curettes if the isthmic space of the laminar is narrow to prevent fracture of isthmus or inferior articular process. The hypertrophied ligamentum flavum in spinal stenosis is composed of several layers. However, the ligamentum flavum can be roughly divided into two layers. The outer layer of ligamentum flavum is attached to the cranial portion of lamina of the lower vertebra. The outer layer can be easily detached from the medial portion of superior articular process to the upper portion of the lamina using angled curettes (Fig. 8.3a). After removing the outer layer of the ligamentum flavum, the cranial portion of the lower lamina is thinned using an endoscopic drill until the distal part of inner layer of ligamentum flavum is freely detached. Then piecemeal or en-block removal of ipsilateral inner layer of ligamentum flavum can be done safely. The medial portion of the superior articular process should be removed to expose the medial margin of pedicle. Adhesions between ventral dura and posterior longitudinal ligament should also be released. In case of severe lateral recess bony stenosis, the authors recommend the usage of a small osteotome instead of a Kerrison

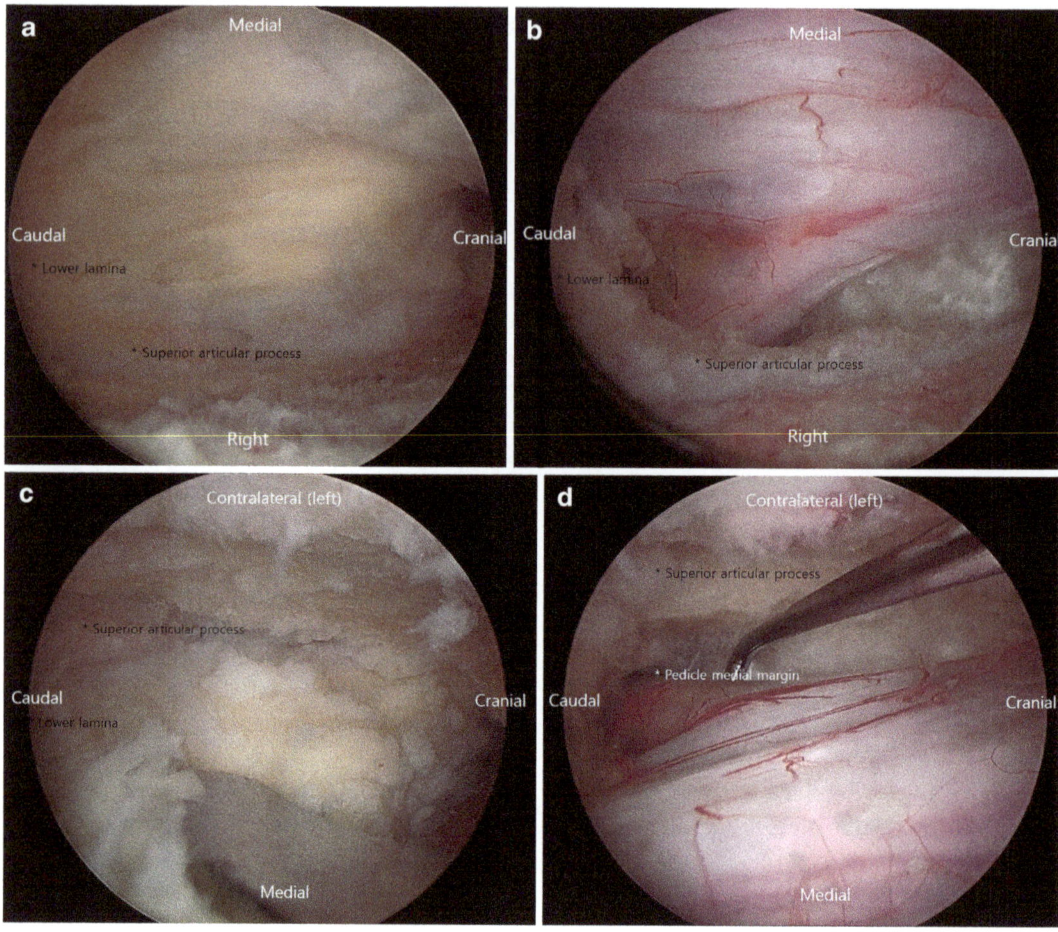

Fig. 8.3 Endoscopic intraoperative view (bilateral decompression right approach) (**a**) Exposure of ipsilateral superior articular process. (**b**) Ipsilateral decompression to medial pedicle margin. (**c**) Exposure of contralateral medial portion of superior articular process. (**d**) Contralateral decompression to medial pedicle margin

punch to prevent dura injury or direct compressive nerve root damage. Ideal decompression should be performed on the medial margin of the lower vertebra pedicle. (Fig. 8.3b).

8.5.4 Contralateral Sublaminar Decompression

The process of contralateral decompression is initiated after detaching the contralateral ligamentum flavum from the ventral side of the opposite lamina using freer or curettes. Contralateral sublaminoplasty should be extended more cranially from the medial side to the lateral side until the edge of ligamentum flavum is freely detached. If the main cause of lumbar stenosis is hypertrophied ligamentum flavum, detachment and removal of ligamentum flavum might be main decompressive procedures. Gentle detachment of ligamentum flavum from the ventral side of lamina should be performed until the medial side of the opposite superior articular process is seen. If there are combined narrow spinal canals from bony structures or spondylolisthesis, ventral lamina of contralateral side should be removed to achieve adequate decompression. Contralateral sublaminoplasty can be performed using endoscopic drills and osteotomes. After exposing the contralateral medial part of the superior articular process, the outer layer of the contralateral ligamentum flavum can be removed from the lateral side to the medial side on the upper portion of the lower lamina (Fig. 8.3c). The head of the endoscopic drill should be placed on the space between the ventral surface of lamina and the dorsal surface of ligamentum flavum to prevent unintended dura or neural structure injuries. Bone works using endoscopic drills should be completed before removing the full layer of ligamentum flavum. After removing the full layer of ligamentum flavum, lateral recess can be fully decompressed using curettes, straight and curved osteotomes, or Kerrison punches. Epidural adhesion between the nerve root and ventral dura surface should be released using angled hooks (Fig. 8.3d). The authors try to decompress until the medial border of the contralateral pedicle is seen.

8.5.5 Bleeding Control and Closure

Epidural bleeding from dissected soft tissue and muscles is easily controlled by RF ablation. The exposed cancellous bone should be sealed using bone wax to prevent prolonged oozing after stopping saline irrigation. A drainage catheter is inserted through the working port with a stay suture to prevent postoperative epidural hematoma. Subcutaneous layers are approximated with absorbable suture material. Skin layers are closed with non-absorbable material or skin tape.

8.6 Illustrated Cases

8.6.1 Case 2 Description: L4-5 Stenosis (Right Unilateral Laminotomy Bilateral Decompression) (Video 8.2)

A 67-year-old male patient visited with the symptoms of both posterior thigh pain and neurogenic intermittent claudication. Preoperative simple radiographs showed degenerative lumbar spondylosis (Fig. 8.4a). Preoperative T2 sagittal and axial MRI scans showed L4-5 central and lateral recess spinal stenosis (Fig. 8.4b, c). The patient received right ULBD using UBE spine surgery and endoscopic view showed well decompression of spinal central canal and lateral recess (Fig. 8.4d). MRI scans obtained on postoperative day 2 showed well decompression of stenotic lesion at the L4-5 level without any other radiologic complications (Fig. 8.4e, f). Facet joints were relatively well preserved. The patient's leg symptoms were relieved immediately after surgery, and postoperative back pain was also dissolved within several weeks after UBE surgery.

8.6.2 Case 1 Description: L4-5 Stenosis (Left Unilateral Laminotomy Bilateral Decompression) (Video 8.3)

A 78-year-old male patient presented with severe buttock pain and neurogenic intermittent claudication. Preoperative T2 sagittal and axial MRI scans revealed severe L4-5 central and lateral recess spinal stenosis (Fig. 8.5a, b). Symptoms of this patient did not respond to conservative management such as physiotherapy, medications, or spinal blockade. The author performed left ULBD through UBE surgery. Intraoperative endoscopic images showed well decompression of spinal canal (Fig. 8.5c–e). MRI scans obtained on postoperative day 2 showed well decompression of stenotic lesion at the L4-5 level (Fig. 8.5f, g). The patient's symptoms resolved without additional medications.

8.7 Complications: Prevention & Managements

8.7.1 Incidental Durotomy

The current spinal endoscopic view on the monitor is mainly a two-dimensional image, which may increase the risk of incidental durotomy or nerve root injury during endoscopic drilling or other decompressive procedures using the Kerrison punch. The authors recommend that most bone works using endoscopic drills should be completed before complete removal of ligamentum flavum to reduce the risk of incidental

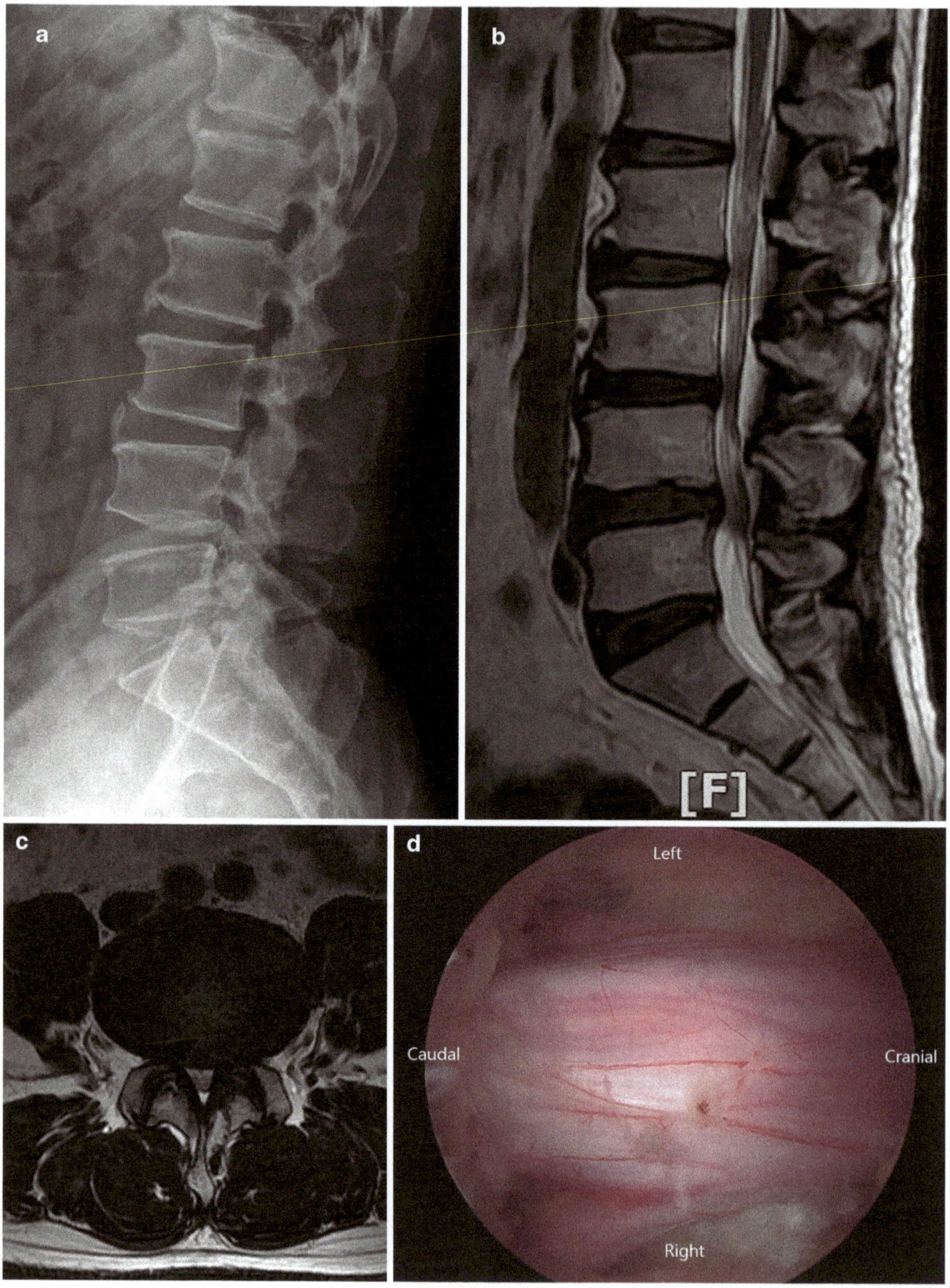

Fig. 8.4 (**a**) Degenerative spondylosis was seen in simple lateral radiograph. (**b** and **c**) magnetic resonance T2-weighted images showed severe lumbar central and lateral recess stenosis on L4-5 level. (**d**) Intraoperative endoscopic view revealed well decompression of spinal canal with 2–3 mm free margin. (**e** and **f**) Postoperative magnetic resonance T2-weighted sagittal and axial images showed well decompression of stenotic lesion at L4-5 level

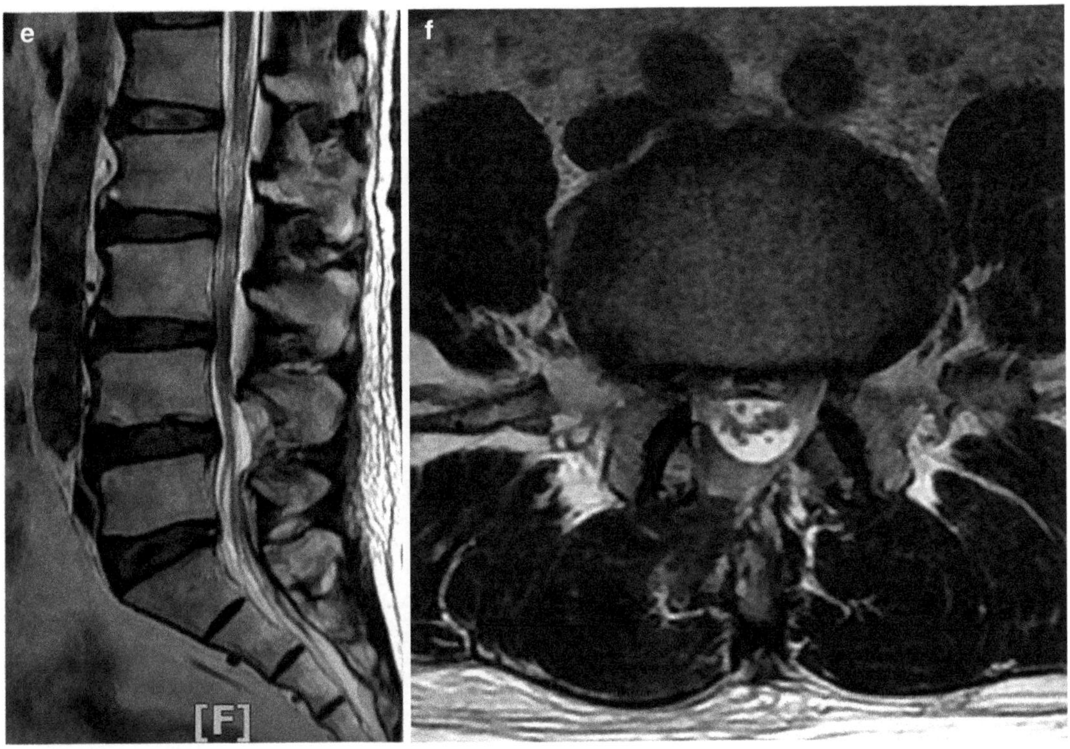

Fig. 8.4 (continued)

durotomy. If further bone work is needed after complete removal of ligamentum flavum, the usage of small osteotomes or angled Kerrison punch is less risky than the usage of a drill. When incidental durotomy occurred during surgery, most cases with a small durotomy can be treated using collagen fibrin patches without conversion to open surgery. However, cases with a large dural defect should consider open direct suture of the defect site. Non-penetrating vascular clips combined with sealing of collagen fibrin patches can also be used to manage incidental durotomy.

8.7.2 Epidural Hematoma

Continuous saline irrigation offers a clean surgical field by washing out bone dust and bleed clots. Hydrostatic pressure on the epidural space can enhance bleeding control during surgical procedures. However, hidden bleeding may occur after cessation of continuous saline irrigation and hydrostatic pressure effect on a working space. After stopping the continuous irrigation, the surgeon should observe the occurrence of bleeding from exposed cancellous bone or epidural space when decompressive procedures are finished [8]. Exposed surface of cancellous bone should be sealed using bone wax. Epidural bleeding from venous plexus can be controlled by ablation of RF. A drainage catheter on the epidural space without root irritation should be adequately inserted under an endoscopic view.

8.7.3 Nerve Root Injury

Blurred surgical field can cause neural structure injury. Kerrison punch and endoscopic drill should be used under a clean surgical view through fluent continuous irrigation. Especially, bone work through endoscopic drill should be ended before removal of ligamentum flavum. RF can also cause neural tissue injury. When RF is used around a neural structure, the current time of RF should be ended shortly. The

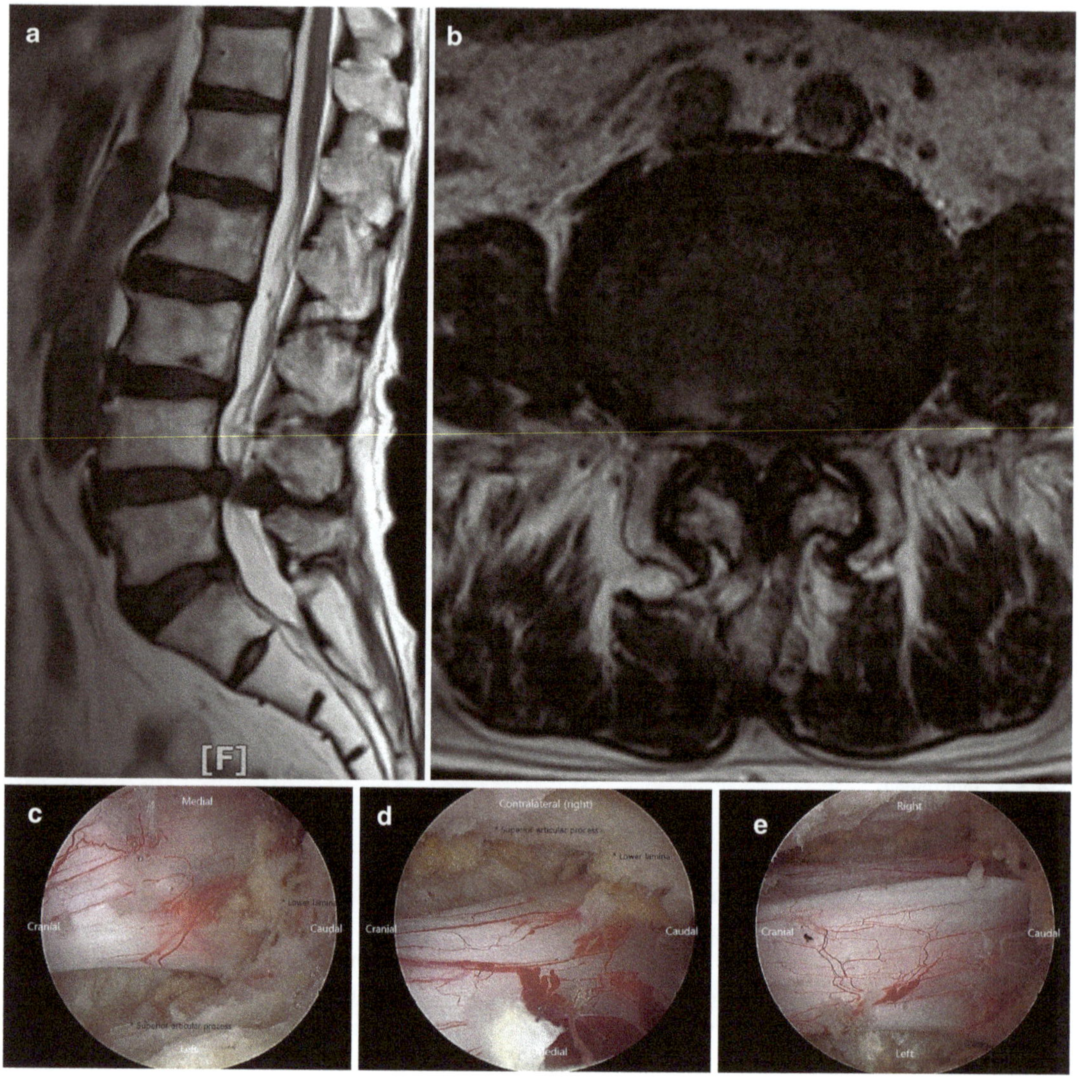

Fig. 8.5 (**a** and **b**) Preoperative magnetic resonance T2-weighted images showed severe lumbar central and lateral recess stenosis on L4-5 level. (**c**, **d**, and **e**) Intraoperative endoscopic view revealed well decompression of central spinal canal and both lateral recesses. (**f** and **g**) Postoperative magnetic resonance T2-weighted sagittal and axial images showed well decompression of stenotic lesion at L4-5 level

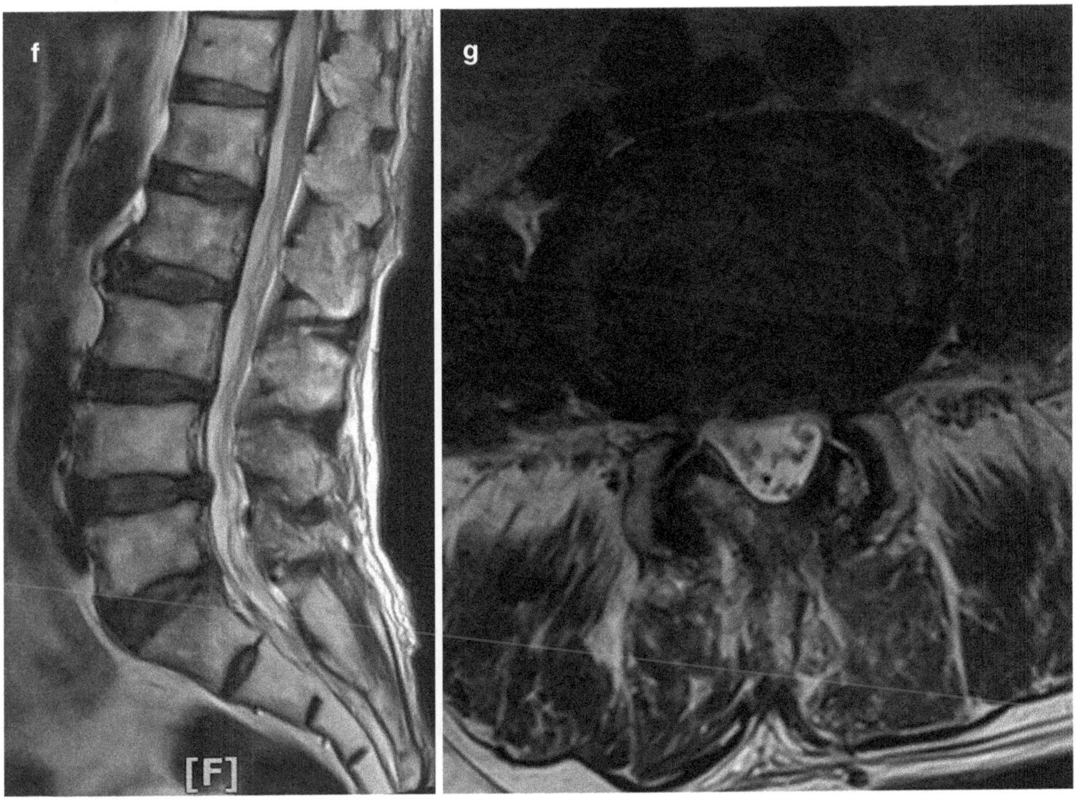

Fig. 8.5 (continued)

RF system has tips with variable degrees of tip angle. It may be helpful to use RF ablation safely around the neural tissue. During a lateral recess decompression, if there is severe lateral recess stenosis combined with calcified lesion or bony structure, the authors recommend the usage of an endoscopic straight or curved osteotome instead of a Kerrison punch to prevent direct compressive nerve root injury.

8.8 Surgical Tips & Pitfalls

8.8.1 Exposure of Distal and Medial Portion of Superior Articular Process

When the surgeon determines the degree of laminotomy for adequate canal decompression, the medial portion of the superior articular process can be a guide point. The medial margin of the superior articular process is located within the medial pedicle margin. Therefore, distal and medial portions of the superior articular process should be removed for adequate decompression of central and lateral recess stenosis. If the medial portion of the superior articular process is not exposed, adequate decompression may not be achieved. Moreover, the outer layer of the ligamentum flavum can be easily detached and removed from the medial side of the facet joint to the upper portion of the lower lamina using angled curettes after exposing the medial portion of the superior articular process. However, isthmus is frequently located within the medial margin of the superior articular process. Thus, bone works toward lateral and superior sites of lamina to expose the superior articular process should be performed carefully.

8.8.2 Decompression: More Is Better

To achieve long-term favorable outcomes after decompression for lumbar central and lateral recess stenosis, adequate decompression is very important. The authors recommend over 3 mm laterally from dura lateral margin during continuous irrigation because dura will shrink under a hydrostatic pressure. The true lateral margin of dura at a natural state might be located more laterally compared to the endoscopic view. It may also help prevent the development of dynamic stenosis by spinal motion. The authors always confirm medial margin of pedicle on lateral recess level to make sure that it enables traversing of the nerve root freely and flexibly without compression.

8.8.3 Release of Adhesion Between Ventral Dura and Epidural Small Ligaments

Epidural adhesion between ventral dura surface and epidural fibrotic tissues (ligaments) should be released using an angled hook. After this procedure, traversing nerve root and dura could be easily retracted medially without resistance after removing the adhesion. This may play an important role in obtaining favorable outcomes.

References

1. Young S, Veerapen R, O'Laoire SA. Relief of lumbar canal stenosis using multilevel subarticular fenestrations as an alternative to wide laminectomy: preliminary report. Neurosurgery. 1988;23(5):628–33.
2. Guha D, Heary RF, Shamji MF. Iatrogenic spondylolisthesis following laminectomy for degenerative lumbar stenosis: systematic review and current concepts. Neurosurg Focus. 2015;39(4):E9.
3. Williams RW. Microlumbar discectomy: a conservative surgical approach to the virgin herniated lumbar disc. Spine (Phila Pa 1976). 1978;3(2):175–82.
4. Costa F, Sassi M, Cardia A, Ortolina A, De Santis A, Luccarell G, et al. Degenerative lumbar spinal stenosis: analysis of results in a series of 374 patients treated with unilateral laminotomy for bilateral microdecompression. J Neurosurg Spine. 2007;7(6):579–86.
5. Kim M, Kim HS, Oh SW, Adsul NM, Singh R, Kashlan ON, et al. Evolution of spinal endoscopic surgery. Neurospine. 2019;16(1):6–14.
6. Hahn BS, Park JY. Incorporating new technologies to overcome the limitations of endoscopic spine surgery: navigation, robotics, and visualization. World Neurosurg. 2021;145:712–21.
7. Heo DH, Quillo-Olvera J, Park CK. Can percutaneous biportal endoscopic surgery achieve enough canal

decompression for degenerative lumbar stenosis? Prospective case-control study. World Neurosurg. 2018;120:e684–e9.
8. Hwa Eum J, Hwa Heo D, Son SK, Park CK. Percutaneous biportal endoscopic decompression for lumbar spinal stenosis: a technical note and preliminary clinical results. J Neurosurg Spine. 2016;24(4):602–7.
9. De Antoni DJ, Claro ML, Poehling GG, Hughes SS. Translaminar lumbar epidural endoscopy: anatomy, technique, and indications. Arthroscopy. 1996;12(3):330–4.
10. Kim J, Heo DH, Lee DC, Chung HT. Biportal endoscopic unilateral laminotomy with bilateral decompression for the treatment of cervical spondylotic myelopathy. Acta Neurochir. 2021;163(9):2537–43.
11. Min WK, Kim JE, Choi DJ, Park EJ, Heo J. Clinical and radiological outcomes between biportal endoscopic decompression and microscopic decompression in lumbar spinal stenosis. J Orthop Sci. 2020;25(3):371–8.
12. Pao JL, Lin SM, Chen WC, Chang CH. Unilateral biportal endoscopic decompression for degenerative lumbar canal stenosis. J Spine Surg. 2020;6(2):438–46.
13. Park SM, Park J, Jang HS, Heo YW, Han H, Kim HJ, et al. Biportal endoscopic versus microscopic lumbar decompressive laminectomy in patients with spinal stenosis: a randomized controlled trial. Spine J. 2020;20(2):156–65.
14. Pranata R, Lim MA, Vania R, July J. Biportal endoscopic spinal surgery versus microscopic decompression for lumbar spinal stenosis: a systematic review and meta-analysis. World Neurosurg. 2020;138:e450–e8.
15. Heo DH, Lee DC, Park CK. Comparative analysis of three types of minimally invasive decompressive surgery for lumbar central stenosis: biportal endoscopy, uniportal endoscopy, and microsurgery. Neurosurg Focus. 2019;46(5):E9.
16. Chen T, Zhou G, Chen Z, Yao X, Liu D. Biportal endoscopic decompression vs. microscopic decompression for lumbar canal stenosis: a systematic review and meta-analysis. Exp Ther Med. 2020;20(3):2743–51.

The Paraspinal Approach with Unilateral Biportal Endoscopy for Lumbar Foraminal Lesions

9

Kwan-Su David Song, Nam Lee, and Jwo Luen Pao

9.1 Introduction

Degenerative change of the vertebral disc can induce hypertrophy of the facet joints, thickening of the ligament flavum, and resultant narrowing of the neural foramen. These degenerative changes lead to symptomatic lumbosacral radiculopathy and account for approximately about 10% of lumbar degenerative diseases that required surgical intervention [1, 2].

Before the concept of minimally invasive spine surgery was introduced, lumbar fusion surgery was probably the one and only surgical solution for lumbar foraminal lesions. However, as the endoscopic spine surgical techniques have matured, many lumbar foraminal pathologies can be well treated by just simple decompression [3–5].

Supplementary Information The online version contains supplementary material available at [https://doi.org/10.1007/978-981-16-8201-8_9].

K.-S. D. Song (✉)
Department of Neurosurgery, Him-Plus Hospital, Suncheon-si, Jeollanam-do, Republic of Korea

N. Lee
Department of Neurosurgery, Yonsei-cheok Hospital, Busan, Republic of Korea

J. L. Pao
Department of Orthopaedic Surgery, Far-Eastern Memorial Hospital, New Taipei, Taiwan

In particular, the unilateral biportal endoscopy (UBE) technique allows for minimally invasive surgical access, has no restrictions on the use of surgical instruments, and has a relatively short learning curve by providing a more familiar surgical anatomy based on the classic Wiltse approach.

Furthermore, the endoscopic lens, the so-called "operative eye," can be advanced very close to the lesion, and capture clear and magnified video images of the lesion and its surrounding structures. Visualization of the deep neural structures and pathologies would no longer be limited by the anatomical structures [6].

In this chapter, we provide a step-by-step description of the surgical procedure of the paraspinal approach with the UBE technique using video and pictures. The paraspinal approach for L5–S1 is described separately, because compared to the other levels, it has special anatomical considerations.

9.2 Indications and Contraindications

The surgical indications and contraindications are the same as the microscopic lumbar foraminotomy via Wiltse approach [7].

D. H. Heo et al. (eds.), *Unilateral Biportal Endoscopic Spine Surgery*,
https://doi.org/10.1007/978-981-16-8201-8_9

9.2.1 Indications

1. Chronic mono-radiculopathy resistant to conservative treatment.
2. Para-sagittal and axial magnetic resonance images (MRI) showing foraminal or extra-foraminal lesions. Stenosis, herniated disc, or hypertrophic osteophyte, etc.

9.2.2 Contraindications

1. Definite segmental instability.
2. Degenerative or isthmic spondylolisthesis over grade 1.

9.3 Anesthesia and Position

The surgery can be performed under general anesthesia or epidural anesthesia, depending on the estimated surgical time, and the patient's conditions. The patient is placed in a prone position on the radiolucent Wilson frame with mild flexion of the lumbar spine and proper padding at the patient's axilla and under his/her knees. To avoid soaking and hypothermia of the patient, the draping must be waterproof (Fig. 9.1).

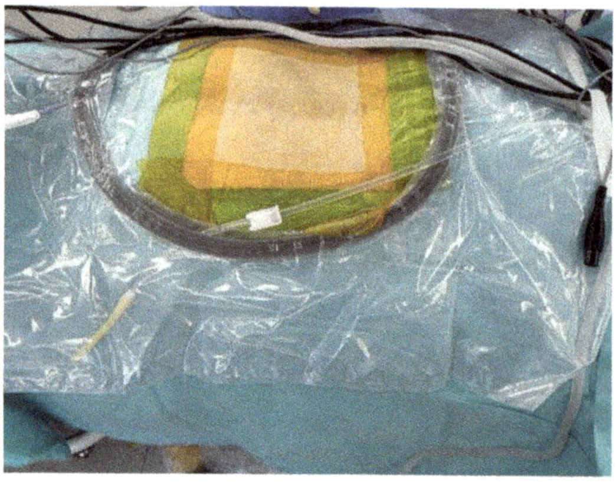

Fig. 9.1 A waterproof surgical drape is draped around the operative field to ensure that saline is smoothly drained during the surgery, does not soak the patient, and does not flood the floor

9.4 Surgical Steps

9.4.1 [L1–5 Level]

9.4.1.1 Skin Marking and Incision

Under the guidance of C-arm fluoroscopy, two skin incisions are made to form the viewing and working portals. The length of the skin incision is about 0.5 cm, and each skin incision is located above the ipsilateral lateral margin of the transverse processes. The interval between the two portals is about 2 cm to 2.5 cm (Fig. 9.2a).

The docking point of the endoscope and the instrument is the isthmus. The distance of the skin incisions away from the midline can be determined preoperatively on the MRI to make the trajectory of 30 degrees to 40 degrees (Fig. 9.2b–d). This angle is the most ideal approach angle, because foraminotomy can be done through undercutting with the lowest risk of an iatrogenic isthmic fracture. In patients with severe disc space narrowing, it is almost impossible to identify the isthmus. In such cases, the alternative docking point will be the tip of the superior articular process (SAP).

The fascia is opened perpendicularly to the skin incision with a No.15 blade for better saline outflow. Serial dilators are used to separate the back muscle and create the initial operative space. After inserting the cannula, a 0° endoscope is inserted through the scope portal. The authors prefer to use a natural gravity drainage system (about 70 cm high above the operation table) for saline irrigation. But if the use of the saline pumping system is preferred, the recommended hydrostatic pressure is about 30 mmHg. This pressure setting is safe, without risks of increasing the intracranial pressure. After triangulation with the endoscope and instrument on the isthmus or the tip of the SAP, the small bleeding can be effectively controlled using the radiofrequency (RF) wand.

9.4.1.2 Foraminotomy/Discectomy (Video 9.1)

To confirm the surgical anatomy, the RF wand and automated shaver are used to clear the soft

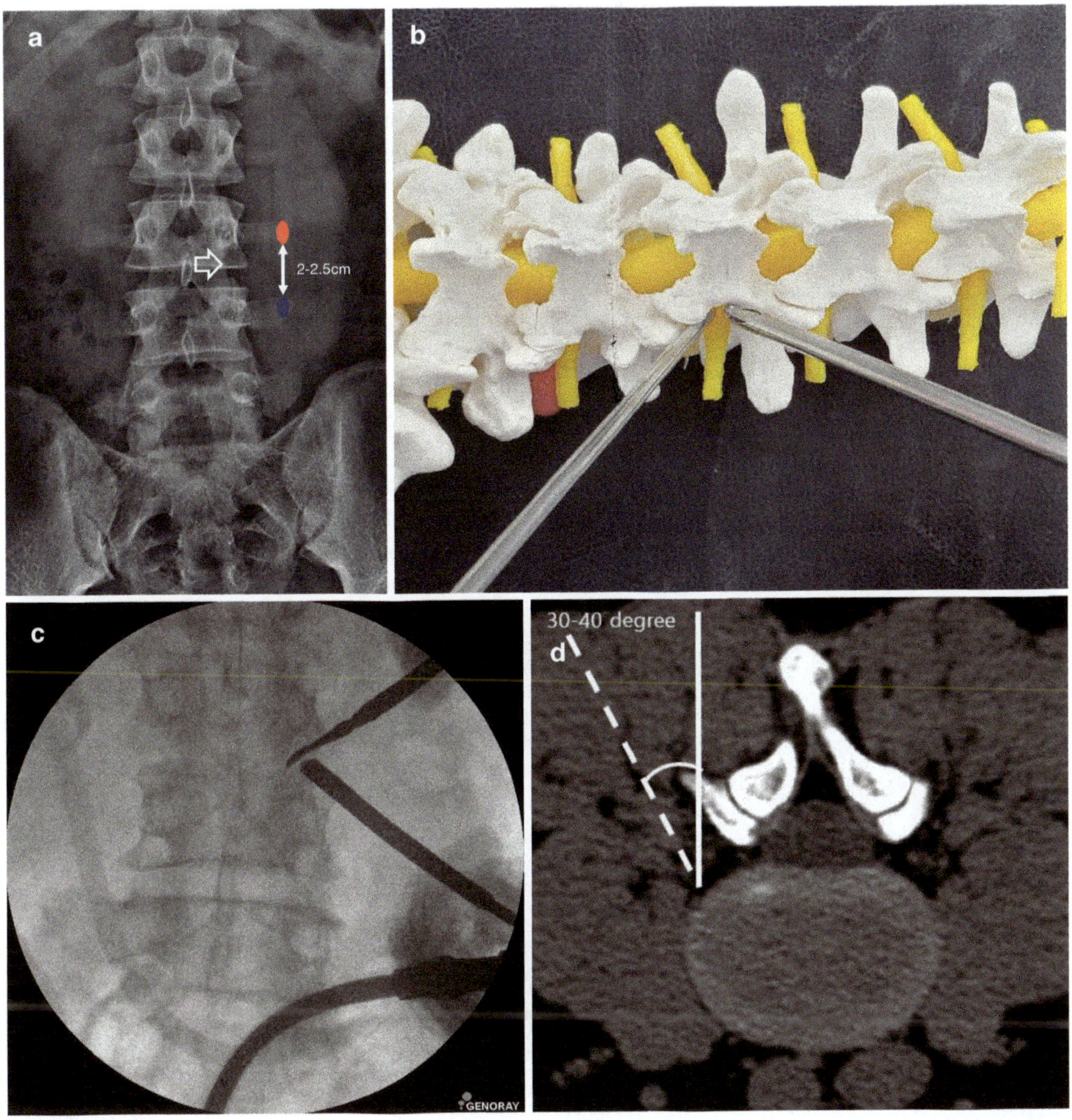

Fig. 9.2 Skin incisions for the scope portal (Blue circle) and the working portal (Red circle) and a docking point (Open white arrow) are illustrated on the X-ray anteroposterior (AP) view (**a**). Endoscope and instruments are triangulated on the isthmus of the artificial lumbar spine model (**b**). Triangulation of endoscope and instruments at the docking point under the C-arm fluoroscopic view (**c**). The appropriate trajectory for the paraspinal approach (white line and white dashed line) is 30 degrees to 40 degrees (**d**)

tissue remnants overlying the lamina and the base of the transverse process. The surgical landmarks, including the lateral aspect of the isthmus, inferior border of the upper transverse process, and lateral aspect of the SAP, should be clearly identified before proceeding to the next step (Fig. 9.3).

A diamond spherical bur is used to drill the lamina. Drilling starts at the lateral border of the isthmus and continues in an under-inside direction. Then the lateral portion of the ligament flavum and the inferior aspect of the pedicle at the base of the transverse process can be exposed (Fig. 9.4a).

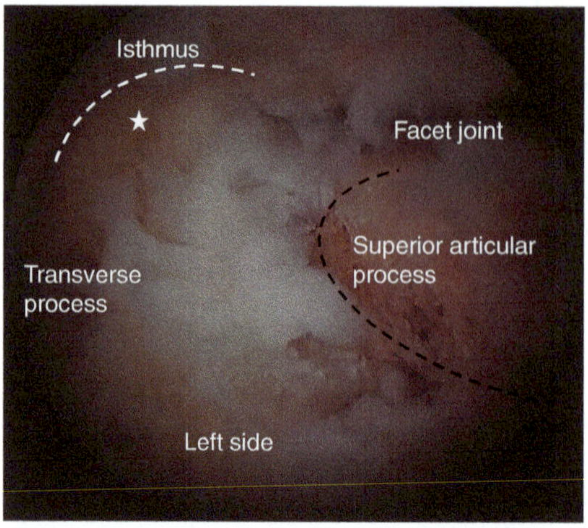

Fig. 9.3 The intraoperative endoscopic image shows the lateral margin of the left isthmus (white dashed line), ligament (asterisk), and facet capsule (black dashed line)

The ligament flavum around the foramen is removed using a curette and Kerrison's punches (Fig. 9.4b). After completion of the flavectomy, the exiting nerve root with its overlying adipose tissue can be exposed (Fig. 9.4c).

If more extent of foraminal decompression is indicated, the cranial tip of the SAP can be resected from the hypertrophic facet joint using a chisel or the diamond bur. If the offending pathology is a lumbar disc herniation, additional discectomy can now be performed, usually from the axilla area of the exiting root (Fig. 9.4d).

After adequate decompression of the exiting root is confirmed, epidural bleeding can be controlled by coagulation with RF wands. A drain is inserted, and after removal of the instruments and the endoscope, the surgical wounds are closed

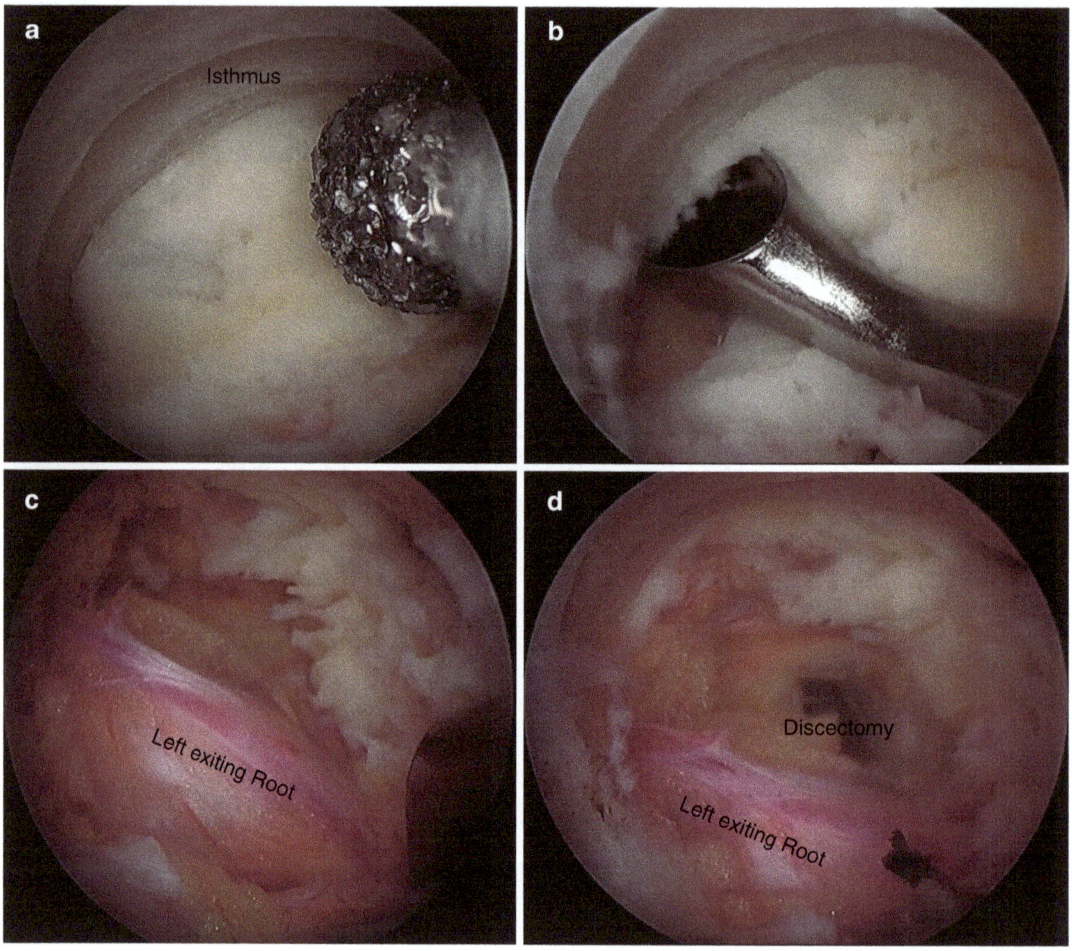

Fig. 9.4 Intraoperative endoscopic view. The starting point of drilling is the lateral margin of the isthmus (**a**). The angled curette is useful in detaching the ligament flavum (**b**). The exiting root is exposed after bleeding control (**c**). Discectomy was done at the axillary portion of the exiting root (**d**)

with a skin stapler. The suction drain is usually kept for 24 h after the surgery, until spontaneous bleeding is controlled.

9.4.2 [L5–S1 Level]

The paraspinal approach at the L5–S1 level has a very limited surgical field. In addition, there are some special and different anatomical features from other lumbar levels. These may include prominent iliac crest, oblique pedicles, and more coronally oriented facet joints. Therefore, it is difficult to create a surgical trajectory to the medial direction of the L5 isthmus.

9.4.2.1 Skin Marking and Incision

Under the guidance of C-arm fluoroscopy, two skin incisions are made to form the viewing and working portals. The length of the skin incision is about 0.5 cm, and each skin incision is located above the ipsilateral lateral margin of the L5 transverse process and sacral alar. The interval between the two portals is about 2 cm (Fig. 9.5a).

Different from other lumbar levels, the isthmus of L5 is very narrow, and the docking point of the endoscope and the instrument is determined by the osseous triangle consisting of the lateral border of the SAP, the sacral alar, and the base of the L5 transverse process (Fig. 9.5b, c). Exposing the boundary of this osseous triangle

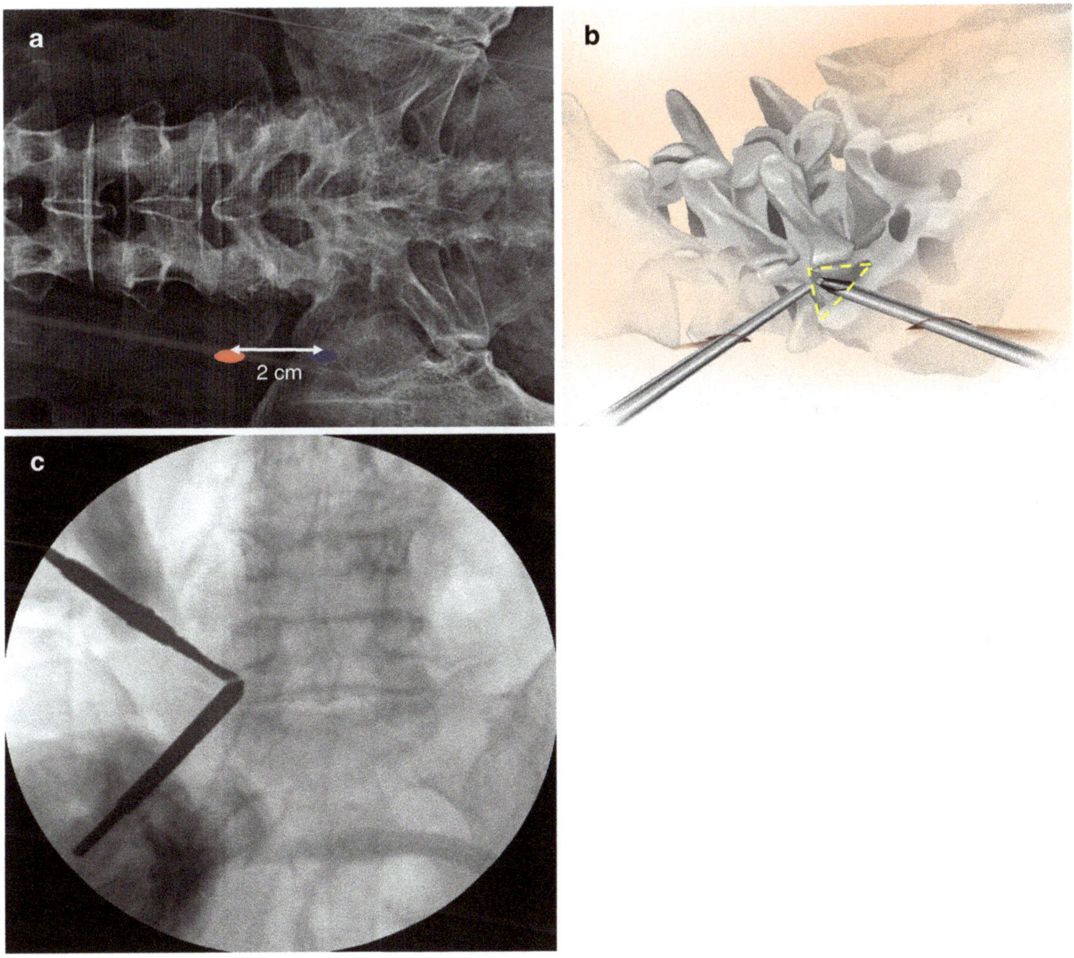

Fig. 9.5 Skin incisions for the scope portal (Red circle) and the working portal (Blue circles) for the paraspinal approach for L5–S1 are illustrated on the X-ray AP view (**a**). The osseous triangle is drawn by the yellow dashed lines on the schematic, and the endoscope and instruments are triangulated on the right osseous triangle (**b**). Triangulation of endoscope and instruments at the osseous triangle under the C-arm fluoroscopic view (**c**)

makes it easier to understand the complex anatomic structures around the L5–S foramen. The recommended trajectory angle is the same as for the other lumbar levels.

9.4.2.2 Foraminotomy/Discectomy (Video 9.2)

To confirm the surgical anatomy, the RF wand and automated shaver are used to clear the soft tissue remnants overlying the osseous triangle (Fig. 9.6a).

After the small bleeders are controlled and the remnant soft tissue around the osseous triangle is cleared, the base of the L5 transverse process and the cranial and lateral aspect of SAP are first drilled out (Fig. 9.6b).

Then, the remaining SAP that is located deep in the foramen is removed. At this point, the remaining SAP is too deep and too steep to be reached by the bur. Angled instruments, such as a hockey stick chisel and angled pituitary clamp, are useful in these situations (Fig. 9.6c). While all of these tasks can be accomplished with a 0° scope, sometimes a 30° scope is more useful to provide a wider vision, especially in obese patients.

After drilling out the bone, the ligament flavum is removed using a curette and Kerrison's punches (Fig. 9.6d). After flavectomy, the L5 exiting root, the perineural fat, and the disc space can be checked (Fig. 9.6e).

If there are offending pathologies at the extra-foraminal area, such as a far lateral disc or marginal osteophytes arising from the vertebral body, it is a good option to drill out the sacral alar before removing the ligament flavum. Removing a part of the sacral alar provides sufficient space to manipulate the endoscope and the surgical instruments. This also allows more space between the L5 exiting root and the disc. This space makes it easier and safer to manipulate the root and remove the herniated disc or the osteophytes (Fig. 9.6f).

After adequate decompression of the L5 exiting root is confirmed, epidural bleeding is controlled by coagulation with RF wands.

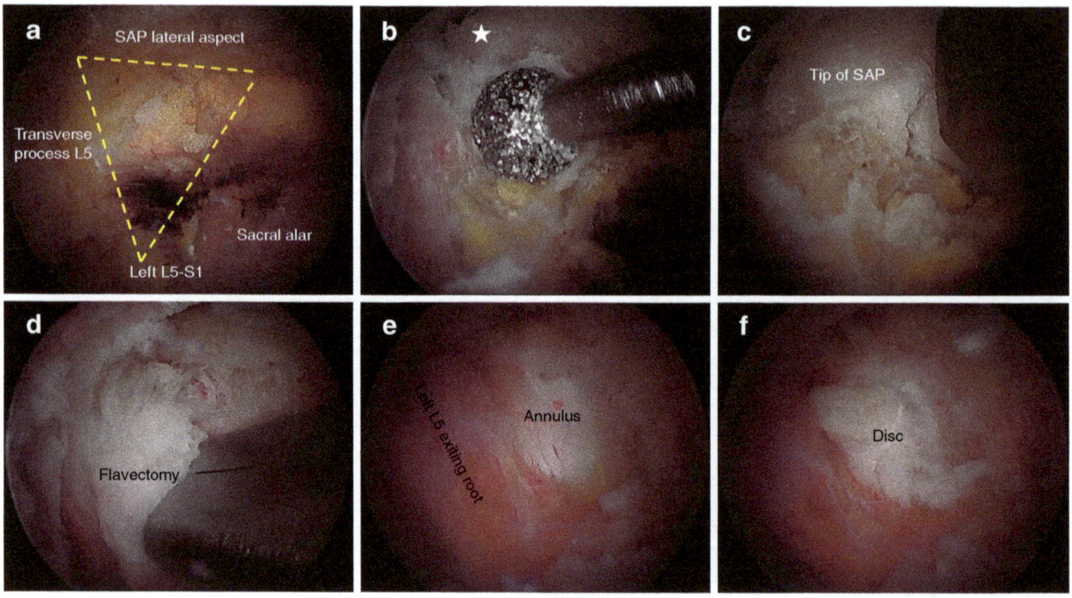

Fig. 9.6 Intraoperative endoscopic view. The osseous triangle (yellow dashed line) consists of the lateral aspect of SAP, the L5 transverse process, and the sacral alar (**a**). The base of the L5 transverse process and the tip of the SAP (asterisk) are drilled out (**b**). The hockey stick chisel is useful for resecting the deep portion of the SAP tip (**c**). Flavectomy is done by Kerrison's punches (**d**). L5 exiting root, perineural fat, and disc space are shown after flavectomy (**e**). A discectomy is done at the axillary portion of the exiting root. If the space is too narrow for discectomy, additional bone-work must be done at the sacral alar (**f**)

9.5 Illustrated Cases

9.5.1 Case 1: Paraspinal Foraminotomy at L3–4 Right Side Approach

A 68-year-old male patient complained about L3 pattern radiation pain in his right leg. The symptoms had been noted for 12 months, and he had difficulty walking because of the pain. The straight leg raising (SLR) test was normal. The neurological intermittent claudication was less than 300 meters to 400 meters. He had motor weakness on the right ankle dorsiflexion (grade 4). The Visual Analogue Scale (VAS) for his right leg pain was 7. Preoperative MRI and computed tomography (CT) scan showed right-side foraminal stenosis at the L3–4 level with a bony spur on the right L4 SAP (Fig. 9.7a, b, f).

A paraspinal foraminotomy using the UBE technique under general anesthesia was performed. Under the endoscope, the right L3 exiting root was decompressed, and the bony spur of the SAP was removed (Fig. 9.7e). Postoperative MRI and CT scan confirmed that the right L3–4 foramen was sufficiently decompressed (Fig. 9.7c, d, g). After the surgery, his symptom disappeared immediately.

9.5.2 Case 2: Paraspinal Discectomy with Resection of the SAP Tip at L3–4 Left

A 56-year-old male patient suffered from left side anterior thigh pain. The pain was distributed along the left L3 dermatome. The pain started 5 days ago, and because of the severe pain, he could not walk. The SLR test was negative on the right leg, and 30 degrees on the left leg. The neurological intermittent claudication was less than 200 meters to 300 meters. The manual muscle test for hip flexion was grade 3 on the left side. The VAS of the left leg pain was 9. Preoperative MRI and CT scan showed a left-side foraminal herniated disc with foraminal stenosis at the L3–4 level (Fig. 9.8a–d).

A paraspinal foraminotomy and discectomy using the UBE technique were performed under general anesthesia. Under the endoscope, the ruptured disc mass was found in the axillar portion of the left L3 exiting root (Fig. 9.8e). After discectomy, the tip of the SAP was removed by a chisel for foraminal decompression. Postoperative MRI and CT scan confirmed that the left L3–4 foramen was sufficiently decompressed (Fig. 9.8f–h). After surgery, his leg pain was immediately improved, and after 1 month, the motor weakness was recovered.

9.5.3 Case 3: Paraspinal Discectomy at L3–4 Left Side Approach

An 84-year-old female patient visited the hospital with severe left lateral thigh pain. The pain was distributed along the left L3 dermatome. The symptoms started 2 months ago, and because of the pain, she could not sit. The SLR test was negative on the right leg, and 10 degrees on the left leg. The manual muscle test of hip flexion and ankle dorsiflexion were both grade 3 on the left side. The VAS of the left leg pain was 9. Preoperative MRI showed an upward migrated disc herniation at the left L3–4 foramen (Fig. 9.9a, b).

A paraspinal discectomy using the UBE technique was performed under epidural anesthesia. Under the endoscope, the ruptured disc was found beneath the left L3 exiting root. After discectomy, the left L3 exiting root was released, and the engorgement of the root also disappeared (Video 9.3). The postoperative MRI and CT scan showed that the left L3–4 foramen was sufficiently decompressed (Fig. 9.9c, d). After surgery, the VAS of the leg pain was improved from 9 to 1. Motor weakness was not recovered till 3 months after the surgery.

9.5.4 Case 4: Paraspinal Foraminotomy at L5–S1 Right Side Approach (Video 9.4)

A 62-year-old male patient suffered from right buttock pain. Symptoms had been noted for one

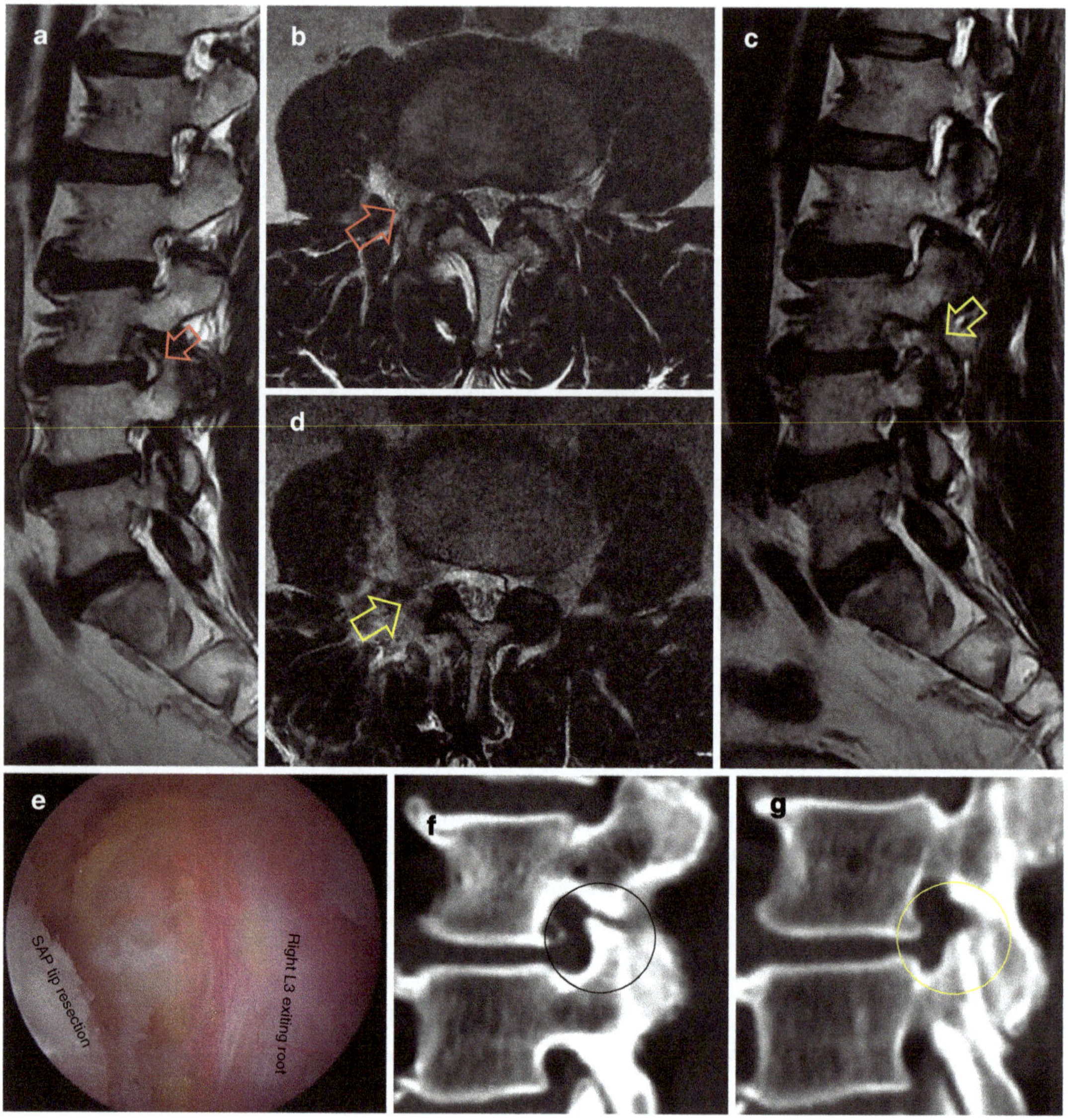

Fig. 9.7 Case 1. The preoperative right para-sagittal (**a**) and T2-weighted MR axial image (**b**) show that the right L3 exiting root is compressed by the bony spur of the SAP (red open arrows). The postoperative right para-sagittal (**c**) and T2 weighted MR axial image (**d**) show that the right L3 exiting root is decompressed, and the right L3–4 foramen is widened (yellow open arrows). The intraoperative endoscopic view shows that after resection of the SAP tip, the right L3 exiting root is released (**e**). The preoperative (**f**) and postoperative CT scan (**g**) show the partial resection (yellow circle) of the cranial tip of the right L4 SAP and bony spur (black circle) without instability

year, and in recent months had gradually worsened. Gradually, the limping phenomenon began to appear when walking. He had tried the conservative treatment for eight months with no significant improvement. The VAS for his left leg pain was 6. The SLR test was negative. The neurological intermittent claudication was less than 400 meters to 500 meters. The motor function was normal.

Preoperative MRI and CT scan showed right side foraminal stenosis at the L5–S1 level without segmental instability (Fig. 9.10a–c).

A paraspinal foraminotomy using the UBE technique was performed under epidural anesthe-

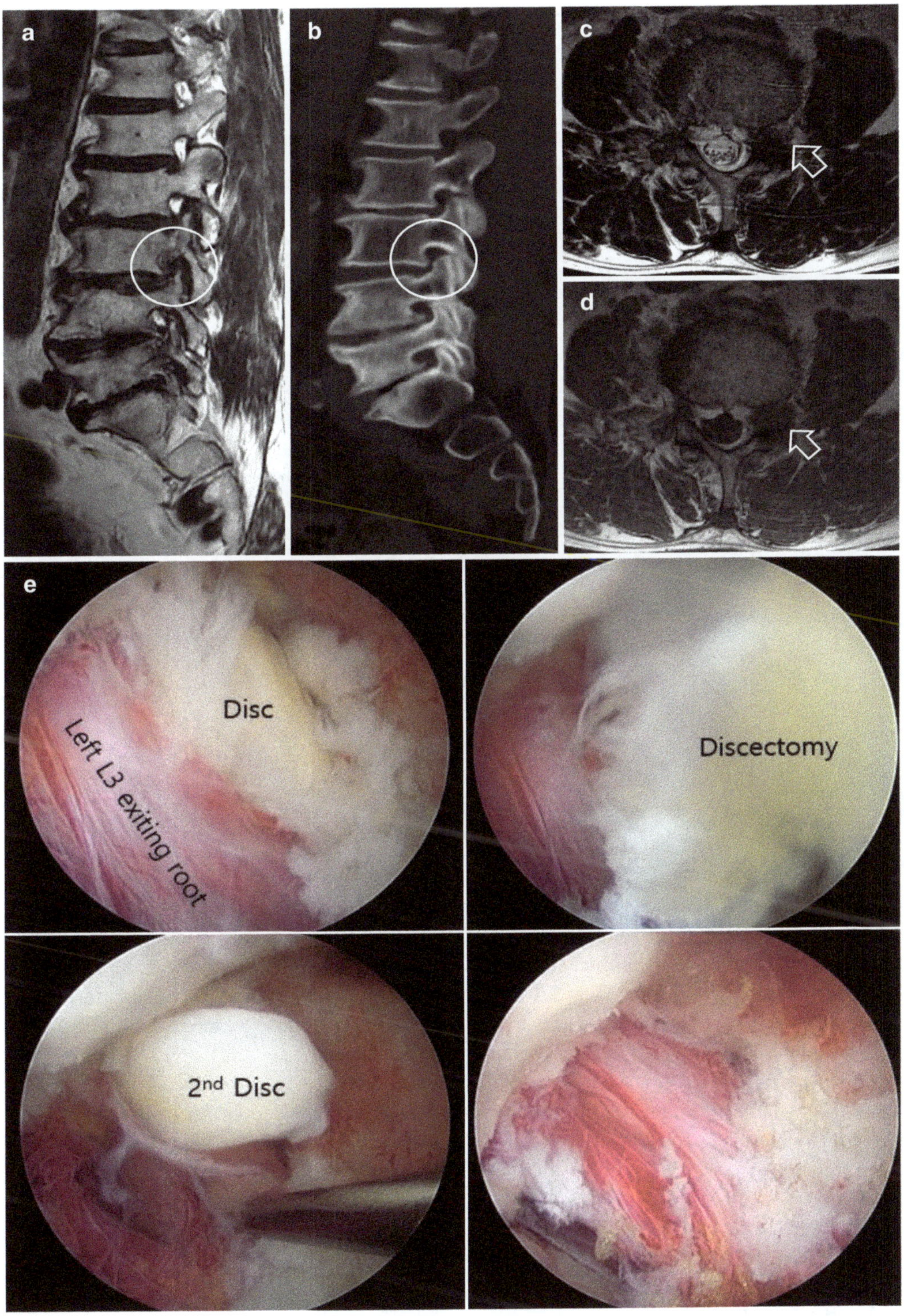

Fig. 9.8 Case 2. The preoperative left para-sagittal T2 weighted MRI (**a**) and CT scan (**b**) reveal severe foraminal stenosis (white circles) with hypertrophic facet joint at the L3–4 left side. The T2 (**c**) and T1 (**d**) weighted MR axial images show that the left L3 root is swollen (white open arrows). The intraoperative endoscopic view shows that the ruptured disc particles are located beneath the left L3 exiting root (**e**). The postoperative left para-sagittal (**f**) and axial T2 weighted MRI (**g**) show that the swelling of the left L3 exiting root is improved (yellow open arrows). The left para-sagittal CT scan (**h**) reveals the resection of the tip of the left L4 SAP (white circle) (**h**)

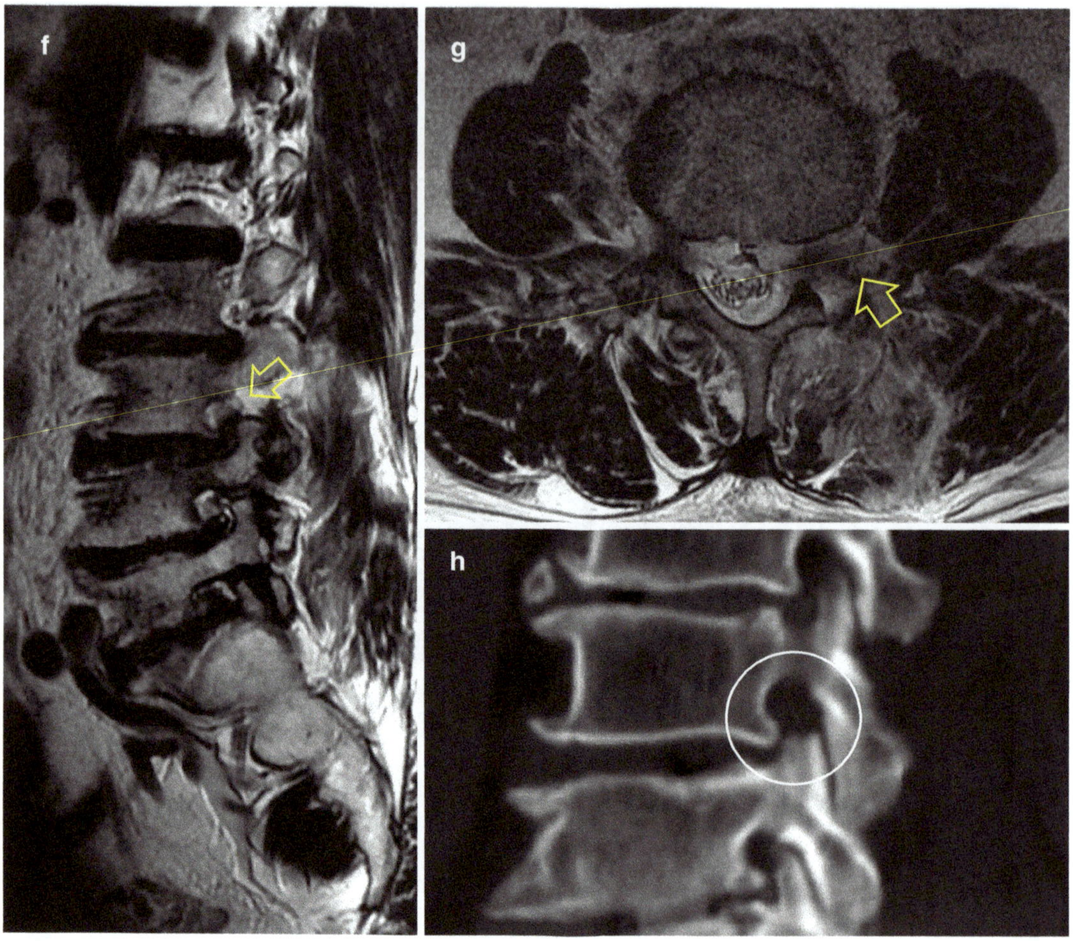

Fig. 9.8 (continued)

sia. Under the endoscope, the neural foramen was compromised, due to a bulging disc and hypertrophy of the foraminal ligament (Fig. 9.10d).

The postoperative MRI and CT scan confirmed that the right L5-S1 foramen was sufficiently decompressed (Fig. 9.10e–g). After surgery, his symptom was improved, and the abnormal gait was recovered immediately.

9.6 Complications and Their Management

9.6.1 Bleeding

Occasionally, radicular arterial bleeding can create many difficulties in performing surgery by obscuring the endoscopic visual field due to massive bleeding. The best way is to coagulate the small vessels using the RF wand before bleeding occurs. The alternative hemostatic technique is to ligate the small vessels using a vessel clip.

If bleeding is so severe as to interfere with the surgery, the scope can be advanced as close as possible toward the possible bleeding focus, and the water pressure temporarily increased to wash out the bleeding, find the bleeding focus, and coagulate the bleeding using a small size RF wand (Video 9.5).

Bleeding from the laminotomy surface can be effectively controlled using bone wax. After the surgery, a suction drain tube is mandatory to drain out the oozing from the perineural plexus and muscles, to prevent epidural hematoma.

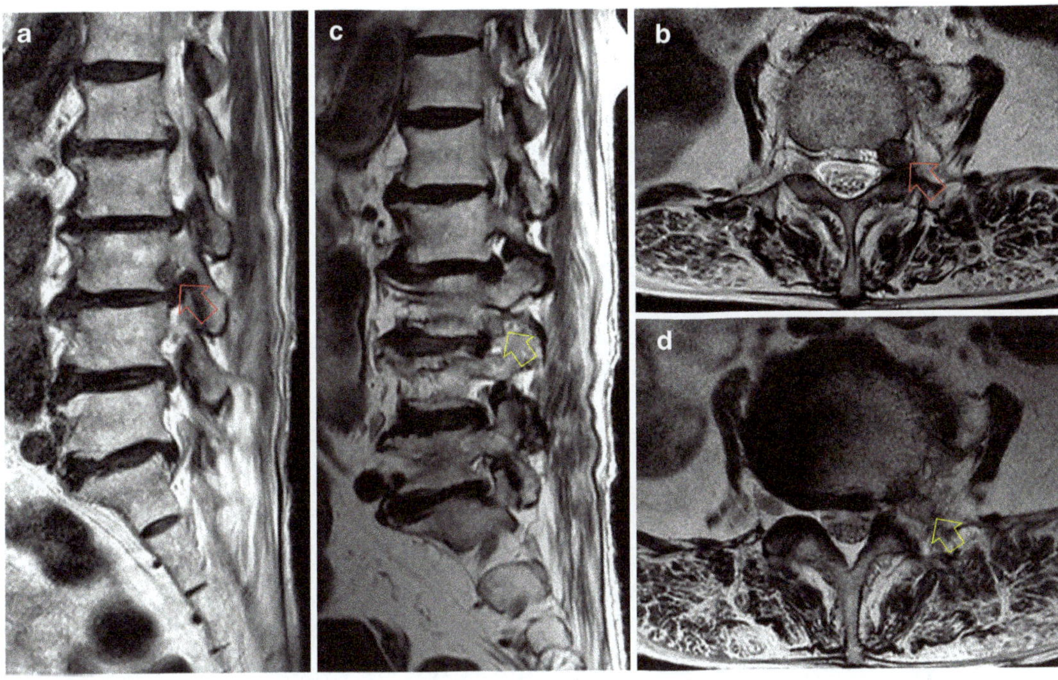

Fig. 9.9 Case 3. The preoperative left para-sagittal T2 weighted MRI (**a**) and T2 weighted MR axial image (**b**) reveal the up-migrated disc herniation at the left foraminal L3–4 level (red open arrows). The postoperative left para-sagittal (**c**) and axial T2 weighted MRI (**d**) show that even though the disc has been removed, the left L3 exiting root is still swollen (yellow open arrows)

9.6.2 Dural Tear/Root Irritation

Dura tear is not a common complication, because the surgery is performed around the exiting root. Rather, postoperative numbness and paresthesia may occur due to excessive manipulation of the root, especially when the operation is done around the dorsal root ganglion. Therefore, this problem can be prevented by gentle manipulation of the root.

9.7 Surgical Tips and Pitfalls

There are several surgical technical tips and tricks.

First, if the anatomy is confusing, discography can be helpful.

Second, make the approaching angle of the endoscope and instrument 30 degrees to 40 degrees. So, portal incision must be made on the lateral tip of the lower and upper transverse process.

Third, the cranial tip of the SAP can be removed to provide space for additional bone working.

Fourth, when performing partial resection of the SAP tip, the scope retractor is useful for protecting the exiting root.

Fifth, some surgeons do not perform enough SAP resection, because they worry that excessive removal of SAP may predispose them to instability. However, this may result in insufficient neural decompression with persistent symptoms. According to biomechanical studies, less than 75% resection does not induce segmental instability [8, 9]. Because of subsequent articular regeneration, the importance of sufficient neural decompression should over-weigh preserving the integrity of the facet joint.

Finally, radicular artery ligation is needed to maintain a clear operative view.

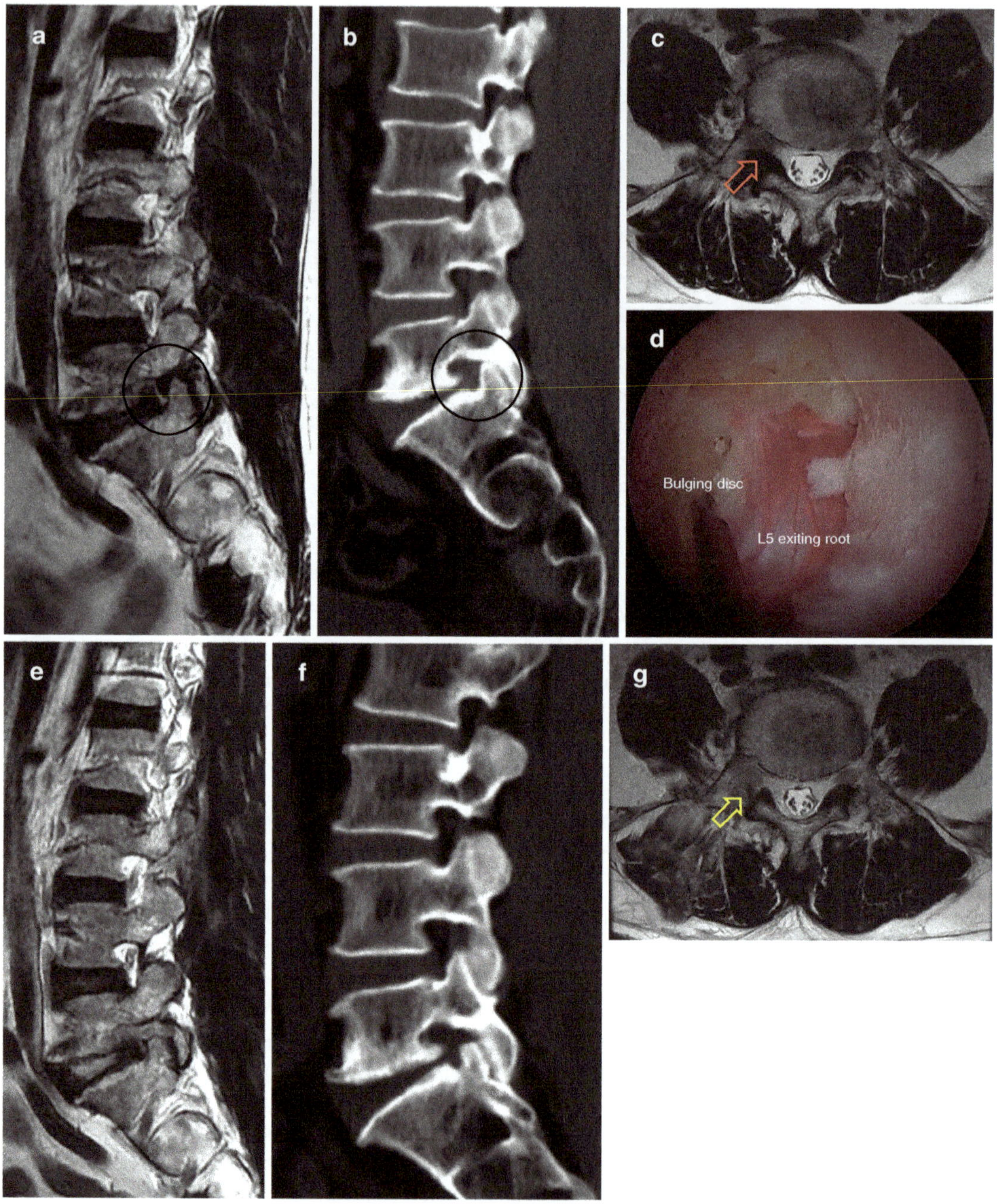

Fig. 9.10 Case 4. The preoperative right para-sagittal T2 weighted MRI (**a**) and CT scan (**b**) reveal the right side foraminal stenosis at the L5–S1 level (black circles). The preoperative T2 weighted MR axial image (**c**) shows the hypertrophic foraminal ligament around the right L5 exiting root (red open arrow). The intraoperative endoscopic view shows the decompressed L5 exiting nerve root and annuloplasty in the bulging disc (**d**). The postoperative right para-sagittal (**e**) and CT scan (**f**) show that the foraminal ligament is removed (white circle) and the tip of SAP is partially resected (yellow dashed circle). The postoperative T2 weighted MR axial image (**g**) reveals the decompression around the right L5 exiting nerve root after the foraminal ligament is removed (yellow open arrow)

References

1. Bose K, Balasubramaniam P. Nerve root canals of the lumbar spine. Spine (Phila Pa 1976). 1984;9(1):16–8.
2. Youn MS, Shin JK, Goh TS, Lee JS. Clinical and radiological outcomes of endoscopic partial facetectomy for degenerative lumbar foraminal stenosis. Acta Neurochir. 2017;159(6):1129–35.
3. Choi G, Lee SH, Bhanot A, Raiturker PP, Chae YS. Percutaneous endoscopic discectomy for extraforaminal lumbar disc herniations: extraforaminal targeted fragmentectomy technique using working channel endoscope. Spine (Phila Pa 1976). 2007;32(2):E93–9.
4. Heo DH, Sharma S, Park CK. Endoscopic treatment of extraforaminal entrapment of L5 nerve root (far out syndrome) by unilateral biportal endoscopic approach: technical report and preliminary clinical results. Neurospine. 2019;16(1):130–7.
5. Kim JE, Choi DJ. Bi-portal arthroscopic spinal surgery (BASS) with 30 degrees arthroscopy for far lateral approach of L5-S1 - technical note. J Orthop. 2018;15(2):354–8.
6. Lee CW, Yoon KJ. The usefulness of percutaneous endoscopic technique in multifocal lumbar pathology. Biomed Res Int. 2019;2019:9528102.
7. Takeuchi M, Yasuda M, Shima H, Funai M, Osuka K, Takayasu M. Surgical method for lumbar foraminal stenosis. No Shinkei Geka. 2012;40(4):319–23.
8. Teo EC, Lee KK, Qiu TX, Ng HW, Yang K. The biomechanics of lumbar graded facetectomy under anterior-shear load. IEEE Trans Biomed Eng. 2004;51(3):443–9.
9. Zhou Y, Luo G, Chu TW, Wang J, Li CQ, Zheng WJ, et al. The biomechanical change of lumbar unilateral graded facetectomy and strategies of its microsurgical reconstruction: report of 23 cases. Zhonghua Yi Xue Za Zhi. 2007;87(19):1334–8.

10 Unilateral Biportal Endoscopy for Decompression of Foraminal (Extraforaminal) Stenosis Through the Contralateral Sublaminar Approach

Ji Yeon Kim, Dong Hwa Heo, Hyun Jin Hong, and Cheol Woong Park

10.1 Introduction

The exiting nerve roots (ENR) at the lumbar spinal levels pass through the neuroforamen below the pedicle and the superior articular process (SAP), and then curve downward in the far-out area. ENR entrapment in the foraminal and extraforaminal areas is usually caused by hypertrophied ligamentum flavum (LF) [1] and enlarged facet joints. In these cases, entrapped ENR can be effectively decompressed by removing the hypertrophied LF and the tip of the SAP. The herniated disc and coexisting prominent syndesmophytes also compress the ENR from the ventral foraminal area and distort the natural course of the nerve root in the far-out area. In these cases, ventrally located lesions should be identified and removed for optimal neural decompression to restore the smooth downward angulation of the nerve root.

Spinal endoscopic decompression of lumbar foraminal stenosis and combined lateral recess or extraforaminal stenosis have been tried via contralateral sublaminar approach. Uniportal endoscopic system has the advantage that the small-diameter endoscope and fine surgical equipment can pass through the foraminal space, almost parallel to the intervertebral disc, making foraminal and extraforaminal nerve root decompression even in the prominent disc herniation without nerve root retraction [2–4]. Biportal endoscopic surgery also accessed the foraminal area and achieved favorable outcomes with a contralateral sublaminar approach to treat lateral recess and foraminal stenotic pathologies [5–7]. Furthermore, with the development of instruments and techniques, the biportal endoscopic system can access the extraforaminal area through the contralateral sublaminar approach overcoming the crowing of the endoscopy with instruments in the narrowed foraminal space [8] (Fig. 10.1). Therefore, we can treat the coexisting stenosis in the lateral recess and foraminal and extraforaminal areas through the contralateral sublaminar approach using biportal endoscopy.

Supplementary Information The online version contains supplementary material available at [https://doi.org/10.1007/978-981-16-8201-8_10].

J. Y. Kim · H. J. Hong
Department of Neurosurgery, Spine Center, Wiltse Memorial Hospital, Anyang, South Korea

D. H. Heo (✉)
Department of Neurosurgery, Spine Center, Seoul Bumin Hospital, Seoul, South Korea

C. W. Park
Department of Neurosurgery, Spine Center, Daejeon Woori Hospital, Daejeon, South Korea

D. H. Heo et al. (eds.), *Unilateral Biportal Endoscopic Spine Surgery*,
https://doi.org/10.1007/978-981-16-8201-8_10

10.2 Indications and Contraindications

- Indication
  - Unilateral lumbar foraminal and extraforaminal stenosis
  - Unilateral lumbar foraminal and extraforaminal stenosis with bilateral central or lateral recess stenosis
  - Unilateral coexisting lumbar lateral recess, foraminal stenosis, and extraforaminal stenosis
- Extended indication
  - Recurrent foraminal stenosis after foraminotomy transforaminal approaches
  - L5-S1 lesions of indicated cases
- Relative contraindication
- Recurrent extraforaminal stenosis after decompression surgery with paraspinal approach
- Contraindication
  - Dominant mechanical back pain
  - Instability with degenerative or spondylolytic spondylolisthesis
  - Bilateral symptomatic foraminal-extraforaminal stenosis
  - L5-S1 extraforaminal stenosis of the lumbosacral transitional vertebrae

We recommend this technique to treat radiculopathy due to compressing the ENR in the narrowed foraminal-extraforaminal area and traversing nerve root at the lateral recess area rather than for patients with dominant back and buttock pain.

This technique may be challenging for the L5–S1 level, which has a wide facet joint and inclination of the disc space [9]. It is impossible to sufficiently decompress the dorsal part of extraforaminal stenoses, such as L5-S1 lumbosacral transitional vertebrae. Paraspinal biportal endoscopic surgery or fusion operation is preferred in this case.

If the patients have symptomatic foraminal and extraforaminal stenosis without definite lateral recess stenosis, paraspinal biportal endoscopic surgery is usually preferred to avoid unnecessary disruption of the ipsilateral unaffected structures.

10.3 Special Instruments (See Detailed Figures in Chapters for Instruments)

The endoscopy and instruments pass over the thecal sac to access the narrow foraminal area during operation with this technique. Fine instruments with proper access angle and neural protection are essential for successful decompression.

1. 3.5-mm and 3.0-mm endoscopic diamond drill for intimate bone drilling along the ENR.
2. Working cannulas to keep proper direction to the contralateral side through sublaminar space.
3. Scope self-retractor to protect the nerve and vessels from rolling up to the high-speed drill.
4. Hockey-shaped chisel to remove the SAP.

10.4 Anesthesia and Position

Biportal endoscopic surgery was performed with patients in the prone position under general endotracheal anesthesia or epidural anesthesia. Prone position with back flexed position induces wider interlaminar area and narrowed foraminal space. Flexed position reduces the extent of sublaminar bone removal and decreases the pressure on the compressed ENR during foraminotomy.

10.5 Surgical Steps of Lumbar Contralateral Sublaminar Approach for Foraminal-Extraforaminal Lesions (Fig. 10.1)

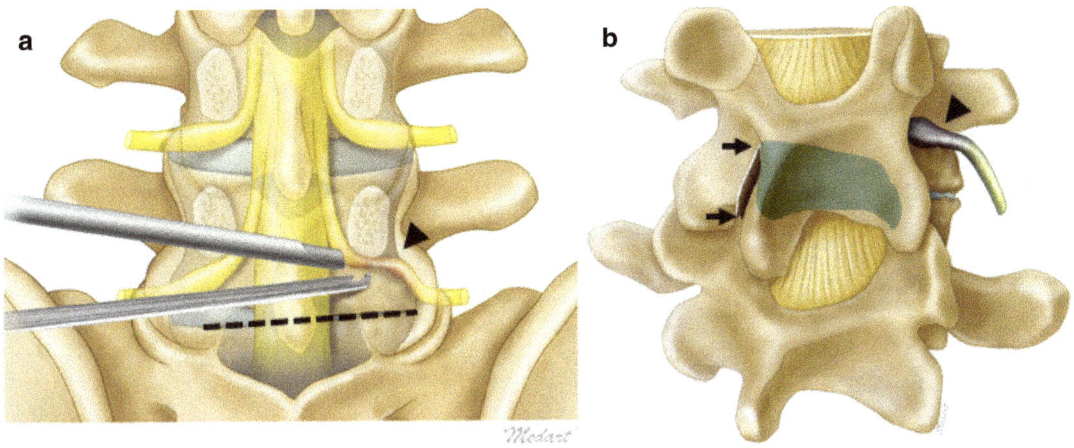

Fig. 10.1 Overview of biportal endoscopic contralateral sublaminar approach for right foraminal-extraforaminal stenosis via left-sided portals. The exiting nerve root is severely compressed and distorted in the foraminal and extraforaminal area (black arrowhead) by the hypertrophied facet joint and herniated disc with prominent syndesmophytes (**a**). Ipsilateral laminotomy (black arrows) and contralateral sublaminar bony drilling (green area) is necessary when the endoscope and instruments access the contralateral foraminal area (**b**). The instrument should pass the sublaminar space nearly parallel to the disc space (black dotted line) to reach the extraforaminal space safely

10.6 Surgical Steps Left-sided Approach for Right-sided Contralateral Lesions

10.6.1 Making Two Portals

Under image intensification, fluoroscopic confirmation of the level is performed with the insertion of spinal needles at the target area. Generally, two skin incisions were created over the ipsilateral medial pedicular area (Fig. 10.2a, b). If we perform the surgery at the L4-L5 level, unilateral two skin incisions were made on the L4 and L5 medial pedicular area to decompression the contralateral lateral recess and foraminal stenosis. Caudocranial access angle of instruments facilitates efficient foraminal decompression (Fig. 10.2b). However, if the contralateral extraforaminal decompression is necessary, a working portal should be created close to the lower endplate of the L4-L5 intervertebral disc to obtain the optimal extraforaminal approach angle nearly parallel to the disc space (Figs. 10.1a and 10.2c, d). Serial dilators were inserted at a working portal. Subsequently, a working sheath was inserted along the dilator for proper drainage of infused saline.

10.6.2 Contralateral Sublaminar Bony Decompression until the Medial Border of Foramen (Video 10.1 and Fig. 10.3)

For decompression of the right lumbar ENR, we first performed left-sided laminotomy and drilling of the spinolaminar junction until the proximal end of the bilateral LF is exposed. After identifying the Y-shaped proximal origin of the LF (Fig. 10.3a), contralateral sublaminar bony decompression was performed by drilling of the inner cortex and partially cancellous bone toward the contralateral side to obtain working space for the procedure (Fig. 10.3b, c). Contralateral sublaminar bony drilling was performed while confirming the bony margin of the lamina and SAP after detachment of the LF (Fig. 10.3d, e). Bony drilling was extended craniolaterally to the pedicle until

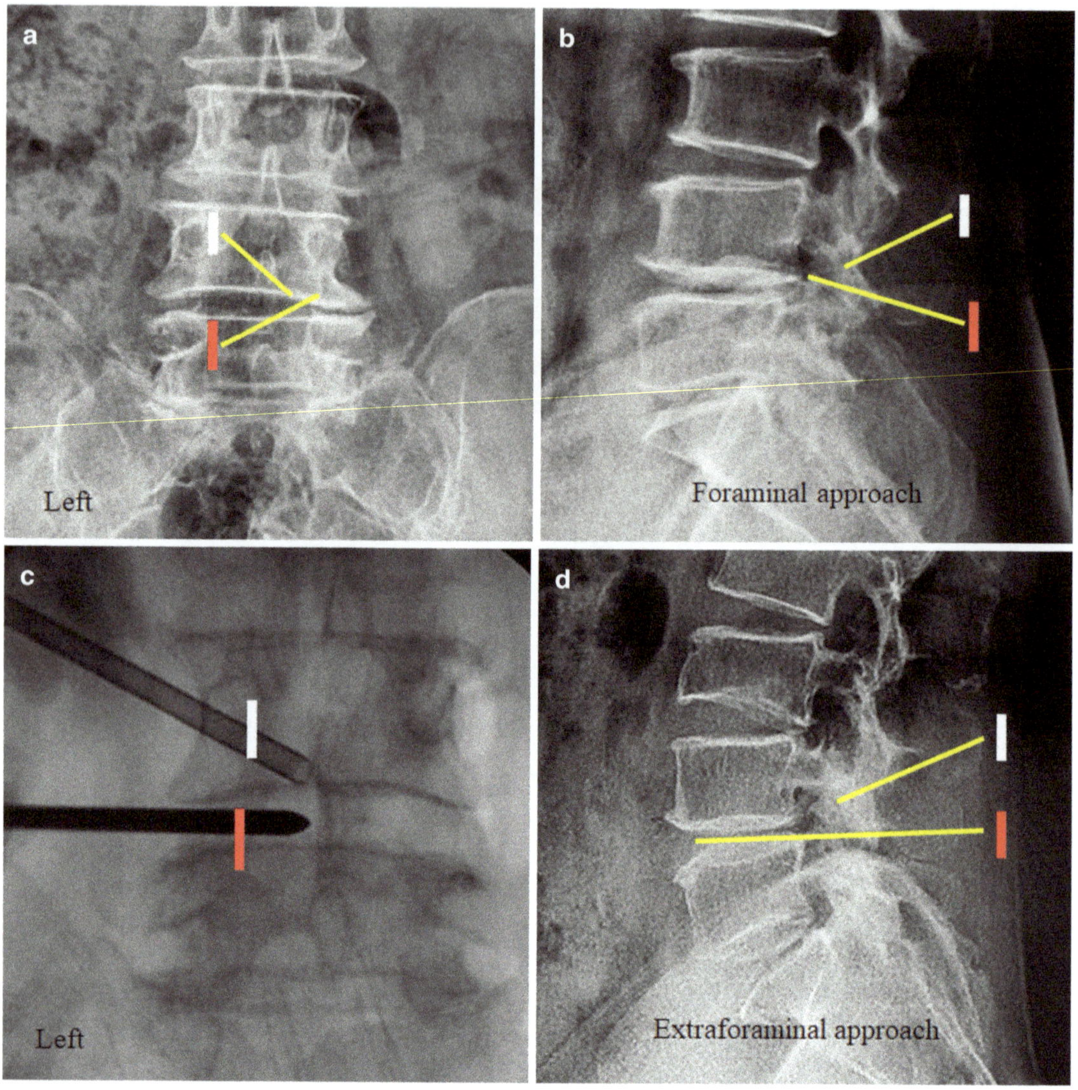

Fig. 10.2 Skin incision points of two portals (white line: endoscopic portal, red line: working portal) with a left-sided approach for the contralateral foraminal decompression (**a** and **b**) and foraminal-extraforaminal decompression (**c** and **d**) at the L4-L5 level. Contralateral foraminal decompression is usually performed using the portals on the L4 and L5 medial pedicle areas (**a** and **b**). The working portal should be placed close to the lower endplate of the L4-L5 intervertebral disc (**c**) to access the extraforaminal area using an optimized approach angle, almost parallel to the disc space (**d**)

the LF edge was freed (Fig. 10.3e). The medial border of the facet joint and pedicle should be clearly exposed after sublaminar bony decompression while preserving the LF (Fig. 10.3f).

If the patient had bilateral leg pain due to bilateral lateral recess stenosis or central stenosis, the ipsilateral LF was removed for ipsilateral traversing nerve root decompression.

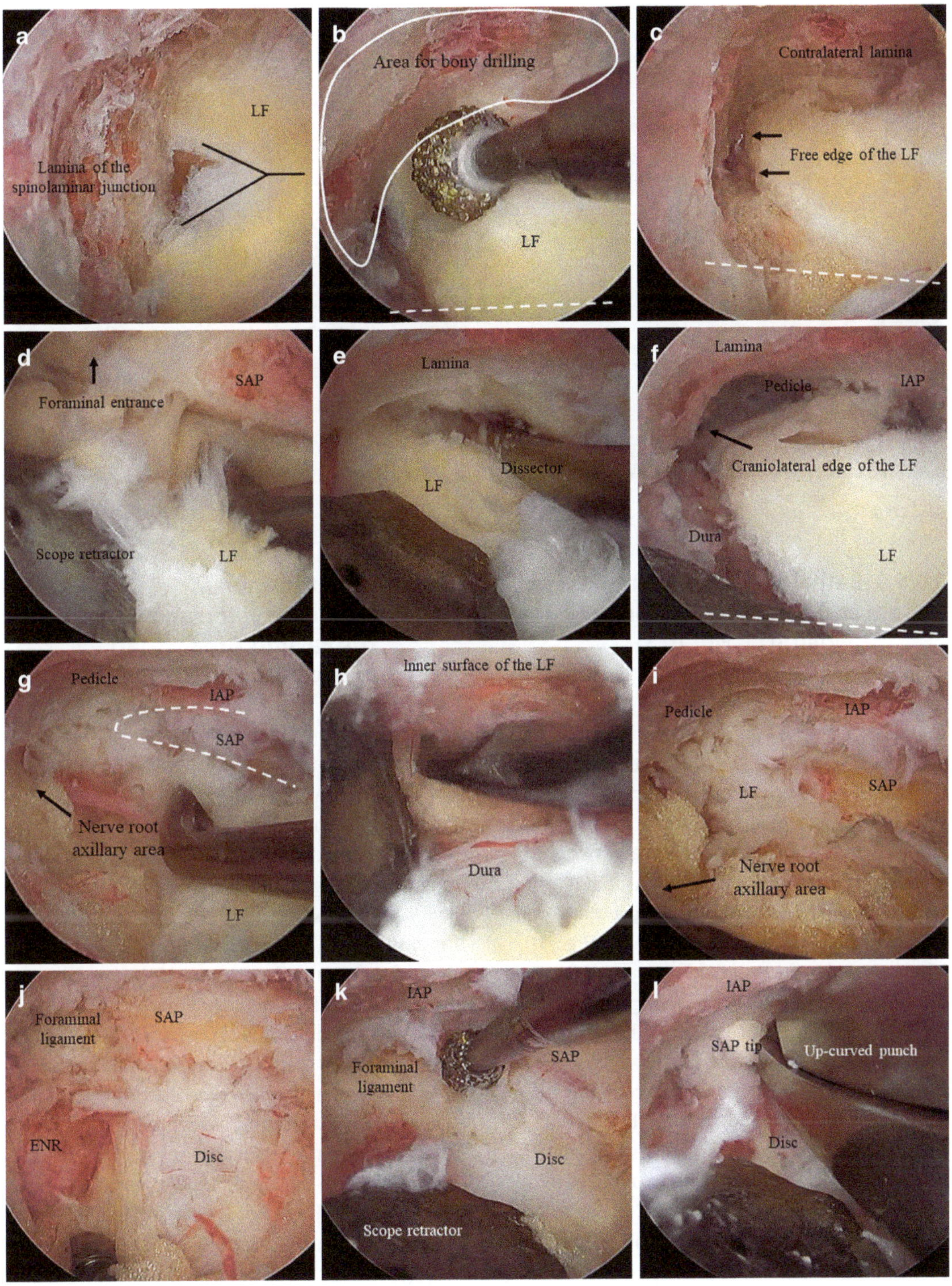

Fig. 10.3 Biportal endoscopic contralateral sublaminar foraminotomy for the right-sided L5-S1 foraminal stenosis and herniated disc via left-sided unilateral approach. Initial ipsilateral laminotomy and spinolaminar junction drilling (**a**). Contralateral sublaminar bony drilling until the medial entrance of the foramen (**b–f**). Ligamentum flavum (LF) and the tip of the SAP were removed to open the narrowed foraminal space (**g–j**). Additional SAP removal and foraminal discectomy were performed for sufficient nerve root decompression (**k, l**). Prominent syndesmophytes compression the nerve root was also drilled (**m**), and sufficiently decompressed nerve root was found (**n**). ENR: exiting nerve root, LF: ligament flavum. SAP: superior articular process, *IAP* inferior articular process

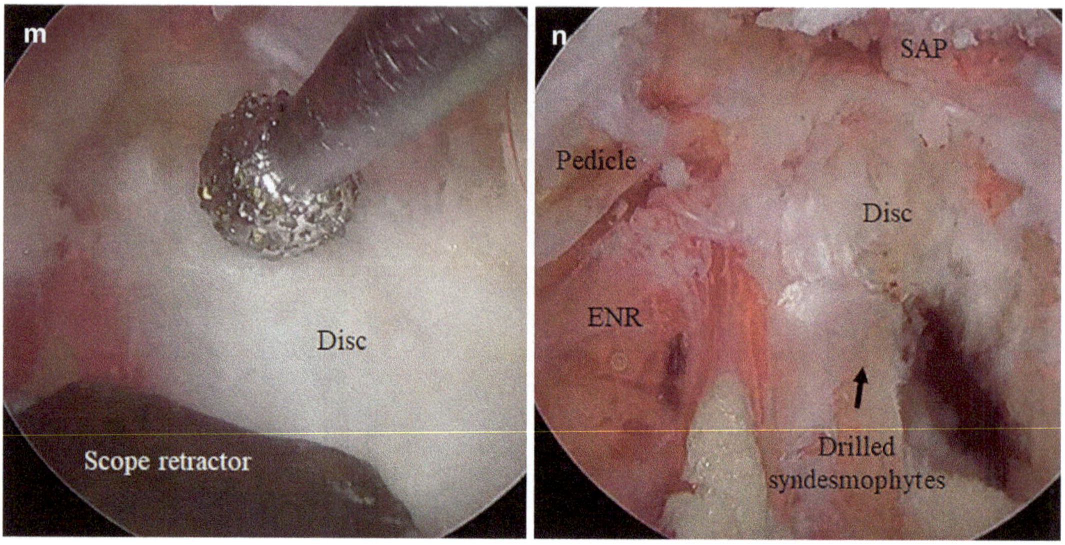

Fig. 10.3 (continued)

10.6.3 Lateral Recess Decompression and Foraminal Decompression (Video 10.1, Fig. 10.3)

The edge of the LF was detached from the foraminal entrance with curettes and double-ended dissectors (Fig. 10.3g), and the contralateral half of the LF was removed after epidural dissection while retraction the LF with a scope retractor (Fig. 10.3h). Additional drilling and punching of the medial part of the inferior articular process and SAP were performed to expose the foramen and decompress the lateral recess (Fig. 10.3i). The tip of the SAP and LF covering foraminal entrance were removed using forceps and punches until the entire disc height and proximal part of ENR was exposed (Fig. 10.3j). Subsequently, we remove the remained tip of SAP and hypertrophied foraminal ligament using a fine drill and up-curved punches (Fig. 10.3k, l). Foraminal herniated disc and prominent syndesmophytes compression the ENR were removed using the fine endoscopic drill and forceps while protecting the nerve root and dura with a scope self-retractor (Fig. 10.3m). Decompressed ENR in the foraminal part is found, and we usually finished the foraminotomy if the patient did not have extraforaminal lesions (Fig. 10.3n).

10.6.4 Extraforaminal Decompression and Opening the Far-out Area (Video 10.2, Fig. 10.4)

If the patient had nerve compressing lesions at the extraforaminal area, we should consider additional extraforaminal decompression for a sufficient nerve root release. Furthermore, if we planned the extraforaminal decompression preoperatively (Fig. 10.1), the working portal should be made close to the disc level to access the extraforaminal and far-out area (Fig. 10.2c, d).

Initial foraminal discectomy and drilling of prominent syndesmophytes enlarged the foraminal space, thereby opening the space between the entrapped ENR and the extraforaminal herniated disc. This created space was critical in enabling access to the extraforaminal region and prevented an increase in the intracanal pressure in the narrowed foramen during manipulation of the extraforaminal disc fragments (Figs. 10.3n and 10.4a). At this point, an up-curved punch was inserted through the open space between the ENR and herniated disc, and the remaining lateral half of the SAP tip was removed, escaping the dorsal root ganglion compression. The extraforaminal herniated disc was then entirely exposed and removed

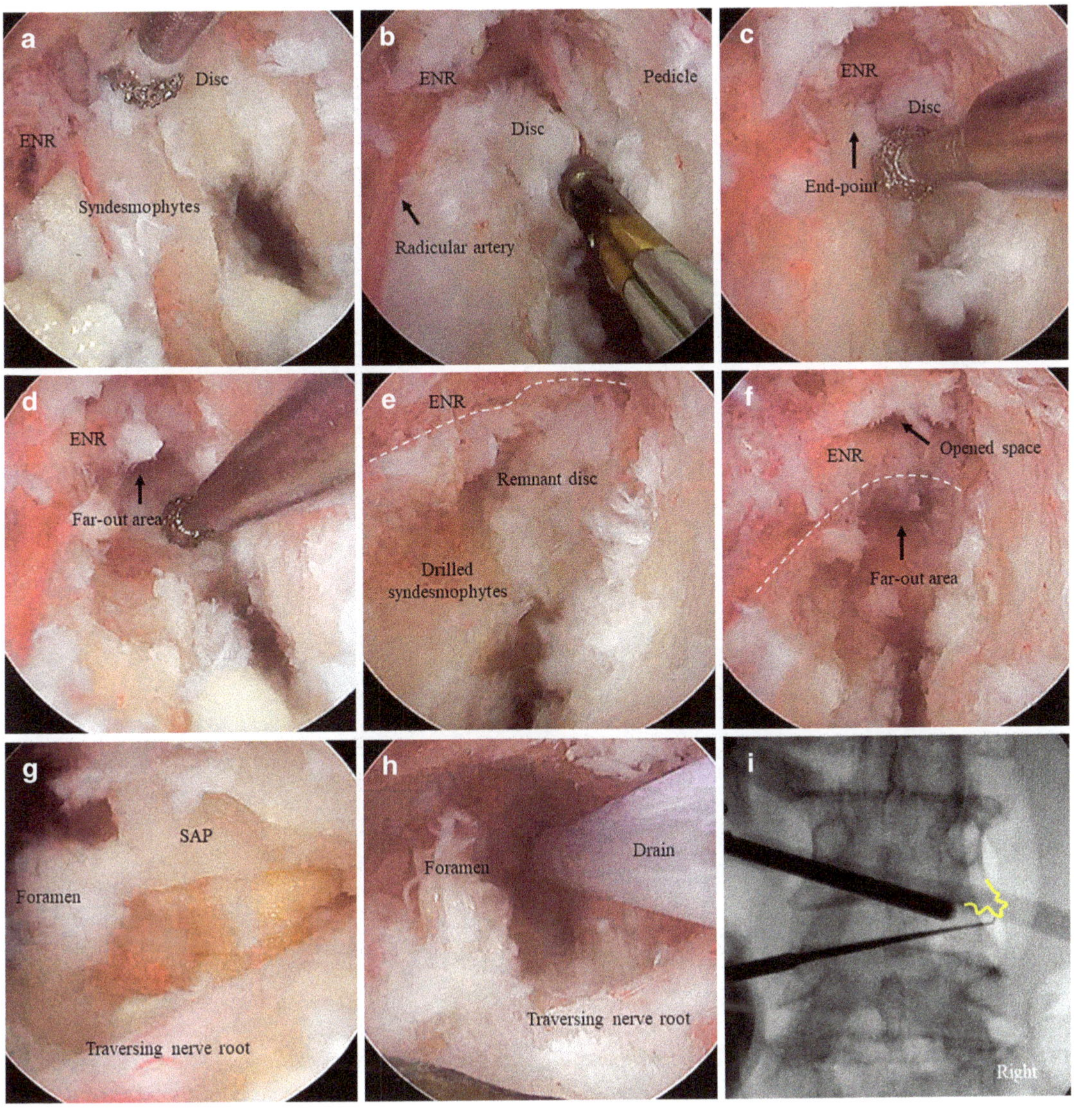

Fig. 10.4 Extraforaminal decompression and opening of the far-out area at the right L5-S1 level after foraminal decompression. Prominent syndesmophytes were drilled to expose the extraforaminal herniated disc (**a**). After removing the extraforaminal herniated disc (**b**), end-point lesions were drilled until the far-out area was exposed (**c** and **d**). The remnant herniated disc, which compressed and distorted the nerve root, was removed with up-curved forceps (**e**). Finally, the exiting nerve root was decompressed entirely from the foraminal area to the far-out area where the nerve root curved downward and restored the natural downward angulation (**f**). Before finishing the operation, traversing nerve root decompression was also confirmed (**g**) and a drainage catheter inserted (**h**). The extent of decompression and end-point (tortuous yellow line) was confirmed using intraoperative X-ray images (**i**). Preoperative MR images revealed lateral recess stenosis and foraminal-extraforaminal stenosis on the right side of the L5-S1 level (**j**). Postoperative MRI images showed successful decompression of the right S1 traversing nerve root and the L5 exiting nerve root while preserving the facet joint (**k**) (White arrow: foraminal area, white arrowhead: extraforaminal area). *ENR* exiting nerve root, *SAP* superior articular process

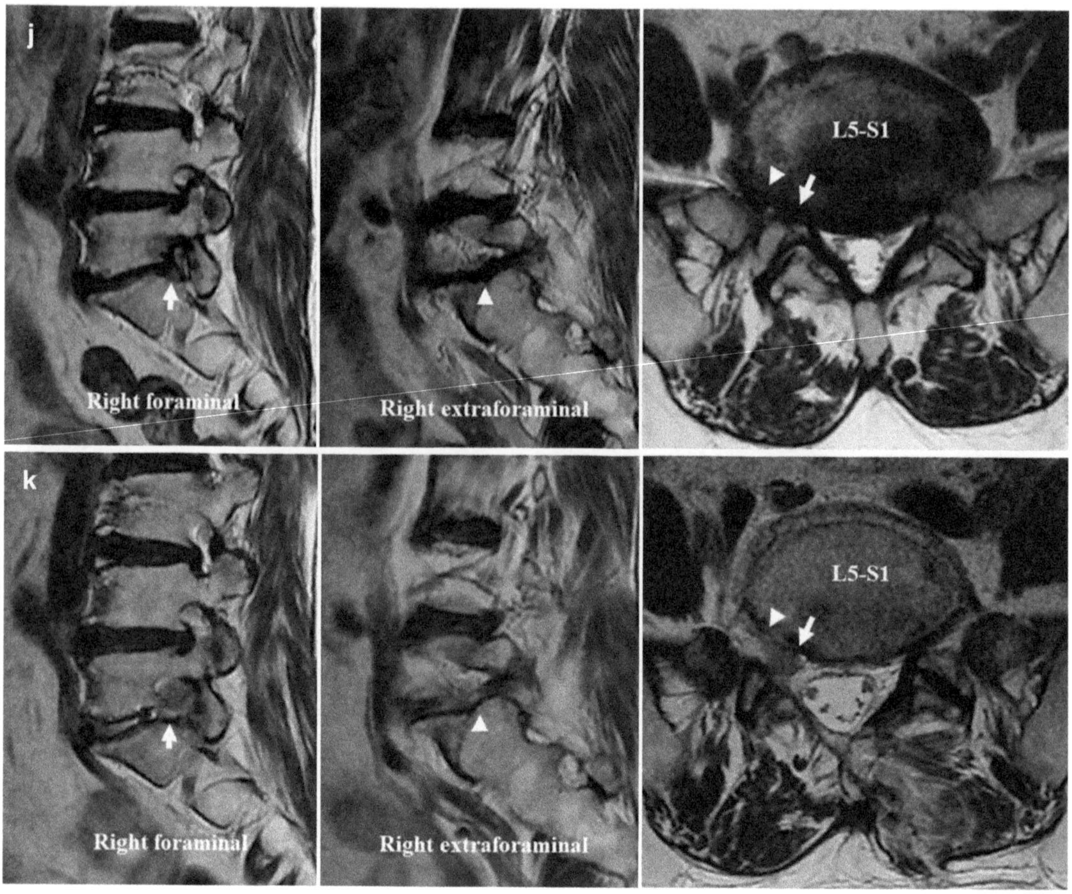

Fig. 10.4 (continued)

using the up-curved forceps while being careful not to injure the segmental artery and nerve root (Fig. 10.4b). Remnant syndesmophytes compressing the ENR at the end-point were removed using a 3-mm endoscopic drill (Fig. 10.4c, d), and the attached residual herniated disc was found nearly far-out area distorting the course of the nerve root (Fig. 10.4e). After removal of remnant herniated disc particles, fully decompressed ENR was found from the foraminal area to the far-out area (Fig. 10.4f). Traversing nerve root was also sufficiently decompressed (Fig. 10.4g). All procedures during foraminal and extraforaminal decompression were performed without dorsal root ganglion retraction, and the patient did not experience postoperative dysesthesia [2]. The extent of decompression was confirmed using intraoperative X-ray images (Fig. 10.4i). A drainage catheter was inserted in the decompressed foraminal space to prevent postoperative hematoma (Fig. 10.4h). The illustrated case showed well decompressed right-side lateral recess and foraminal-extraforaminal area after left sided-approach of biportal endoscopic contralateral lumbar foraminotomy (Fig. 10.4j, k).

10.6.5 End-point and Final Confirmation of Complete Decompression (Video 10.2, Fig. 10.5)

The end-point was in the far-out area where the exiting root began to curve downward with natu-

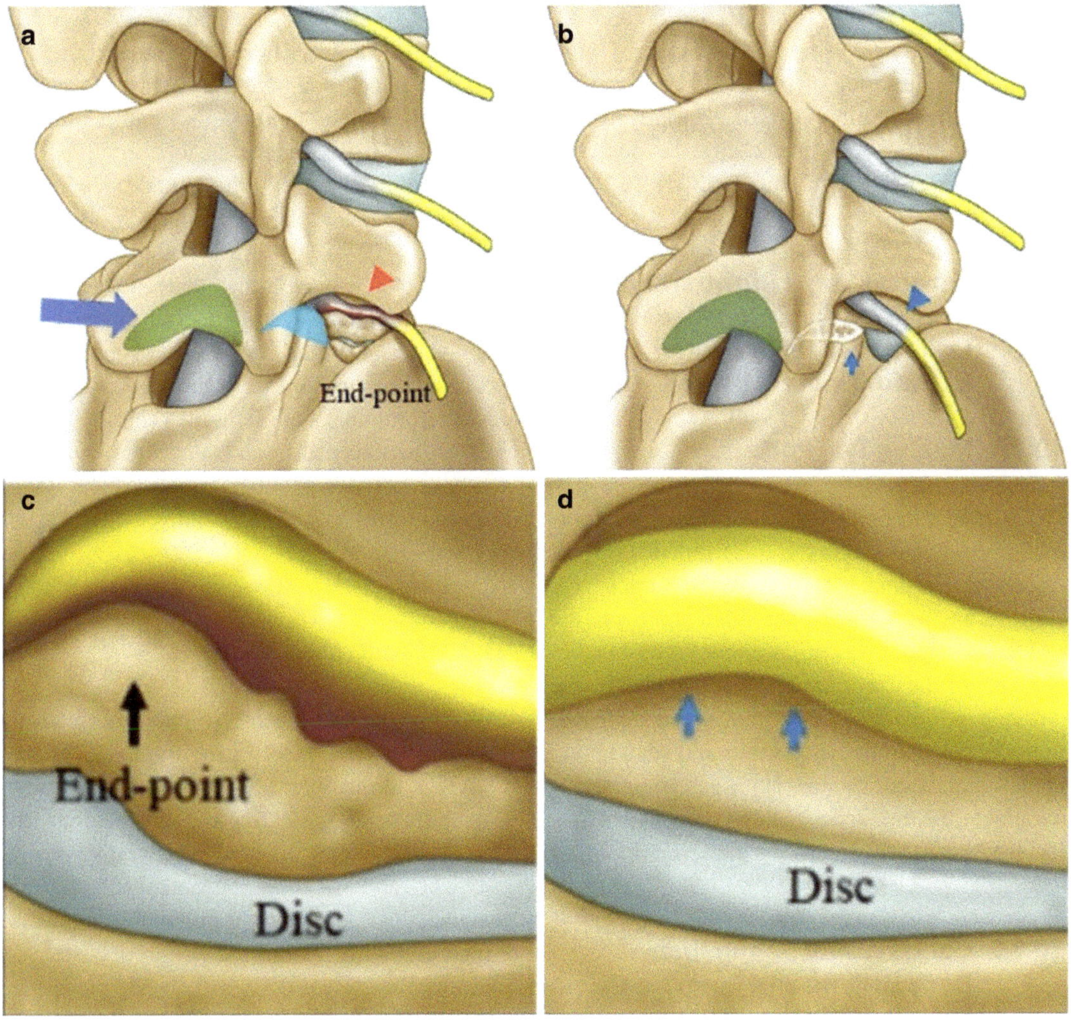

Fig. 10.5 The end-point of biportal endoscopic contralateral lumbar foraminal and extraforaminal decompression surgery. The exiting nerve root was severely compressed and distorted (red arrowhead) at the extraforaminal area by the herniated disc and the superior articular process (SAP). The end-point indicate the prominent bony spur and herniated disc at the caudolateral edge of the upper-level vertebral body (**a, c**). SAP removal (**a**: blue semicircular zone, **b**: blue arrow) and discectomy are necessary for sufficient nerve root decompression (**b**, blue arrowhead). End-point removal is essential to resolve the distorted nerve root in the extraforaminal and far-out area (**b** and **d**)

ral angulation [2, 4] (Fig. 10.5a, c, and e). Adequate decompression was assessed by confirming the pulsating nerve roots, the anemic nerve root turning pink, and the return of natural angulation of the ENR under direct endoscopic visualization (Figs. 10.4f and 10.5b, d).

10.7 Surgical Steps Right-sided Approach for Left-sided Contralateral Foraminal-Extraforaminal Lesions

10.7.1 Making Two Portals

Under image intensification, fluoroscopic confirmation of the trajectory is performed with the insertion of spinal needles at the target area (Fig. 10.6a , b). For the right-sided approach, the endoscopic portal was made on the medial pedicular area of the lower lumbar level. However, the working portals should be placed close to the upper endplate of the intervertebral disc to obtain the optimal extraforaminal approach angle nearly parallel to the disc space (Fig. 10.6c, d). A working sheath was inserted along the serial dilators.

10.7.2 Contralateral Sublaminar Bony Drilling and Foraminal-Extraforaminal Decompression (Video 10.3 and Fig. 10.7)

An endoscope accessed the foraminal area with a caudocranial angle during the right-sided approach and showed a broad and detailed view of foraminal space than the left-sided approach (Fig. 10.7a–f). However, instruments and the endoscopic drill accessed the foraminal space over the axillary area of the nerve root close to the ENR (Fig. 10.7g–j). These procedures increase the risk of incidental hitting and tearing injury of nerve root during the drilling of prominent syndesmophytes under exiting nerve root. We recommend using the chisel to remove the bony spur very close to the ENR, especially in the extraforaminal area (Fig. 10.7k). Furthermore, it is not easy to decompress the end-point due to the craniocaudal access angle of instruments. Various curved instruments such as up-curved punches, up-curved forceps, and curved curettes help decompress the end-point area (Fig. 10.7l). It is challenging to decompress the ventral part of the extraforaminal area at the L5-S1 level via a right-sided approach. Illustrated case (Fig. 10.7p, q) with endoscopic views (Fig. 10.7m–o) showed the successful foraminal and extraforaminal decompression at the L5-S1 level via right-sided contralateral sublaminar approach. Primary stenotic components of foraminal-extraforaminal stenosis were ventrally located calcified herniated disc and syndesmophytes and clearly removed without retraction of the dorsal root ganglion even in the L5-S1 level via right-side approach (Fig. 10.7).

10.8 Illustrated Cases

1. A 59-year-old woman presented with severe pain of abrupt onset in the right leg through the L4 dermatome. She also had left leg radicular pain of gradual progression along the posterior lateral aspect. Preoperative operative CT and MR images revealed right foraminal stenosis and extraforaminal herniated disc and combined bilateral lateral recess stenosis at the L4-L5 level (Fig. 10.8). We performed the biportal endoscopic left-sided unilateral laminotomy and bilateral lateral recess decompression, and contralateral foraminal-extraforaminal decompression. Postoperative MRI showed sufficient decompression of bilateral lateral recess and right-sided foraminal and extraforaminal area (Fig. 10.8). Symptoms of radicular leg pain were remarkably improved after surgery.
2. A 59-year-old woman presented with gradual onset pain in the right leg through L4 and L5 dermatomes. She had left leg radicular pain through the posterior lateral aspect. Preoperative operative CT and MR images revealed right foraminal stenosis (white arrow) and extraforaminal herniated disc (arrowhead) and combined bilateral lateral recess stenosis at the L4-L5 level. The right-

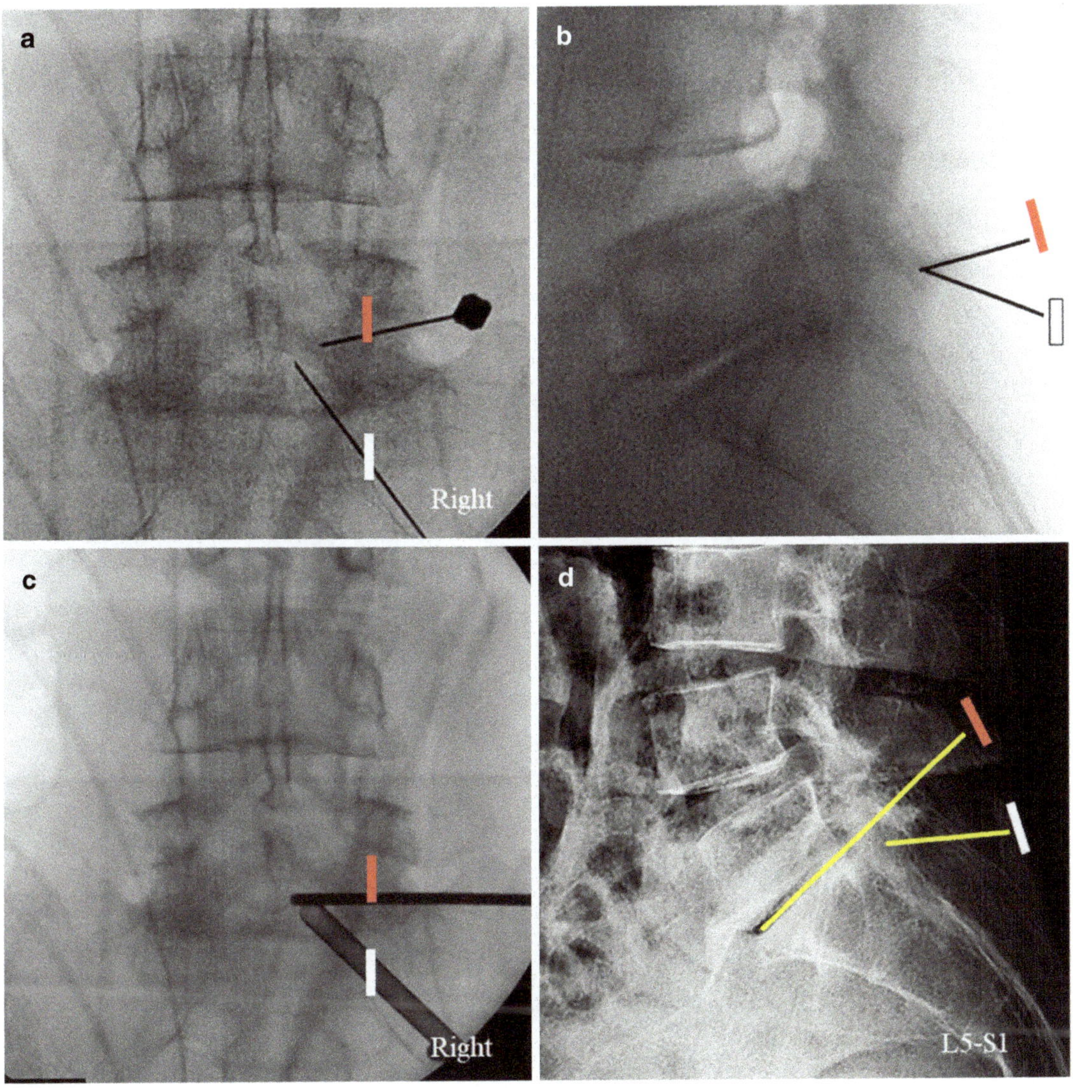

Fig. 10.6 Skin incision points of two portals (white line: endoscopic portal, red line: working portal) with a right-sided approach for the contralateral foraminal-extraforaminal decompression at the L5-S1 level. Confirm the trajectory of the endoscope and instruments using the spinal needle before skin incision. The working portal was created close to the upper endplate of the disc space rather than a pedicular area (**c** and **d**)

side facet joint of the L4-L5 level had a large osteophyte disrupting the paraspinal approach or transforaminal approach to the foraminal area (Fig. 10.9). We performed the biportal endoscopic left-sided unilateral laminotomy and bilateral lateral recess decompression, and contralateral foraminal-extraforaminal decompression. Postoperative MRI and endoscopic photos showed sufficient decompression of bilateral lateral recess and right-sided foraminal and extraforaminal area with well-preserved facet joints. Postoperatively, symptoms of radicular buttock and leg pain were significantly improved (Fig. 10.9).

3. An 87-year-old man presented with abrupt onset pain in the left leg through L3 and L4 dermatome. She also had bilateral radiating buttock pain and motor weakness in the left leg. Preoperative operative CT and MR images revealed left foraminal stenosis and

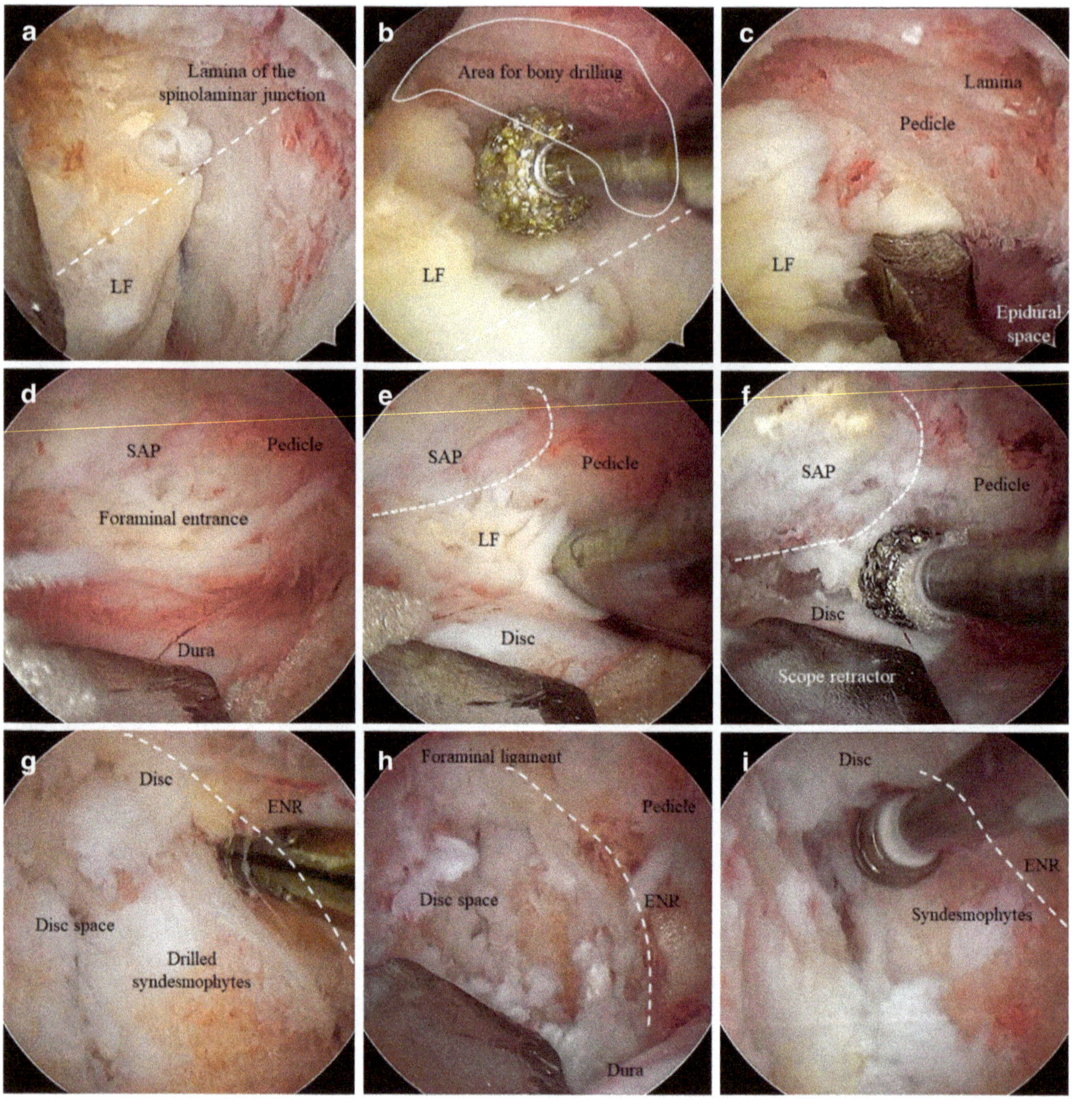

Fig. 10.7 Biportal endoscopic contralateral sublaminar foraminotomy for the left-sided L5-S1 foraminal stenosis and herniated disc via right-sided unilateral approach. Ipsilateral laminotomy and spinolaminar junction drilling (**a**). Contralateral sublaminar bony drilling (**b** and **c**). Removal of the ligament flavum (**d** and **e**). drilling of the superior articular process (**f**). Foraminal decompression (**g** and **h**) Extraforaminal decompression (**i** and **j**). End-point resection using the chisel (**k** and **l**). Entirely decompressed exiting nerve root from the foraminal area to the fart out area while preserving the inferior articular process (**m–o**). Preoperative MR images revealed lateral recess stenosis and foraminal-extraforaminal stenosis on the left side of the L5-S1 level (**p**). Postoperative MRI images showed successful decompression of the left S1 traversing nerve root and the L5 exiting nerve root (**q**). *ENR* exiting nerve root, *LF* ligamentum flavum, *SAP* superior articular process, *IAP* inferior articular process

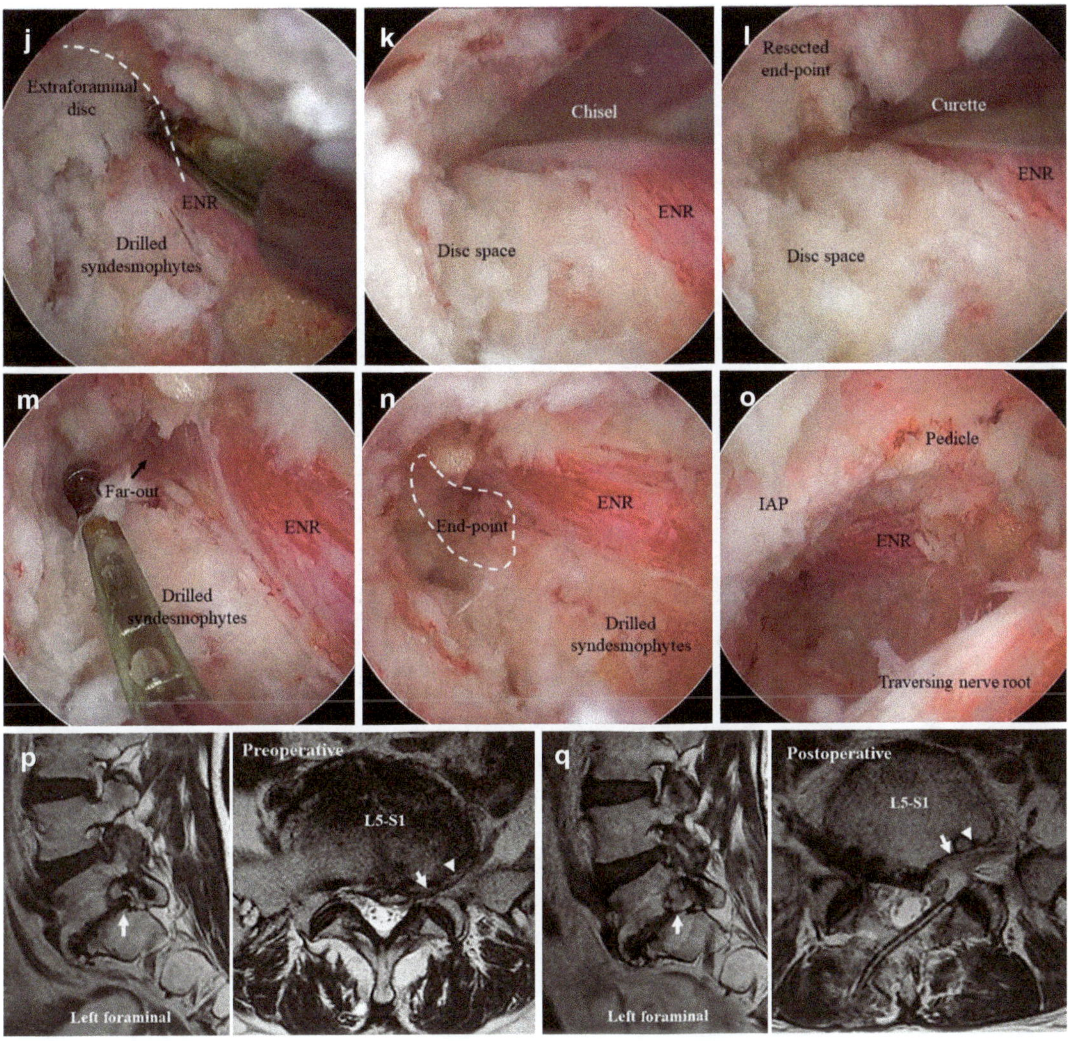

Fig. 10.7 (continued)

extraforaminal herniated disc and combined bilateral lateral recess stenosis at the L4-L5 level (Fig. 10.10). We performed the biportal endoscopic right-sided unilateral laminotomy and bilateral lateral recess decompression, and contralateral foraminal-extraforaminal decompression. Postoperative MRI and endoscopic photos and endoscopic photos revealed sufficient decompression of bilateral lateral recess and left-sided foraminal and extraforaminal areas (Fig. 10.10). Symptoms of neurologic deficits and radicular pain were improved after surgery.

10.9 Complications and Their Management

Sufficient sublaminar space should be created for the free pass of the endoscope and instruments over the thecal sac to the contralateral foraminal area while avoiding incidental hitting of neural structures. There is a rich epidural venous plexus in the nerve root axillary area. Meticulous hemostasis should be performed, although the bleeding vessel is tiny to ensure a clear endoscopic view (Fig. 10.11a). Bone bleeding control, sealing the bone wax on the medial foraminal area, enhance

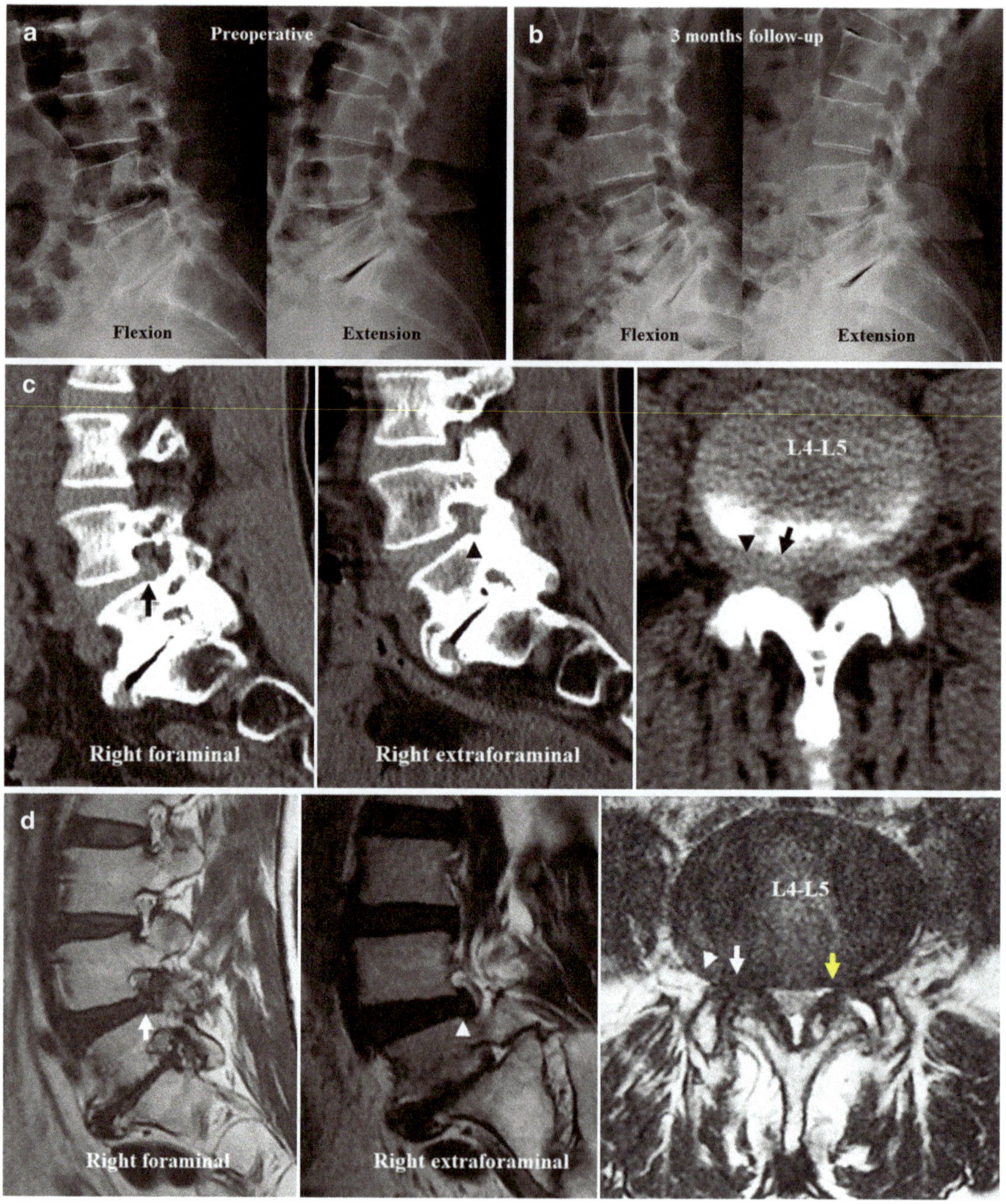

Fig. 10.8 A 59-year-old woman presented with severe pain of abrupt onset in the right leg through the L4 dermatome. There was no definite segmental instability on the preoperative and 3 months follow-up X-ray images (**a** and **b**). Preoperative CT images showed a herniated disc in the foraminal (black arrow) and extraforaminal area (black arrowhead) without a definite bony spur at the right L4-L5 level (**c**). Preoperative operative MR images revealed right foraminal stenosis (white arrow) and extraforaminal herniated disc (white arrowhead) and combined bilateral lateral recess stenosis at the L4-L5 level (yellow arrow) (**d**). Postoperative MRI showed sufficient decompression of the right L4 exiting nerve root (white arrow and arrowhead) and bilateral lateral recess (yellow arrow) while well preserving the facet joints (**e**). Foraminal and extraforaminal herniated discs were removed entirely (**e**)

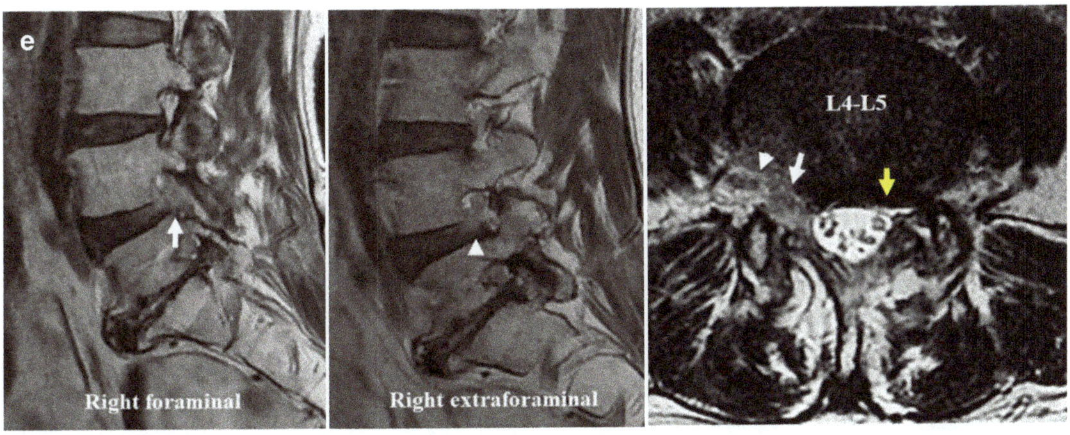

Fig. 10.8 (continued)

the clear endoscopic view during foraminal decompression (Fig. 10.11b).

Radicular artery tearing during discectomy causes the enormous pumping bleeding obscuring the endoscopic view. RF for the injured radicular artery just beneath the ENR may cause nerve heating injury and postoperative dysesthesia. Therefore, careful discectomy after clear identification is essential for safe and successful neural decompression (Fig. 10.11c). If the bleeding in the extraforaminal area was not controlled, a drainage catheter should be inserted deeply in the foraminal space to prevent retroperitoneal hematoma (Fig. 10.4h) [10].

If the ENR is severely impinged under hypertrophied SAP, chiseling on the SAP may induce the crushing injury of ENR. Furthermore, SAP chiseling is not recommended in patients who have neurologically compromised nerve roots due to the severely narrowed foramen. Stepwise removal of SAP using the endoscopic drill and up-curved punches is preferred in these cases.

All the foraminal and extraforaminal area procedures should be done while a scope self-retractor protects the traversing nerve root and thecal sac (Fig. 10.7f, h). This procedure prevents the hitting nerve injury during instrument advancement to the foraminal area and tearing nerve injury during drilling close to the nerve root.

After opening the far-out space, the saline infusion pressure should be reduced to prevent retroperitoneal fluid collection [11].

10.10 Surgical Tips and Pitfall

We have to give the patients about surgery and the potential risks of this technique. In cases of bilateral spinal canal stenosis with unilateral foraminal-extraforaminal stenosis, the benefits of minimal invasiveness as bilateral multifocal compressions can be achieved with a one-direction approach. However, it is weighed against unnecessary decompression and disruption of the ipsilateral unaffected-sided structures. Extraforaminal decompression via the contralateral approach is technically demanding and may result in insufficient decompression. Additional surgery with a paraspinal approach may be required in such cases.

If the contralateral extraforaminal decompression is necessary, working portals should be created close to the upper or lower endplate of the intervertebral disc to obtain the optimal extraforaminal approach angle. The surgical instruments can access the extraforaminal and far-out area when the instruments pass through the narrowed foraminal space nearly parallel to the disc space without blocking by the bony structures.

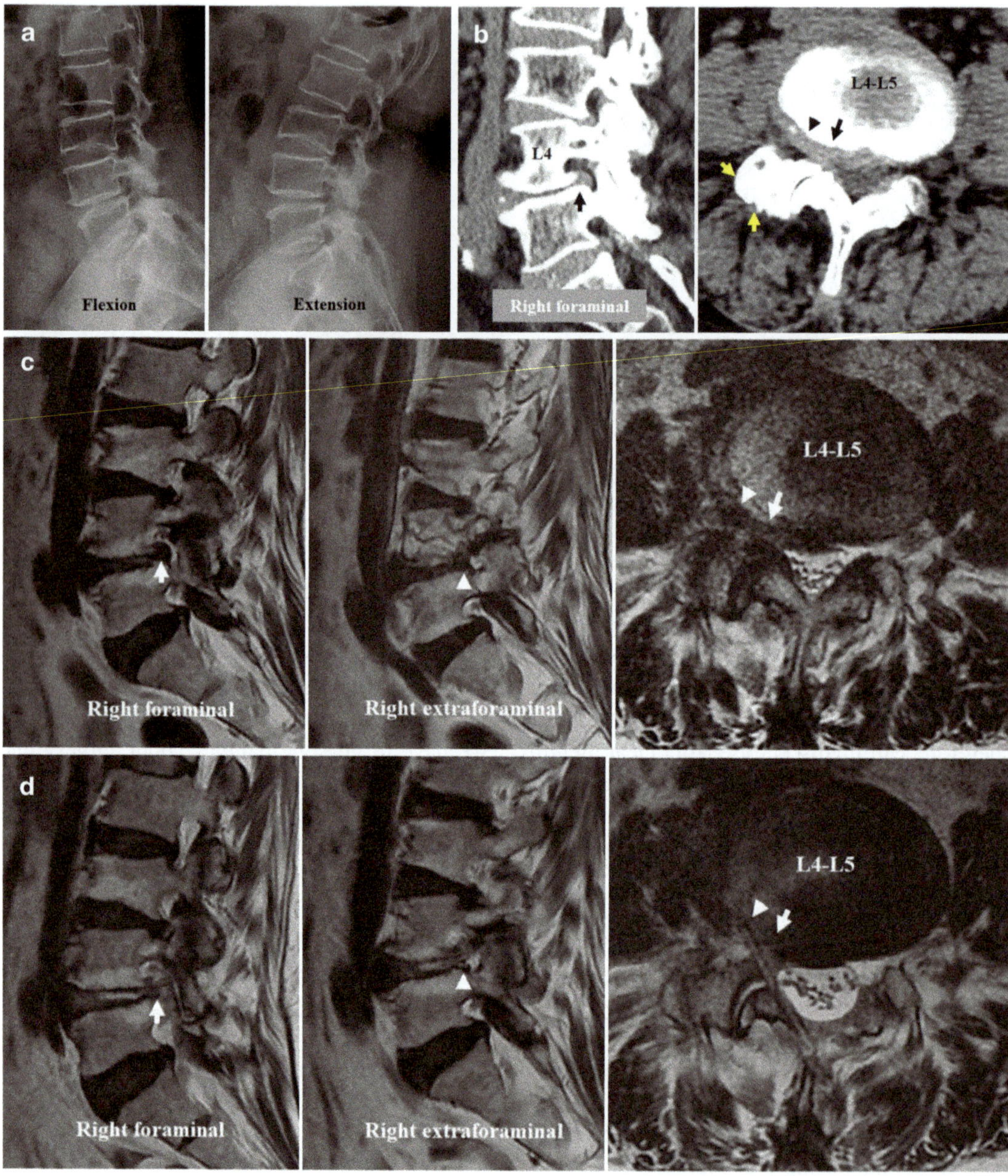

Fig. 10.9 A 59-year-old woman presented with gradual onset pain in the right leg through L4 and L5 dermatomes. There was no definite segmental instability on the preoperative X-ray images (**a**). Preoperative CT images showed a right foraminal (black arrow) and extraforaminal herniated disc (black arrowhead) with prominent syndesmophytes at the L4-L5 level (**b**). The right-side facet joint had a large osteophyte (**b**, yellow arrows). Preoperative operative MR images revealed right foraminal stenosis (white arrow) and extraforaminal herniated disc (white arrowhead) and combined bilateral lateral recess stenosis at the L4-L5 level (**c**). Postoperative MRI showed sufficient decompression of the right L4 exiting nerve root (white arrow and arrowhead) and bilateral lateral recess (**d**). The intraoperative view showed a foraminal herniated disc compressing and distorting the ENR (white dotted line) (**e**). After removing the foraminal and extraforaminal herniated disc, ENR was fully decompressed and restored the natural course of downward angulation at the extraforaminal area (white arrow and dotted line) (**f**). ENR: exiting nerve root

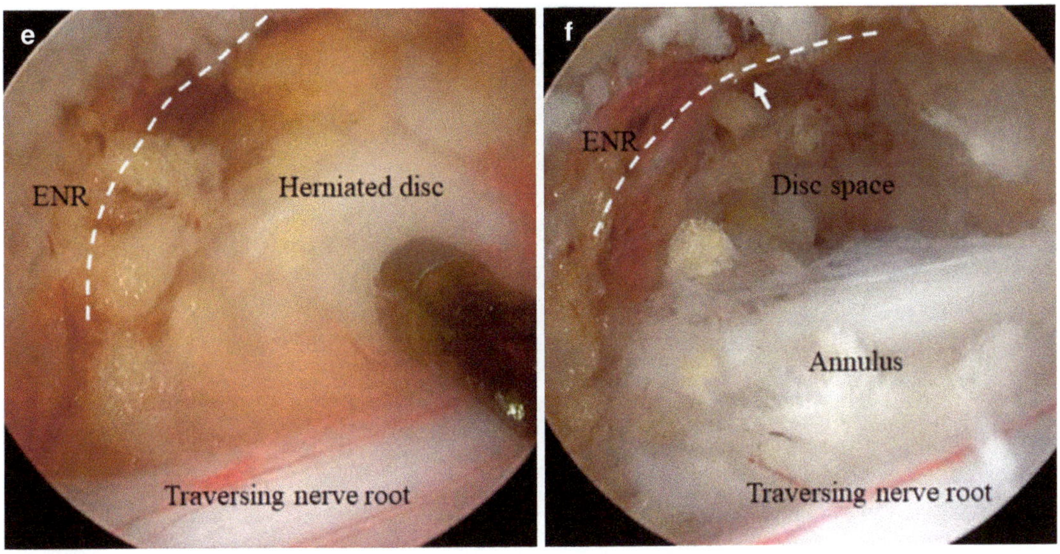

Fig. 10.9 (continued)

Furthermore, the approach of optimized angle saves the unnecessary drilling of the inferior articular process and induces efficient neural decompression along the exiting nerve root without dorsal root retraction. However, moving the working portal is not needed for only contralateral foraminal decompression. We can resolve the foraminal stenosis via the usual location of portals for the posterior lumbar decompression or discectomy surgery (Figs. 10.2 and 10.6).

Removal of prominent foraminal syndesmophytes using a drill or fine angled chisels is essential to create the redundant space for identifying the extraforaminal space and instruments insertion between the ENR and extraforaminal herniated disc. The created foraminal space reduces the risk of tearing the nerve root and a radicular artery during extraforaminal decompression. However, if the ventrally located lesions are not prominent, foraminal and extraforaminal decompression can be performed without violation of the foraminal disc.

Decompression of the end-point in the far-out area restores a smooth downward angulation of the ENR, which may enhance the relief of radicular pain. If the angulated and distorted ENR was found on the oblique sagittal MRI of the far-out area, we recommend removing the end-point lesions that lift and distort ENR for complete decompression of the entire length of ENR.

Biportal endoscopic contralateral sublaminar approach for foraminal and extraforaminal decompression has several advantages, as we showed above and a recently reported technical note [8]. However well-designed study with long-term follow-up is necessary to confirm these findings.

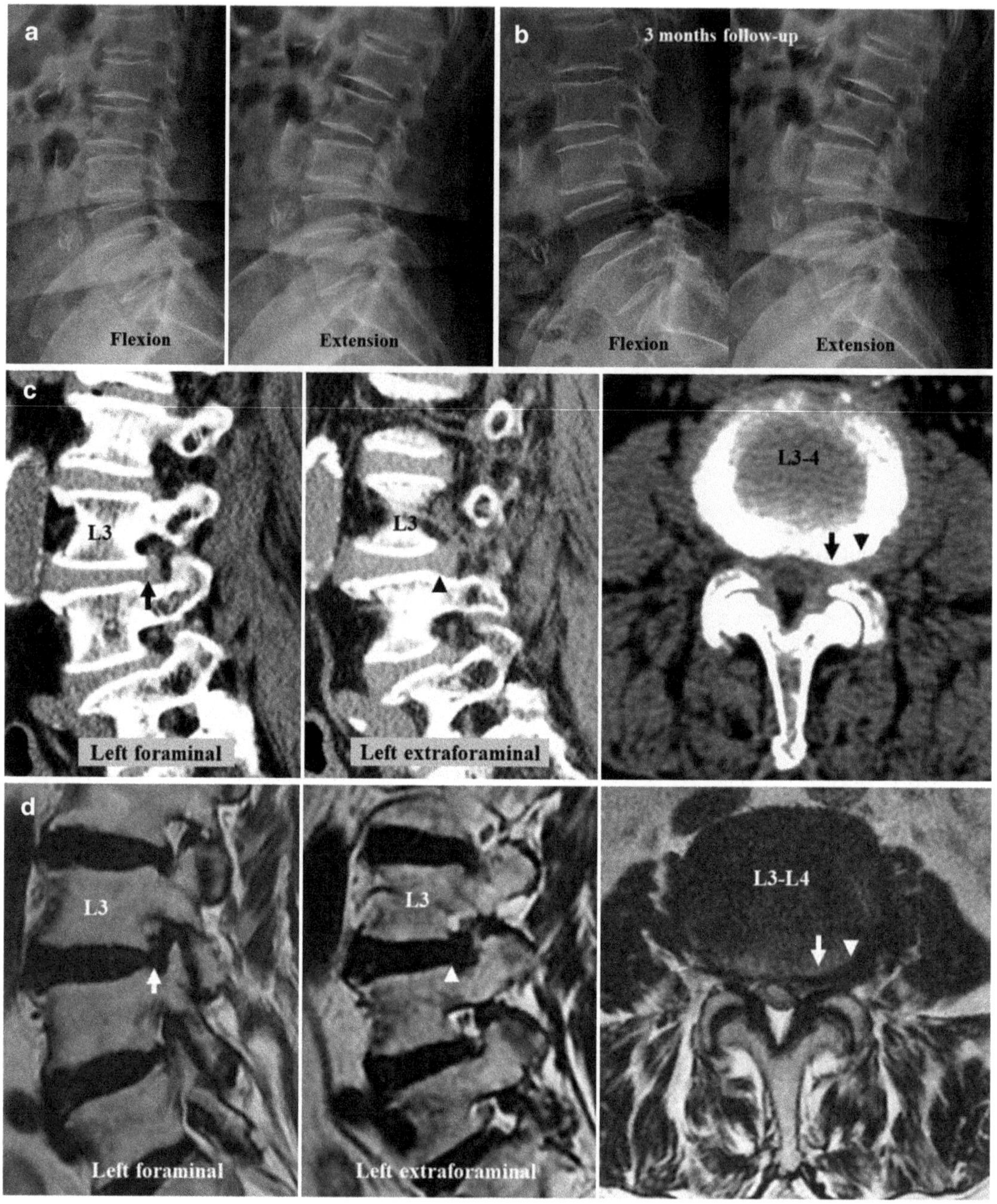

Fig. 10.10 An 87-year-old man presented with abrupt onset pain in the left leg through L3 and L4 dermatome. She also had bilateral radiating buttock pain and motor weakness in the left leg. There was no definite segmental instability on the preoperative and 3 months follow-up X-ray images (**a** and **b**). Preoperative CT images showed a herniated disc in the foraminal (black arrow) and extraforaminal area (black arrowhead) with bony spur at the left L3-L4 level (**c**). Preoperative operative MR images revealed left foraminal stenosis (white arrow) and extraforaminal herniated disc (white arrowhead) and combined bilateral lateral recess stenosis at the L4-L5 level (**d**). Postoperative MRI showed sufficient decompression of the left L3 ENR (white arrow and arrowhead) and bilateral lateral recess. Bilateral facet joints were well preserved (**e**). (**f**) The intraoperative view showed a foraminal herniated disc compressing and distorting the ENR (yellow arrow). Extraforaminal herniated disc was removed after confirming the course of the ENR (**g**). (**h**) Finally, ENR was entirely decompressed and restored the natural course of downward angulation at the extraforaminal area (white arrow and dotted line)

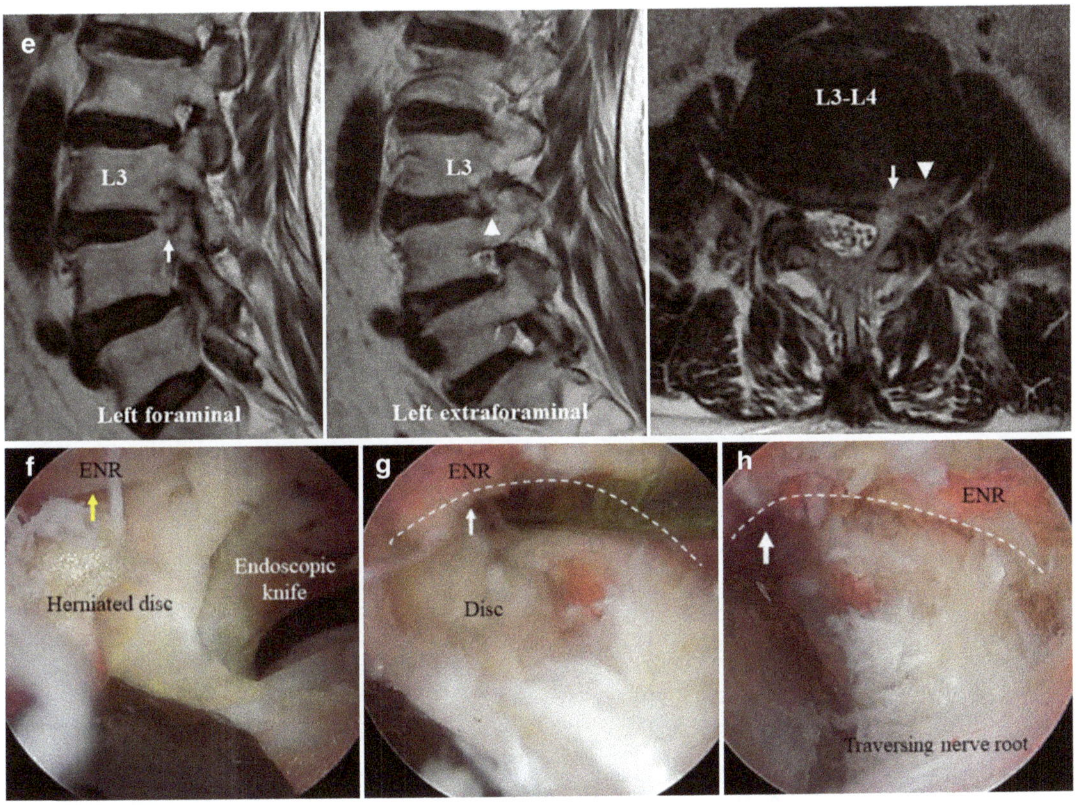

Fig. 10.10 (continued)

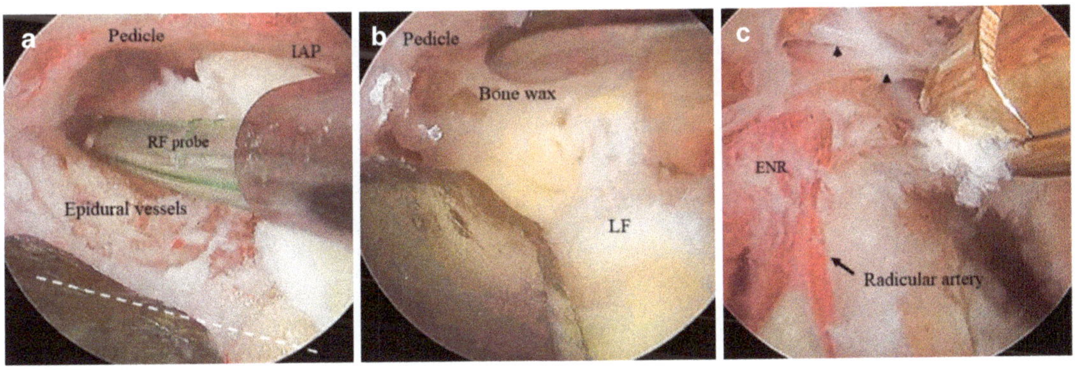

Fig. 10.11 Procedures to prevent complications during surgery. Meticulous bone bleeding control using the bone wax (**b**) and coagulation of epidural vessels in the axillary area of the nerve root (**a**) is essential for a clear endoscopic view. Identification and confirmation of radicular artery and tiny vessels (black arrowheads) are critical during tissue removal closed to the nerve root to prevent vessel injury (**c**)

Acknowledgments None.

Conflicts of Interest The authors declare that they have no competing interests.

Consent to Participate Informed consent was obtained from all patients.

Consent to Publish Not applicable.

Data and/or Code Availability Not applicable.

Funding Statement This study did not receive grants or other financial and material support.

References

1. Olszewski AD, Yaszemski MJ, White AA 3rd. The anatomy of the human lumbar ligamentum flavum. New observations and their surgical importance. Spine (Phila Pa 1976). 1996;21(20):2307–12.
2. Kim HS, Kim JY, Wu PH, Jang IT. Effect of dorsal root ganglion retraction in endoscopic lumbar decompressive surgery for foraminal pathology: a retrospective cohort study of interlaminar contralateral endoscopic lumbar foraminotomy and discectomy (ICELF) versus transforaminal endoscopic lumbar foraminotomy and discectomy (TELD). World Neurosurg. 2021;148:e101–14.
3. Kim HS, Patel R, Paudel B, Jang JS, Jang IT, Oh SH, et al. Early outcomes of endoscopic contralateral foraminal and lateral recess decompression via an interlaminar approach in patients with unilateral radiculopathy from unilateral foraminal stenosis. World Neurosurg. 2017;108:763–73.
4. Wu PH, Kim HS, Jang IT. How I do it? Uniportal full endoscopic contralateral approach for lumbar foraminal stenosis with double crush syndrome. Acta Neurochir. 2020;162(2):305–10.
5. Akbary K, Kim JS, Park CW, Jun SG, Hwang JH. Biportal endoscopic decompression of exiting and traversing nerve roots through a single interlaminar window using a contralateral approach: technical feasibilities and morphometric changes of the lumbar canal and foramen. World Neurosurg. 2018;117:153–61.
6. Heo DH, Kim JS, Park CW, Quillo-Olvera J, Park CK. Contralateral sublaminar endoscopic approach for removal of lumbar juxtafacet cysts using percutaneous biportal endoscopic surgery: technical report and preliminary results. World Neurosurg. 2019;122:474–9.
7. Park JH, Jang JW, Park WM, Park CW. Contralateral keyhole biportal endoscopic surgery for ruptured lumbar herniated disc: a technical feasibility and early clinical outcomes. Neurospine. 2020;17(Suppl 1):S110–s9.
8. Kim JY, Heo DH. Contralateral sublaminar approach for decompression of the combined lateral recess, foraminal, and extraforaminal lesions using biportal endoscopy: a technical report. Acta Neurochir. 2021;163(10):2783–7.
9. Choi KC, Kim JS, Ryu KS, Kang BU, Ahn Y, Lee SH. Percutaneous endoscopic lumbar discectomy for L5-S1 disc herniation: transforaminal versus interlaminar approach. Pain Physician. 2013;16(6): 547–56.
10. Ahn Y, Kim JU, Lee BH, Lee SH, Park JD, Hong DH, et al. Postoperative retroperitoneal hematoma following transforaminal percutaneous endoscopic lumbar discectomy. J Neurosurg Spine. 2009;10(6):595–602.
11. Heo DH, Sharma S, Park CK. Endoscopic treatment of extraforaminal entrapment of L5 nerve root (far out syndrome) by unilateral biportal endoscopic approach: technical report and preliminary clinical results. Neurospine. 2019;16(1):130–7.

11 Far-out Syndrome Decompression Using Unilateral Biportal Endoscopy

Nam Lee, Sang Hyuk Park, and Jin Woo An

11.1 Introduction

Far-out syndrome (FOS) is one type of lumbosacral transitional vertebrae (LSTV). LSTV is a various anatomical variant of lumbosacral junctional area. There are four types of LSTV [1, 2]. Among them, type 2 shows the pseudo-articulation between L5 transverse process and sacral ala, and in addition, the foraminal height is decreased than normal structure. Therefore, FOS is defined as the compression of L5 nerve root in the far-out area by the pseudo-articulation of the L5 transverse process and the sacral ala (Fig. 11.1). The gold standard treatment of FOS is a conventional microscopic decompression surgery or lumbar fusion surgery [3–6]. However, due to the development of endoscopic surgery system, we can treat this lesion sufficiently using unilateral biportal endoscopy (UBE) technique. Basically, this surgical approach is the same as the Wiltse approach that contains enough decompression far laterally [7].

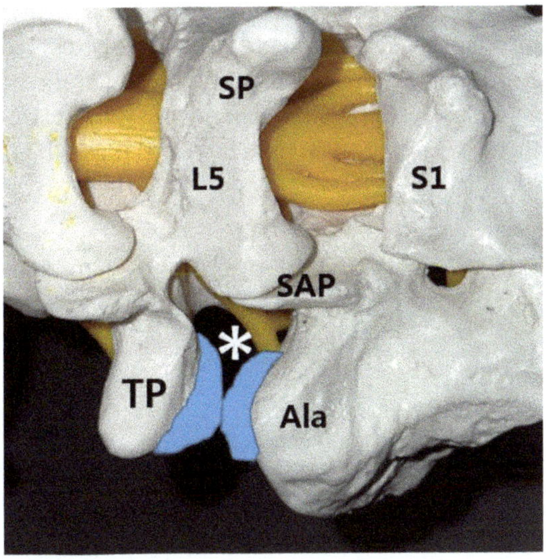

Fig. 11.1 This figure shows the fundamental concept of an extra-foraminal lesion. The blue overlaid areas indicate the pseudo-articulation of the hypertrophied transverse process and sacral ala. The exiting L5 nerve root is compressed in the narrow area (*)

Supplementary Information The online version contains supplementary material available at [https://doi.org/10.1007/978-981-16-8201-8_11].

N. Lee
Department of Neurosurgery, Yonseicheok Hospital, Busan, South Korea

S. H. Park (✉)
Department of Neurosurgery, Yonsei Barowalk Hospital, Kyoungki-Do, South Korea

J. W. An
Department of Orthopedic Surgery, Nanoori Korea by Saudi German Hospital, Dubai, UAE

11.2 Indications and Contraindications

Indication and contraindication are very similar with conventional microscopic decompression surgery. The FOS lesion combined with foraminal

D. H. Heo et al. (eds.), *Unilateral Biportal Endoscopic Spine Surgery*,
https://doi.org/10.1007/978-981-16-8201-8_11

stenosis at L5/S1 level and the recurrent FOS can also be treated by this technique. However, grade 2 or higher spondylolisthesis and segmental instability are contraindicated in this technique.

11.3 Special Instruments

Zero-degree endoscope is most commonly used in UBE surgery. Radiofrequency (Arthrocare®) probe is essential to control intraoperative bleeding. The arthroscopic drill system with saline drain portal and high-speed electrical drill is commonly used to drill out the bony structure (Fig. 11.2). The scope-retractor is also useful in preventing nerve root damage. The curved Kerrison punch is very useful to decompress the foraminal lesion. All conventional surgical instruments are available in this technique (Fig. 11.3).

11.4 Anesthesia and Position

Both endotracheal general anesthesia and epidural anesthesia are available in this surgery. The authors prefer epidural anesthesia because it is a less invasive procedure and less loading on cardio-pulmonary function than general anesthesia. The patient is always placed on a Wilson frame in the prone position. In addition, less lumbar lordosis using elevation of Wilson frame can make the operation comfortable because this induces the widening of foraminal area and it also reduces the intra-abdominal pressure. In addition, the compression stockings prevent thrombosis in the lower extremities during the surgery. The Foley catheter is usually inserted to check the perioperative urine output (Fig. 11.4).

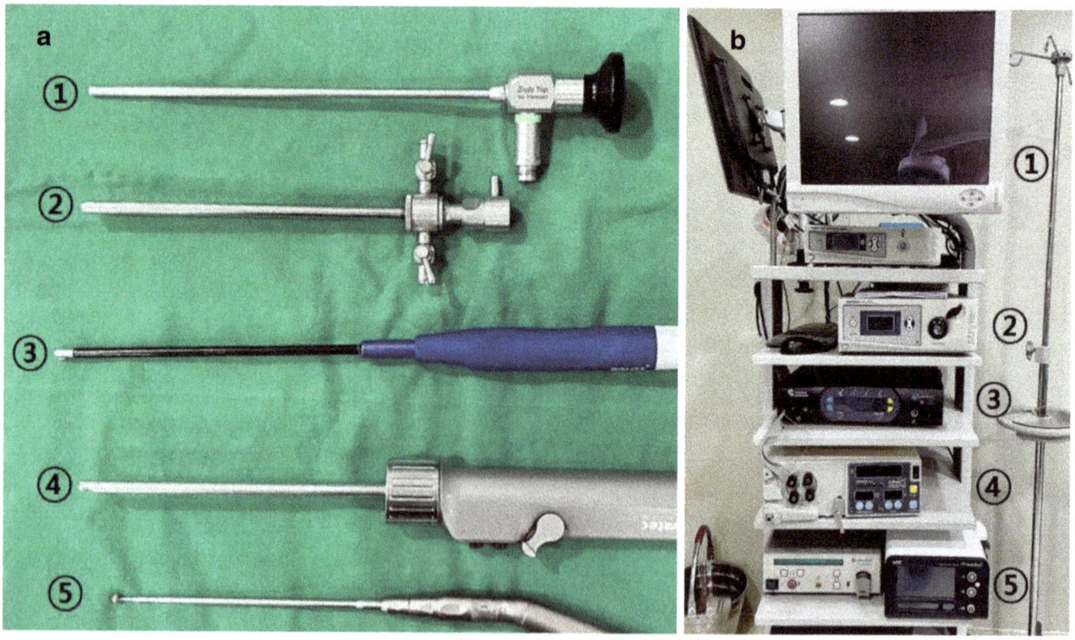

Fig. 11.2 UBE instruments. (**a**): ① Zero-degree endoscope. ② Sheath for endoscope. ③ RF probe device. ④ Arthroscopic drill system with saline drain tube. ⑤ High-speed electrical drill. (**b**): ① Monitor for endoscope. ② Light source generator of endoscope. ③ RF probe device generator. ④ Automatic irrigation pump. ⑤ Electrical drill system

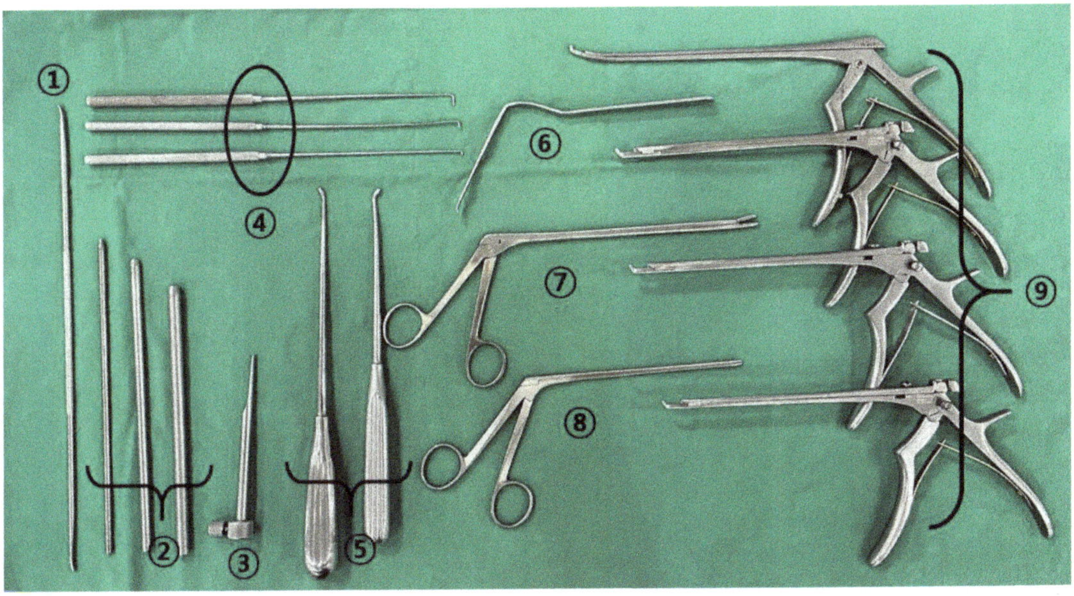

Fig. 11.3 UBE instruments. ① Double-ended dissector. ② Serial dilators #1 ~ #3. ③ Scope retractor. ④ Blunt/ball-hook. ⑤ Angled curettes. ⑥ Root retractor. ⑦ Alligator forceps. ⑧ Pituitary forceps. ⑨ Kerrison punch & curved punch

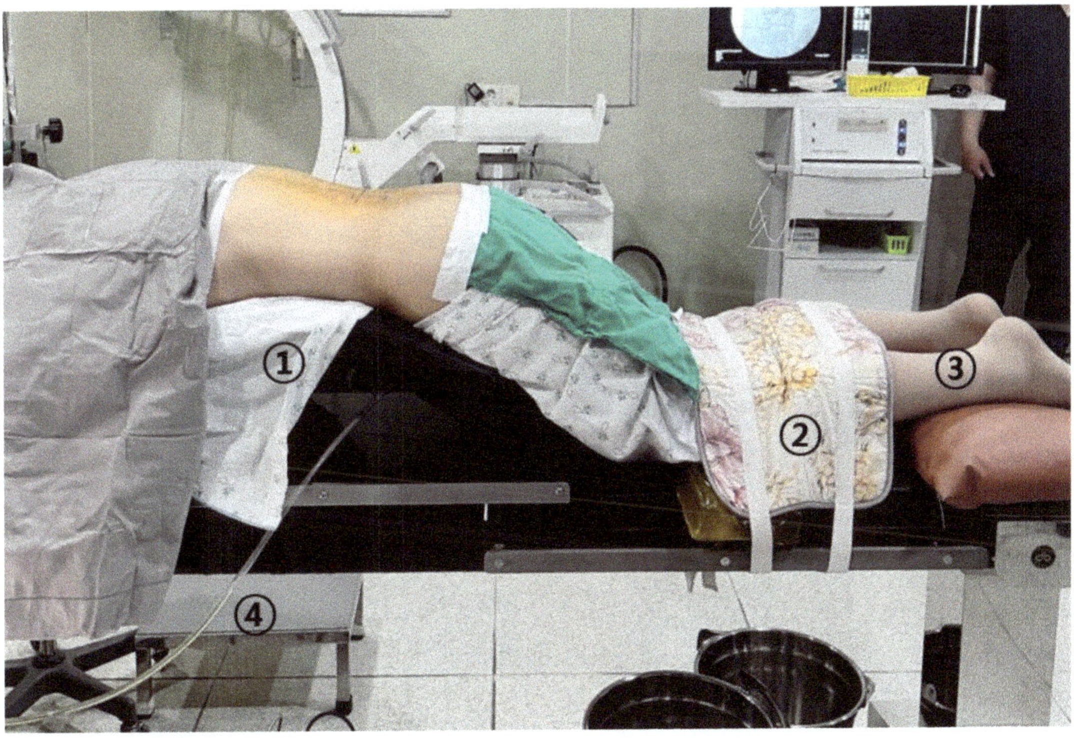

Fig. 11.4 UBE position. ① Wilson frame with elevation. ② Knee band. ③ Compression stockings for anti-thrombosis. ④ Foley catheter is inserted

11.5 Surgical Steps

1. **Identify the location of two portals and make portals (left side approach) (Fig. 11.5)**

   Setting the true anteroposterior (A-P) image under fluoroscopic guidance is the first step for this surgery. Especially, the L5-S1 level has the most lordotic angle, it is very important to apply the fluoroscopic device a cranial angle to get the accurate A-P image (Fig. 11.6). The UBE surgery utilizes two portals, one is an endoscopic portal for endoscope and the other is an instrumental portal for surgical instruments. We describe the surgical steps as the point of view of the left side approach. First, we identify the L5 and S1 pedicles and disc space, and also the lateral margin of vertebral body on A-P view. The skin incision is made 1–2 cm laterally to the lateral margin of vertebral body. This location will be more lateral than UBE paraspinal approach. Because, the target of paraspinal approach is the facet joint or isthmus, on the contrary, the target of FOS surgery is pseudo-articulation of transverse process (TP) - sacral ala. The instrumental portal is made 1 cm below the intervertebral foramen level and the endoscopic portal is made 1 cm above this level. Usually, the distance of two portals is about 2–2.5 cm and the size of incision is

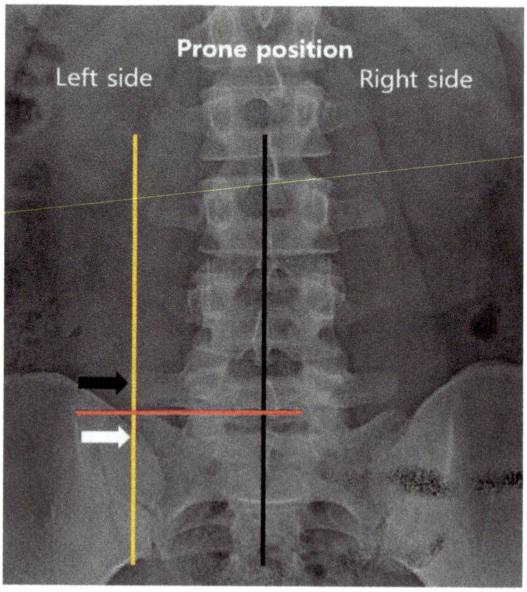

Fig. 11.6 True A-P image of L5-S1 level. Black line: mid vertical line. Red line: intervertebral foramen line at L5/S1. Yellow line: 1–2 cm lateral line from vertebral body. Black arrow: cranial-scope portal (1 cm cranially from red line). White arrow: caudal-instrument portal (1 cm caudally from red line)

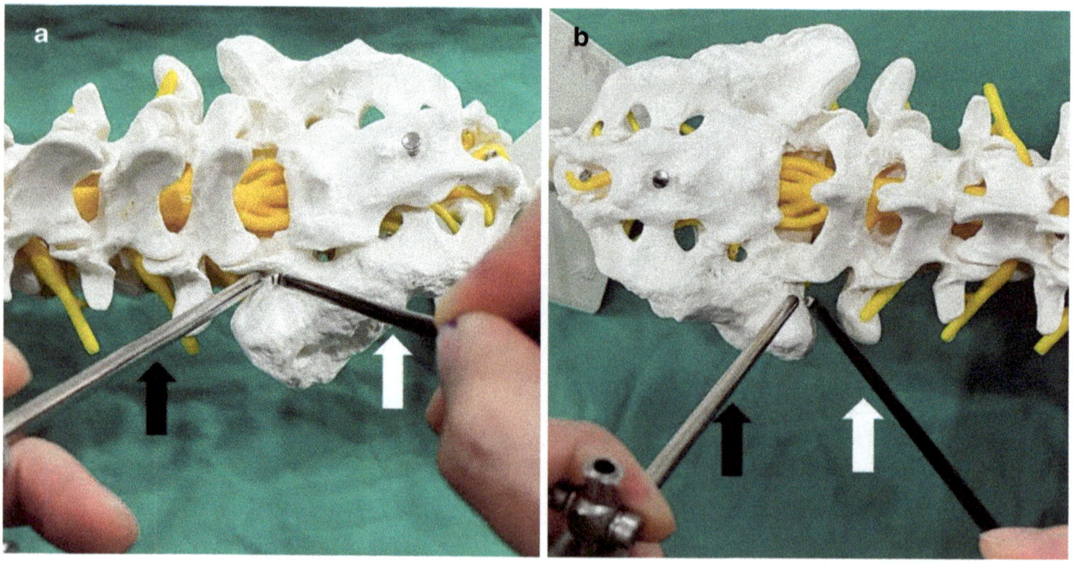

Fig. 11.5 Basic concept of UBE surgery. (**a**): Left side approach for FOS decompression. (**b**): Right side approach for FOS decompression. Zero-degree endoscope (black arrow) and RF probe (white arrow)

about 1 cm. We always make instrumental portal firstly and it is very important that the incision should penetrate the fascial layer to maintain the continuous outflow of the irrigation saline during the surgery. After incision, serial dilators are inserted sequentially. At this point, the landing point of first dilator is very important. The aim of FOS decompression surgery is removal of the pseudo-articulation of TP and sacral ala, the dilator should touch the sacral ala or sacral notch initially where the interspace of superior articular process (SAP) of S1 and sacral ala (Fig. 11.7). After finishing the instrumental portal making, the endoscopic portal is made in the same manner. The first dilator inserted in endoscopic portal should also touch the sacral ala or sacra notch. The triangulation of two portals is a cornerstone of this technique (Fig. 11.8).

2. **Making initial working space**

   To obtain good initial operative visualization, the meticulous dissection and detachment of muscular ending and soft tissue around the surface of sacral alar or sacral notch are essential. The initial working space of FOS decompression surgery is the interspace filled with irrigation saline between the surface of bony structure and soft tissue. This space is very narrow, but we can gradually obtain wider space by ablating or coagulating the soft tissue using RF device. The stage of initial working space is finished until clearly identifying the bony surface of SAP lateral aspect, sacral alar, and lower border of TP. The triangle zone of these three structures is a true working space. In addition, we can also easily identify the lateral aspect of isthmus and sacral notch (Fig. 11.9).

3. **Removal of bony structures and soft tissue**

   After full exposure of these bony structures, we usually start the drilling to sacral alar, lateral aspect of SAP, and inferior border of TP. The exposure of cancellous bone sometimes induces severe bony bleeding and this can be controlled by bone wax or RF probe. When drilling out in the lateral direction of TP and alar, pseudo-articulation is observed. This lesion should be removed as laterally as possible, because the exiting nerve root runs under this pseudo-articulation (Fig. 11.10a). Drilling to the lower portion of L5 TP and lateral aspect of SAP and alar area, combined further removal of soft tissue using RF device allow identification of the ligamentum flavum covering the exiting nerve root (Fig. 11.10b).

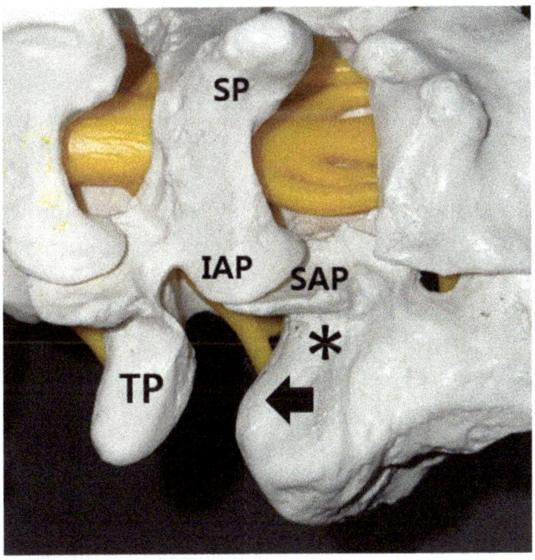

Fig. 11.7 The initial target point of FOS (*): sacral notch. Black arrow: sacral ala. TP: transverse process. IAP: inferior articular process. SAP: superior articular process. SP: spinous process

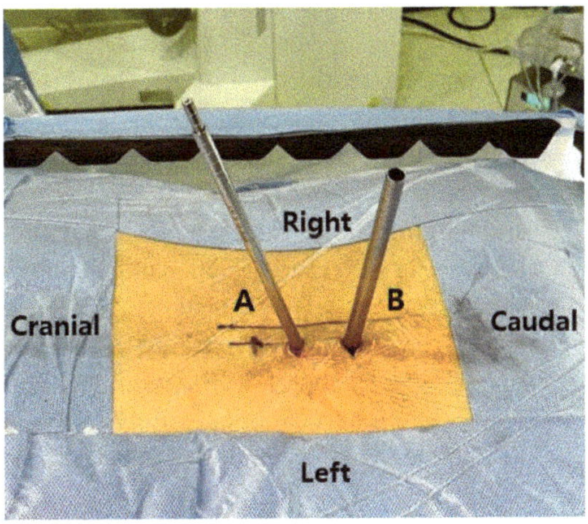

Fig. 11.8 Triangulation of endoscopic portal (**A**) and instrumental portal (**B**)

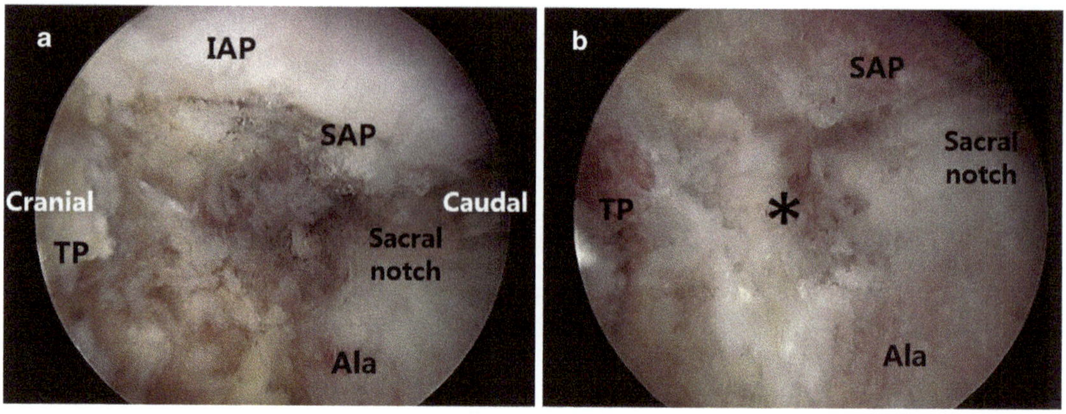

Fig. 11.9 (**a**): Initial endoscopic image. After removal of soft tissue around bony structures, initial working space is acquired. (**b**): Initial working space. The triangle zone (*) of TP, SAP, and Ala is a main field of FOS decompression surgery. TP: transverse process; SAP: superior articular process; IAP: inferior articular process

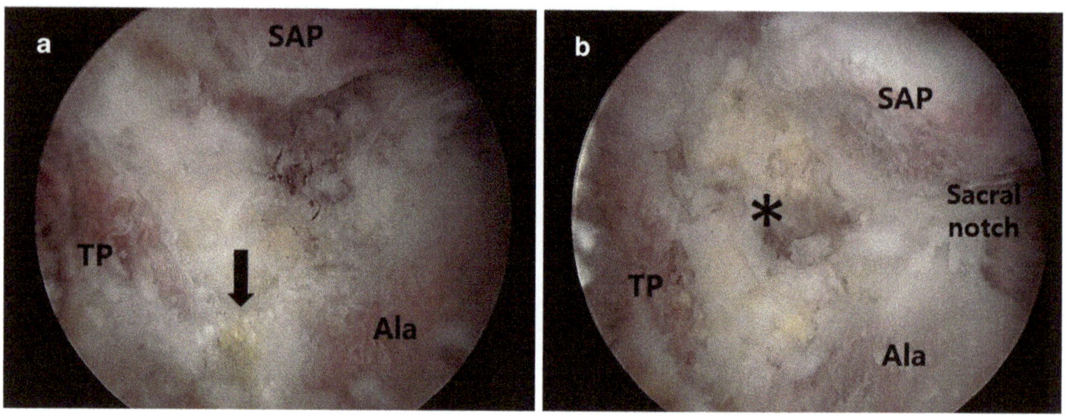

Fig. 11.10 (**a**): Pseudo-articulation (black arrow) is observed at the point of TP and ala encounter. (**b**): After more resection of bony structures and soft tissue, the ligamentum flavum (*) covering the exiting nerve root (L5 root) is identified. TP: transverse process; SAP: superior articular process

4. **Identify the exiting nerve root and alar resection**

   After dissecting the lower part of the TP and along the fissure of the ligament flavum, we can figure out the exiting nerve root immediately (Fig. 11.11a). Then, using a small Kerrison punch or angled curette, the ligamentum flavum can be removed easily and safely (Fig. 11.11b). Now, the foraminal portion of exiting nerve root is entirely exposed. We also identify the annulus of intervertebral disc located just below the nerve root (Fig. 11.12a). In order to completely decompress the extra-foraminal portion of exiting nerve root, the medial part of Alar as well as pseudo-articulation part must be further removed by drilling out or Kerrison punch (Fig. 11.12b).

5. **Finish the decompression and wound closure**

   In the case of severe bulging disc or disc herniation, the discectomy is also performed using pituitary forceps or Kerrison punch for fully ventral decompression of the nerve root. (Fig. 11.13a). It is also very important that clarify the ventral decompression of the nerve root to improve the prognosis after surgery. All decompression procedure is successfully completed when the root confirmed freely passes through alar and enters the abdominal cavity.

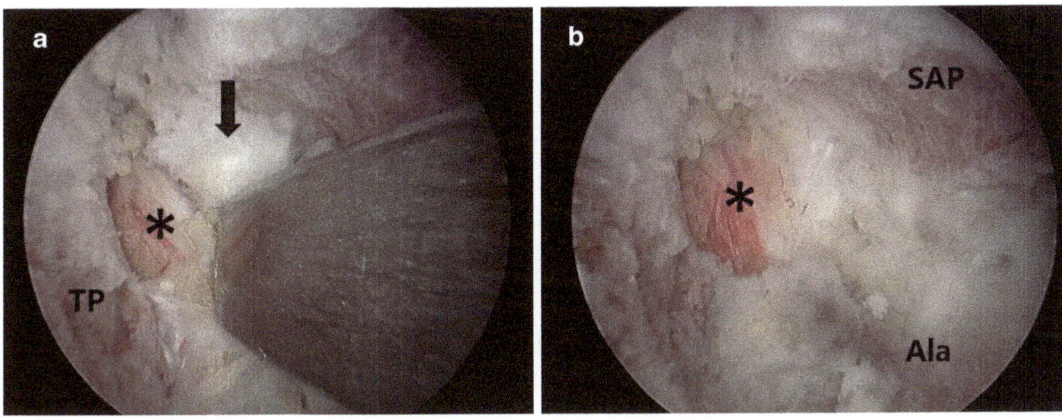

Fig. 11.11 (**a**): The ligamentum flavum (black arrow) covering the exiting nerve root (*). (**b**): After removal of ligamentum flavum, L5 nerve root is identified (*). TP: transverse process; SAP: superior articular process

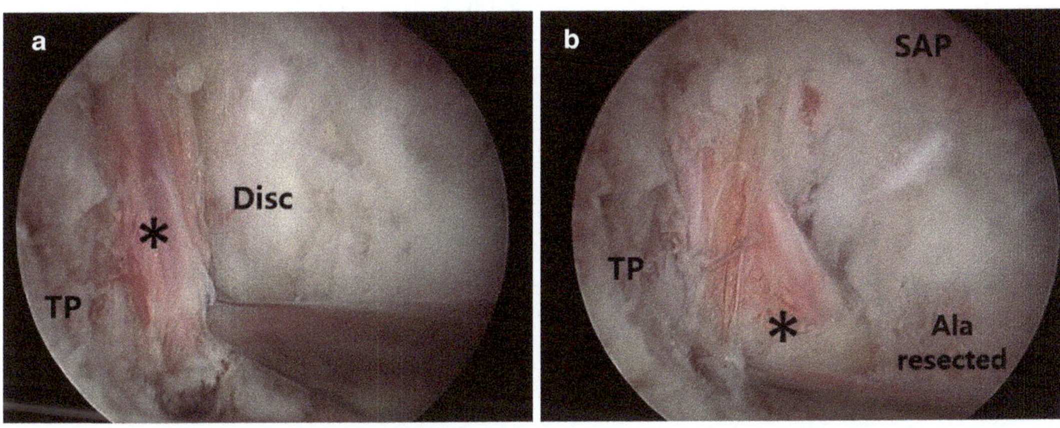

Fig. 11.12 (**a**): The intervertebral disc is located just below the exiting nerve root (*). (**b**): The extra-foraminal portion (*) of exiting nerve root is identified. TP: transverse process; SAP: superior articular process

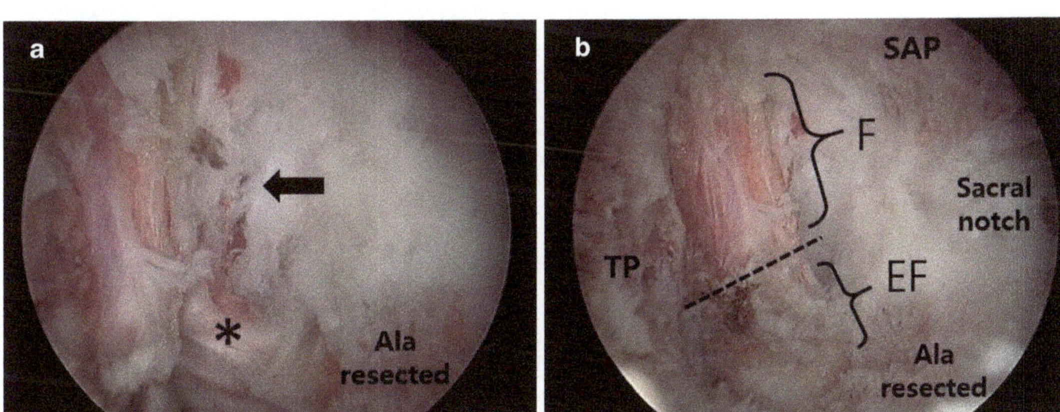

Fig. 11.13 (**a**): The ventral portion of nerve root (*) is exposed. Black arrow indicates the discectomy site. (**b**): Final image. Both foraminal portion and extra-foraminal portion of exiting nerve root is identified (F: foraminal portion, EF: extra-foraminal portion). TP: transverse process; SAP: superior articular process

In the final image, we can check the details including foraminal portion and extra-foraminal portion of exiting nerve root (Fig. 11.13b). A drain catheter is always inserted through the instrumental portal before skin closure (Fig. 11.14). After approximation of subcutaneous layer using absorbable suture material, skin stapler or a point of non-absorbable suture is applied to close the skin.

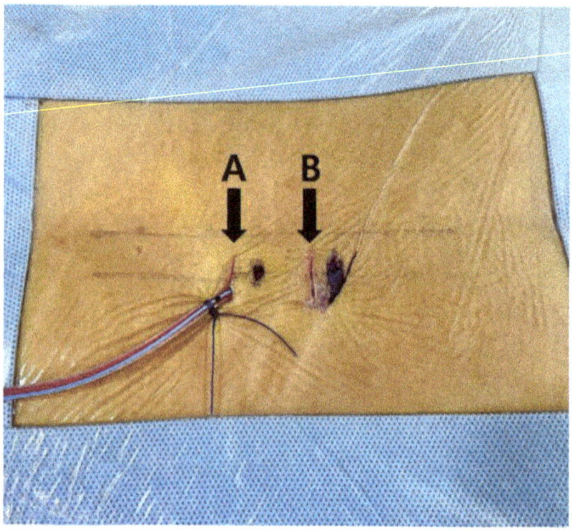

Fig. 11.14 (**a**): Scope portal. (**b**): Instrument portal. A drain catheter is fixed by suture

11.6 Illustrated Case

11.6.1 Case 1 (Left Side Approach, Video 11.1)

A female patient complained of severe radiating pain in the left lower extremities with L5 dermatome. This patient had undergone microscopic lumbar L4/5 decompression surgery 7 years ago at another hospital. Her symptoms have recently worsened and selective nerve block did not improve the symptoms, and she has been unable to lie down due to the pain. Preoperative MRI showed severe extra-foraminal stenosis on the left side of L5/S1, and UBE surgery was performed to relieve the pain (Fig. 11.15). The description of the surgical method is replaced by the main text of the surgical steps in this chapter. The sufficient decompression of the exiting nerve root is well observed in the postoperative MRI images and the final endoscopic image showed full decompression of nerve root from foraminal portion to extra-foraminal portion (Fig. 11.16). The patient was discharged on the fifth day after surgery without any complication.

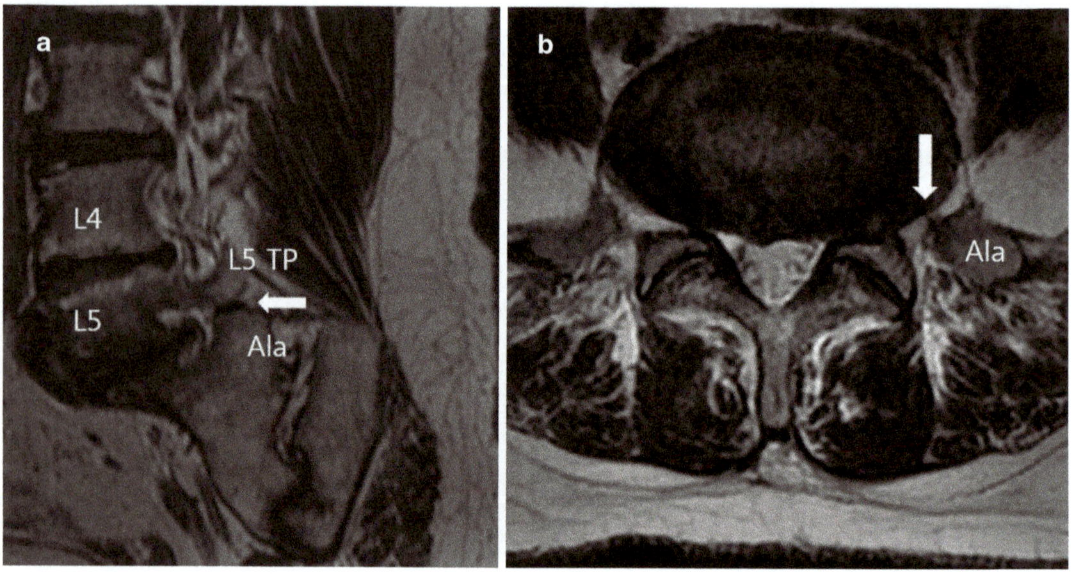

Fig. 11.15 Preoperative MRI T2WI (**a**): Left side oblique view. The pseudo-articulation between L5 TP and sacral ala is indicated with white arrow. (**b**): Axial view. The exiting L5 nerve root (white arrow) is entrapped in the extra-foraminal area surrounded with ala

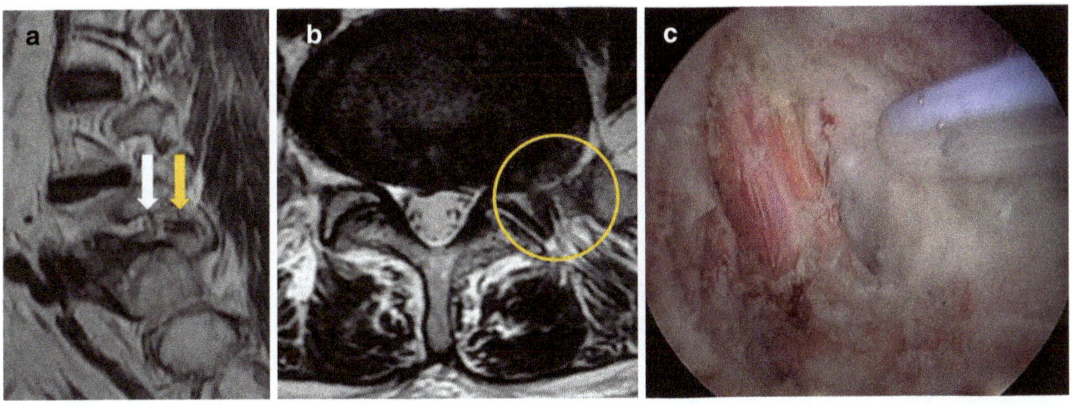

Fig. 11.16 Postoperative MRI T2WI sagittal view (**a**) and axial view (**b**). White arrow indicates decompressed exiting L5 nerve root and yellow arrow indicates the drain catheter. In the yellow circle, partially removed SAP and Ala are observed. (**c**): Final endoscopic image. The drain catheter is inserted

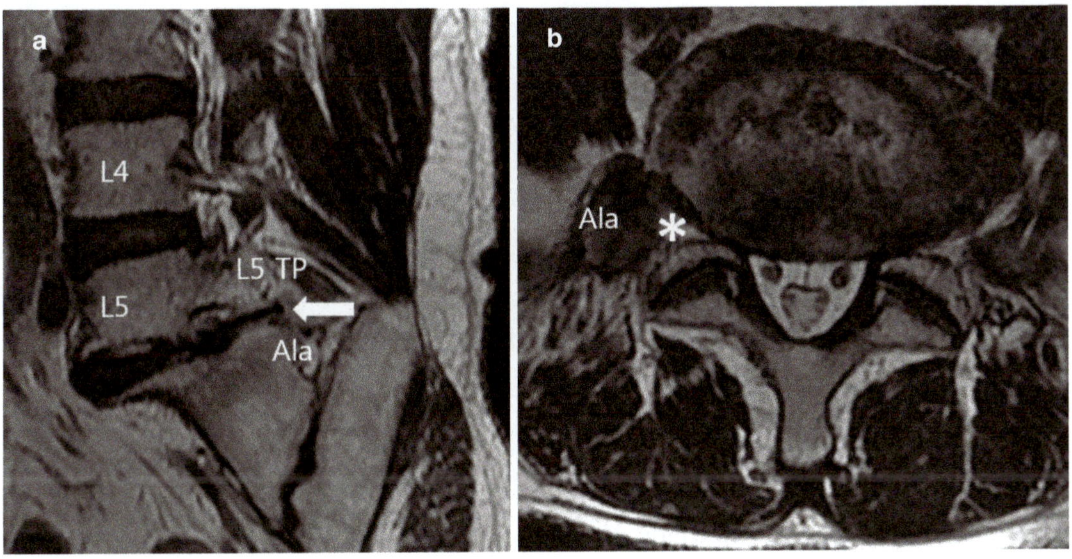

Fig. 11.17 Preoperative MRI T2WI (**a**): Right side oblique view. The pseudo-articulation between L5 TP and sacral ala is indicated with white arrow. (**b**): Axial view. The exiting L5 nerve root is compressed from forminal portion to extra-foraminal portion (*) due to hypertrophied bony structures

11.6.2 Case 2 (Right Side Approach, Video 11.2)

A male patient complained of radiating pain and tingling sensation in the right lower extremities with L5 dermatome. He also complained of neurogenic intermittent claudication (NIC) on left leg, so he could not walk for more than 5 min. There was no response to the selective nerve block and the gait was very uncomfortable, so the UBE decompression surgery was performed. Preoperative MRI showed severe foraminal and extra-foraminal stenosis on the right side of L5/S1 and the exiting L5 nerve root is severely compressed (Fig. 11.17). Under the epidural anesthesia, UBE far-out decompression with right side approach was performed. After identifying the triangle zone in the initial working

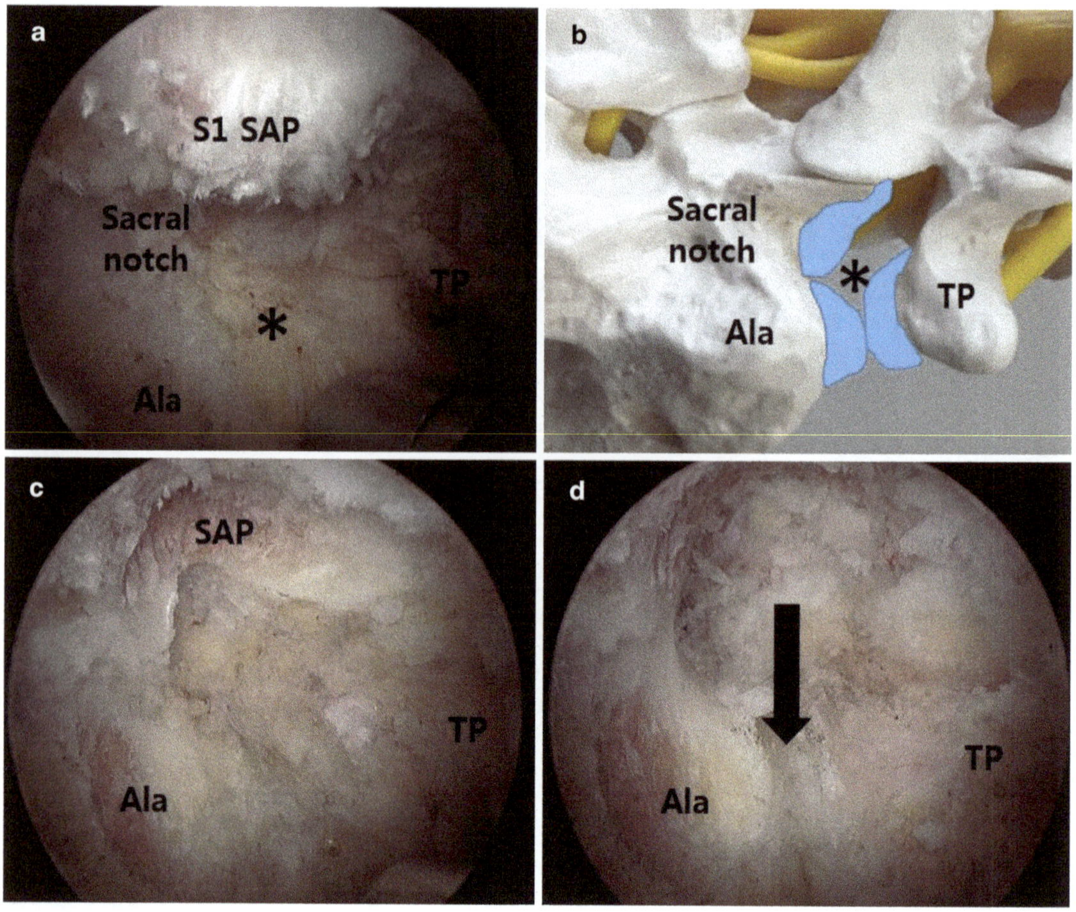

Fig. 11.18 Endoscopic image. Right side approach. (**a, b**): The triangle zone (*) is surrounded with hypertrophied bony structures. (**c, d**): After drilling out the hypertrophied bony structure, the pseudo-articulation is exposed (black arrow)

space, drilling out the bony structures is performed and the pseudo-articulation is well exposed (Fig. 11.18). The exiting nerve root can be identified by uncovering the yellow ligament, and the pseudo-arthosis is sufficiently removed to decompress the extra-foraminal lesion (Fig. 11.19). To decompress the ventral portion of nerve root and foraminal portion, a discectomy could be added. After full decompression along the nerve root from foraminal portion to extra-foraminal portion, the operator confirms that there are no remaining lesions, inserts a drain catheter, and can finish the surgery (Fig. 11.20). Postoperative MRI showed a completely decompression state of far-out lesion and did not show paraspinal muscle edema or hematoma (Fig. 11.21).

11.7 Complications and Their Management

1. Intraoperative bleeding

   The radicular artery around the facet joint is a common cause of intraoperative bleeding [8]. In far-out syndrome, this artery usually runs over the sacral notch. Gentle dissection and approach to sacral notch are very important to prevent

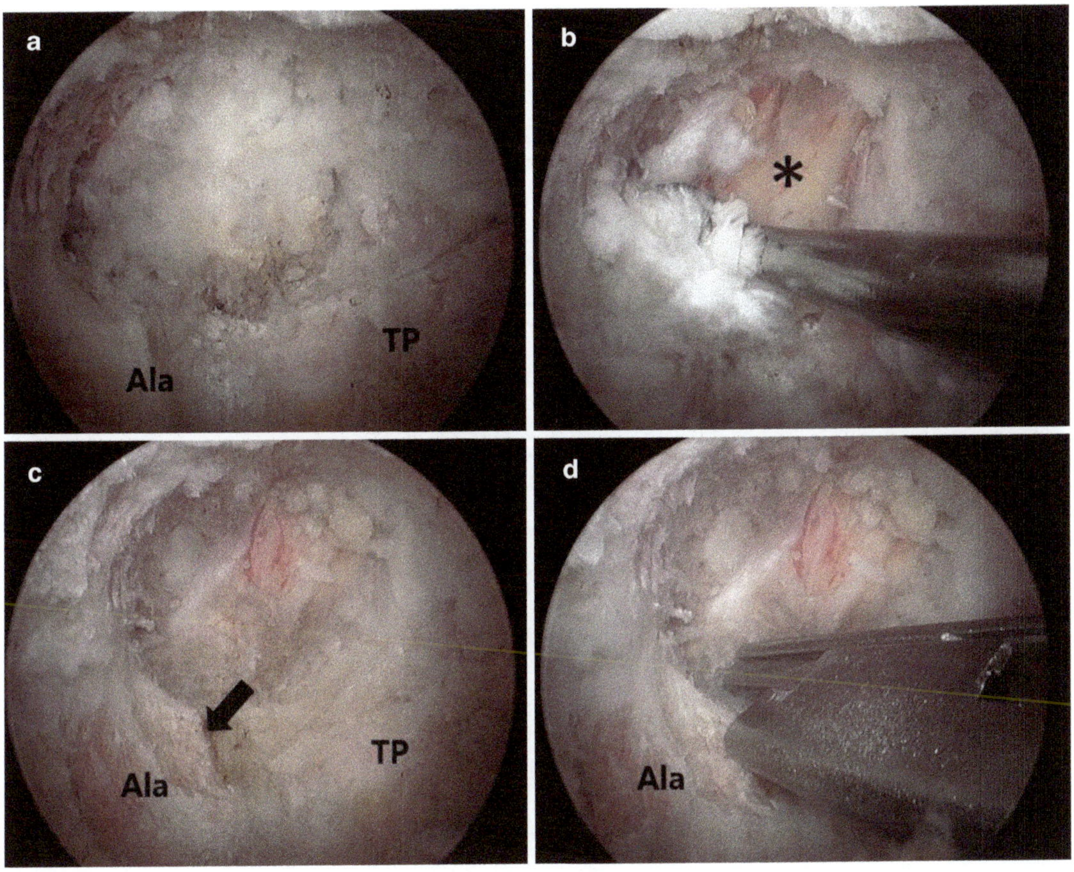

Fig. 11.19 (**a, b**): The yellow ligament covering the nerve root. After removal of ligament, exiting nerve root is exposed (*). (**c, d**): To decompress the far-out lesion, ala and pseudo-articulation should be removed more

arterial bleeding. If arterial vessels are not recognized, severe bleeding may occur. In this case, the endoscope must be closely attached to identify the bleeding site. Thereafter, RF device can be used to control the bleeding (Fig. 11.22).

2. Dural tear or root injury

   Because FOS is an extra-foraminal lesion, the dural tear or damage in spinal canal rarely occurs. However, the exiting nerve root injury can occur. Most of the time, it happens when the Kerrison punch or pituitary forceps are used deeply without the exiting nerve fully identified. In this case, the dura mater surrounding the exiting nerve may be damaged and the nerve rootlets can be exposed (Fig. 11.23a–b). To repair dural defect, the injured area was packed and covered with Tachocomb® (Fig. 11.23c–d).

11.8 Surgical Tips, and Pitfall

1. Postoperative nerve root swelling and dysesthesia

   After UBE decompression surgery, residual symptoms such as radiating pain and paresthesia in the index lower extremities sometimes remain. Young male patient underwent UBE FOS decompression surgery to treat the severe radiating pain in the

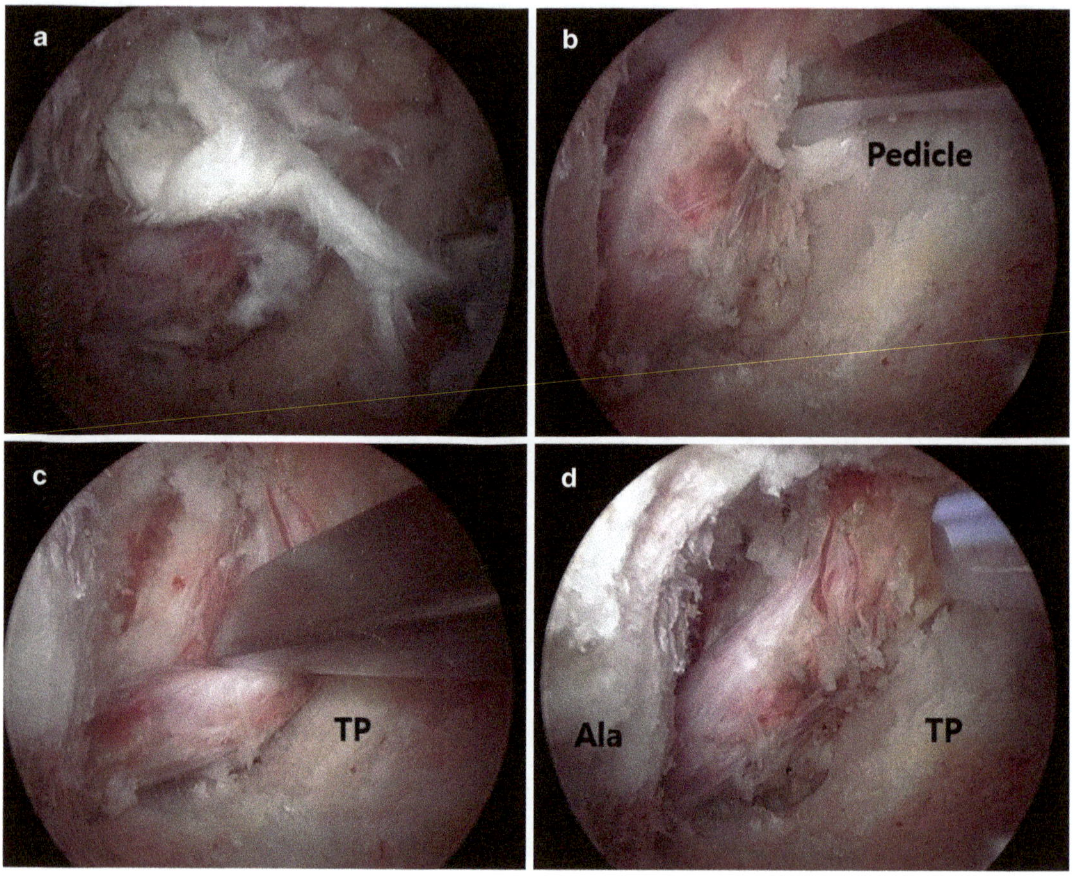

Fig. 11.20 (**a**): Discectomy for ventral decompression of nerve root. (**b, c**): L5 pedicle and vertebral body can be identified after full decompression. (**d**): Final endoscopic image. A drain catheter is inserted

left lower extremities. The lower extremity symptoms improved for a few days after surgery, but the pain worsened again after 1 month, and the MRI study was retaken. It showed significant swelling of nerve root ganglion (Fig. 11.24). Porchet et al reported that in 27% of patients who underwent far-lateral approach for extra-foraminal lumbar disc herniation showed fair or poor outcomes after surgery [9]. In order to reduce these complications, the gentle manipulation of nerve root is very important.

2. Retroperitoneal fluid collection

Continuous saline irrigation is essential to UBE surgery. To treat the far-out syndrome, removal of pseudo-articulation around the ala is most important and this may cause damage to the boundary between the paraspinal muscle and retroperitoneum [10]. Retroperitoneal fluid collection can cause abdominal discomfort and pain and can be diagnosed by abdominal computed tomography (CT) scan. In most cases, it can be resolved with conservative treatment, but sometimes lead to serious complications.

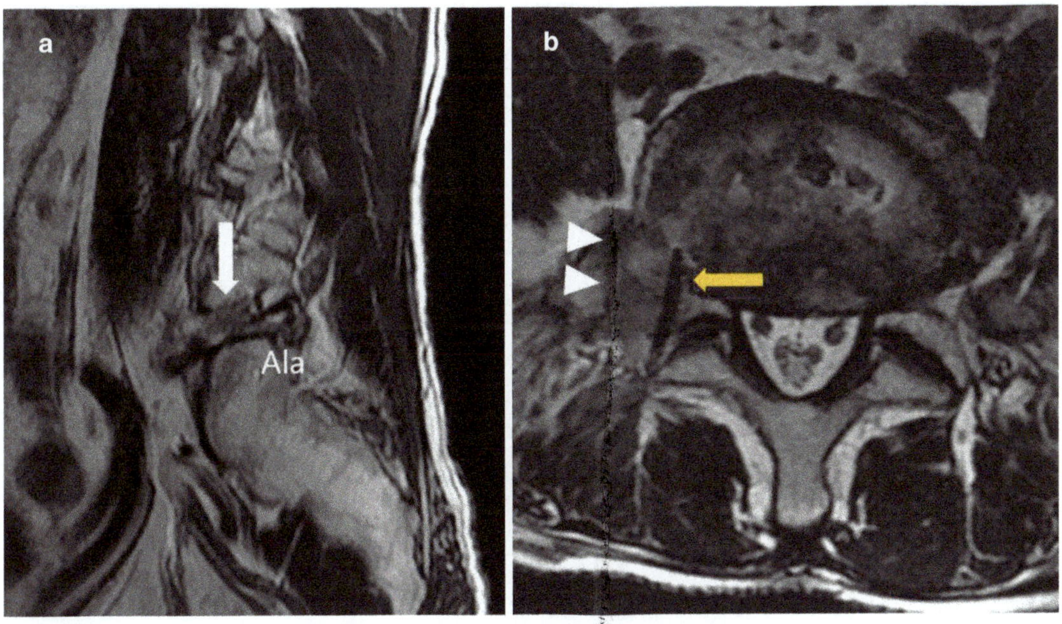

Fig. 11.21 Postoperative T2WI sagittal view (**a**) and axial view (**b**). White arrow indicates decompressed exiting L5 nerve root. In the axial view, ala bone has been sufficiently removed (arrowheads). The drain catheter is inserted (yellow arrow)

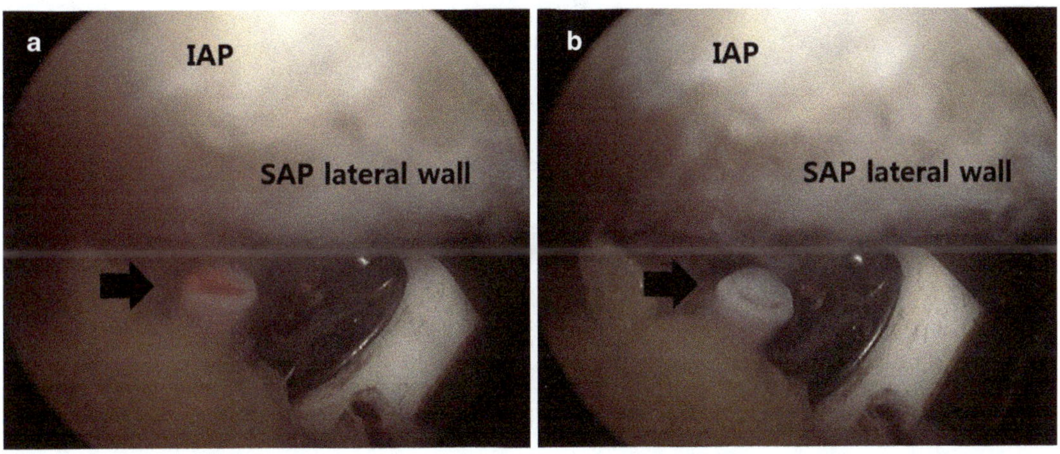

Fig. 11.22 (**a**): The radicular artery (black arrow) is identified at lateral of SAP. (**b**): Coagulated state of radicular artery (black arrow) by RF probe

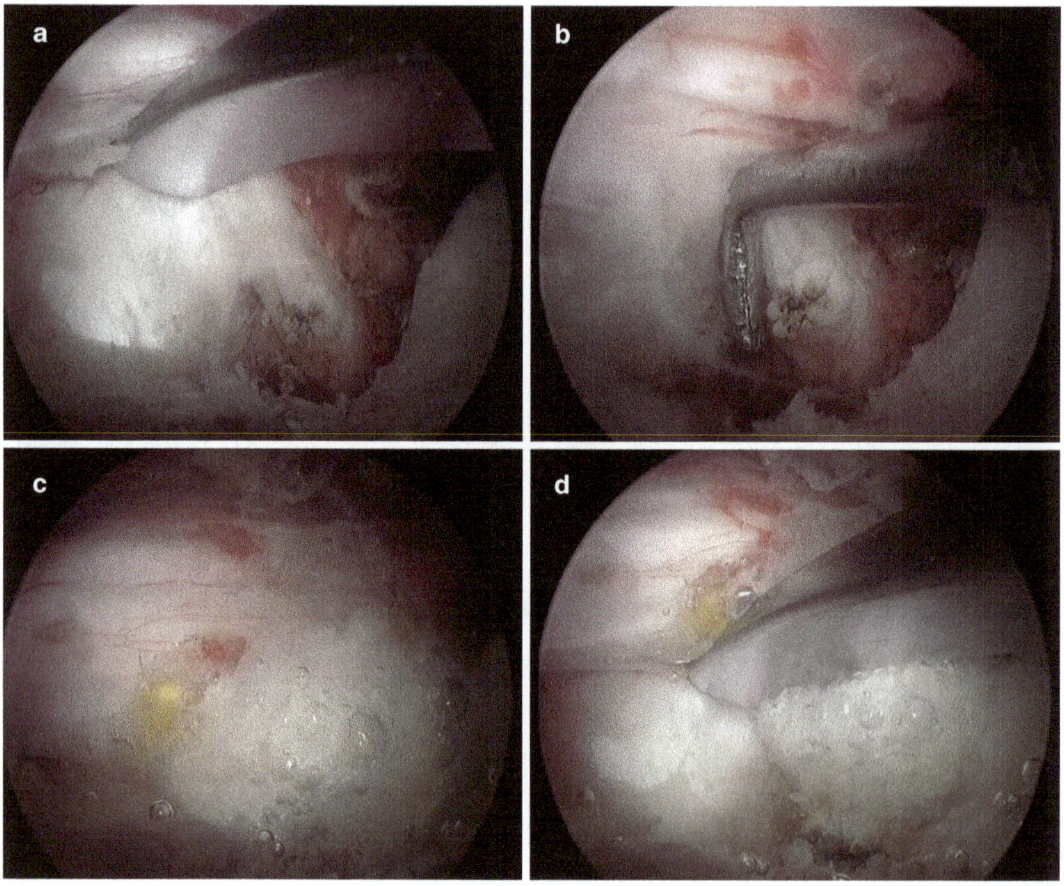

Fig. 11.23 Example case of L5 nerve root injury. (**a, b**): The shoulder portion of L5 nerve root was damaged and the rootlets were exposed. (**c, d**): The damaged area was packed and covered using a Tachocomb®

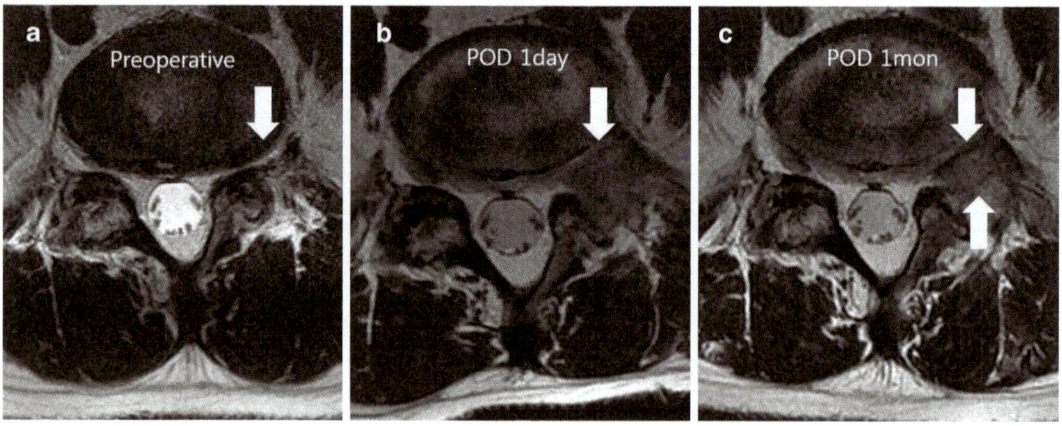

Fig. 11.24 The serial MRI T2WI axial view. (**a**): The extra-foraminal lesion is indicated (white arrow) in preoperative image. (**b**): Well-decompressed state is observed in POD 1 day image. (**c**): A month after surgery, significant swelling of nerve root ganglion is observed

References

1. Jancuska JM, Spivak JM, Bendo JA. A review of symptomatic lumbosacral transitional vertebrae: Bertolotti's syndrome. Int J Spine Surg. 2015;9:42.
2. Holm EK, Bünger C, Foldager CB. Symptomatic lumbosacral transitional vertebra: a review of the current literature and clinical outcomes following steroid injection or surgical intervention. Sicot-J. 2017;3:71.
3. Watanabe K, Yamazaki A, Morita O, Sano A, Katsumi K, Ohashi M. Clinical outcomes of posterior lumbar interbody fusion for lumbar foraminal stenosis: preoperative diagnosis and surgical strategy. Clin Spine Surg. 2011;24(3):137–41.
4. Li Y, Lubelski D, Abdullah KG, Mroz TE, Steinmetz MP. Minimally invasive tubular resection of the anomalous transverse process in patients with Bertolotti's syndrome: presented at the 2013 joint spine section meeting. J Neurosurg Spine. 2014;20(3):283–90.
5. Sasaki M, Aoki M, Matsumoto K, Tsuruzono K, Akiyama C, Yoshimine T. Middle-term surgical outcomes of microscopic posterior decompression for far-out syndrome. J Neurol Surg A Cent Eur Neurosurg. 2014;75(02):079–83.
6. Iwasaki M, Akiyama M, Koyanagi I, Niiya Y, Ihara T, Houkin K. Double crush of L5 spinal nerve root due to L4/5 lateral recess stenosis and bony spur formation of lumbosacral transitional vertebra pseudoarticulation: a case report and review. NMC Case Rep J. 2017;4(4):121–5.
7. Wiltse L, Guyer R, Spencer C, Glenn W, Porter I. Alar transverse process impingement of the L5 spinal nerve: the far-out syndrome. Spine. 1984;9(1):31–41.
8. Yang H-S, Lee N, Park J-Y. Current status of biportal endoscopic decompression for lumbar foraminal stenosis: endoscopic partial facetectomy and outcome factors. J Minim Invasive Spine Surg Tech. 2021;6:157–63.
9. Porchet F, Chollet-Bornand A, de Tribolet N. Long-term follow up of patients surgically treated by the far-lateral approach for foraminal and extraforaminal lumbar disc herniations. J Neurosurg Spine. 1999;90(1):59–66.
10. Heo DH, Sharma S, Park CK. Endoscopic treatment of extraforaminal entrapment of L5 nerve root (far out syndrome) by unilateral biportal endoscopic approach: technical report and preliminary clinical results. Neurospine. 2019;16(1):130.

Part IV

Lumbar Interbody Fusion

12 Lumbar Interbody Fusion by Unilateral Biportal Endoscopy

Man Kyu Park, Sang Kyu Son, and Seung Hyun Choi

12.1 Introduction

Gold standard techniques such as transforaminal lumbar interbody fusion (TLIF) or posterior lumbar interbody fusion (PLIF), conventionally used for the treatment of degenerative lumbar spinal disease, have disadvantages, such as postoperative back pain as well as paraspinal muscle atrophy due to paraspinal muscle dissection or retraction [1, 2].

Recently, a technique for lumbar interbody fusion by unilateral biportal endoscopy (UBE lumbar interbody fusion [ULIF]) has been developed and published by several studies that have demonstrated its various advantages compared with conventional PLIF/TLIF, while reporting competent clinical outcomes as well as fusion rates [3–6]. In this technique, independent movement of the surgical instruments and endoscope is possible because the working portal, and not the working cannula, is utilized for surgical instruments [3]. Consequently, direct neural decompression of the central and foraminal stenosis is possible with less limitation of movement and vision [3, 7]. As the cage is inserted through the working portal, and not through the working cannula, large-sized cages can be inserted into the intervertebral space [3]. Moreover, ULIF can provide a familiar surgical view and high magnification/clearing by continuous irrigation for safe and effective surgery [5]. Additionally, ULIF can achieve meticulous endplate preparation and reduce the probability of bony endplate injury, which can be confirmed under endoscopic view [5, 7]. Furthermore, because of ULIF's advantageous minimal invasiveness, patients have less postoperative back pain [3–5].

In order to safely and effectively perform ULIF, there are surgical tips that need to be taken into account at each stage of the procedure. This chapter aims to describe the surgical technique of ULIF.

Supplementary Information The online version contains supplementary material available at [https://doi.org/10.1007/978-981-16-8201-8_12].

M. K. Park · S. K. Son (✉)
Department of Neurosurgery, Parkweonwook Hospital, Busan, South Korea
e-mail: Bread0309@handmail.net

S. H. Choi
Department of Orthopedic Surgery, Parkweonwook Hospital, Busan, South Korea

12.2 Indications and Contraindications

The indications of ULIF are similar to those for conventional PLIF/TLIF.

The indications for ULIF are as follows:

1. Grade 1 or 2 degenerative or isthmic spondylolisthesis

D. H. Heo et al. (eds.), *Unilateral Biportal Endoscopic Spine Surgery*,
https://doi.org/10.1007/978-981-16-8201-8_12

2. Central or foraminal stenosis with instability
3. Recurrent disc herniation

The contraindications for ULIF are as follows:

1. High-grade spondylolisthesis (grade 3 or 4)
2. Spinal deformity
3. Vertebral fractures
4. Spondylodiscitis

12.3 Special Instruments

Most of the instruments used during ULIF are similar to other surgeries by UBE. However, some instruments specially designed for ULIF are also available and could be safe.

1. Semi-tubular retractor: Semi-tubular retractor keep continuous fluid output and guide the instrument to the operation field during operation (Fig. 12.1a). In addition to semi-tubular retractor, a working sheath can also be used to keep continuous fluid output.
2. Hook radiofrequency probe: It is used for coagulation of focal epidural vessels or annulotomy (Fig. 12.1b).
3. Funnel and Funnel pusher: Insertion of bone graft is performed through a specialized bone graft funnel (Fig. 12.1c).
4. Serial dilator bars (11 mm, 13 mm, 15 mm): Prior to cage insertion, serial dilatation of paraspinal muscle can be achieved by using bar dilators to make it easier for insertion of the cage (Fig. 12.1d).
5. Specilized root retractor: Thecal sac and nerve root can be protected with a specialized root retractor during cage insertion, which is anchored at lower vertebral body edge (Fig. 12.1e).
6. Endplate removers: Specialized various angles of endplate removers are useful for endplate preparation, especially in contralateral side (Fig. 12.1f).

12.4 Anesthesia and Position

Patients are prepared in the prone position under general or epidural anesthesia. Generally, the left side is preferred for a right-handed spine surgeon, as it becomes easy to take surgical instruments from the nurse. However, in the case of high lordotic angle of surgical level, such as L5–S1 level, or when direct neural decompression of right foraminal stenosis is needed, right-side approach is a better alternative.

12.5 Surgical Steps

12.5.1 Skin Marking and Making Portal

Once the patient is positioned, intraoperative fluoroscopy is used to confirm the level of operation. Lower endplate line of upper vertebral body should be parallel under C-arm fluoroscopy guidance. The docking point is identified by using an anteroposterior view of C-arm fluoroscopy as the lower part of the cranial lamina. Two incisions are made, about 3 cm apart, with the center being the lower part of the cranial lamina at the midline of the proximal and distal pedicles. A transverse skin incision is made cranially for the endoscopic portal; another skin incision is made caudally for the working portal (Fig. 12.2a). Skin incisions may need to be further lateral and wide in obese patients. Each incision will be used for percutaneous pedicle screw insertion at the end of operation. If multi-level fusion is planned, the cranial endoscopic portals can be used in the working portal for the next-level ULIF.

Once the skin incision is made, the 15-blade is used to make incision in the lumbosacral fascia, enough to insert the serial tube dilators and the endoscopic sheath. After the fascia is opened, the serial tube dilators and the endoscopic sheath, which make triangulation, are placed at the target lamina. Triangulation of the endoscope and

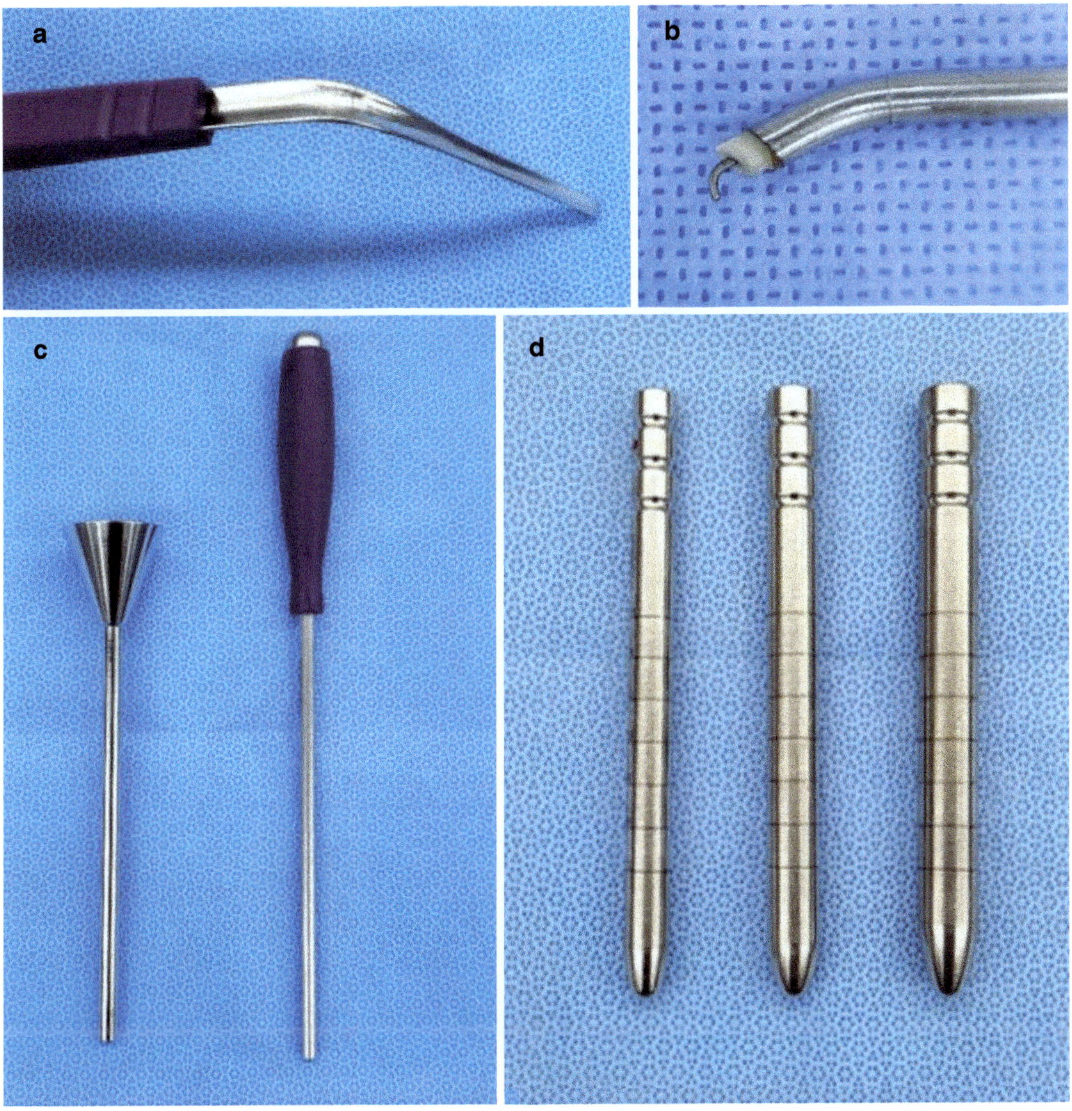

Fig. 12.1 Special instruments for lumbar interbody fusion by unilateral biportal endoscopy. Semi-tubular retractor (**a**), hook radiofrequency probe (**b**), funnel and funnel pusher (**c**), serial dilator bars (**d**), specialized root retractor (**e**), endplate removers (**f**)

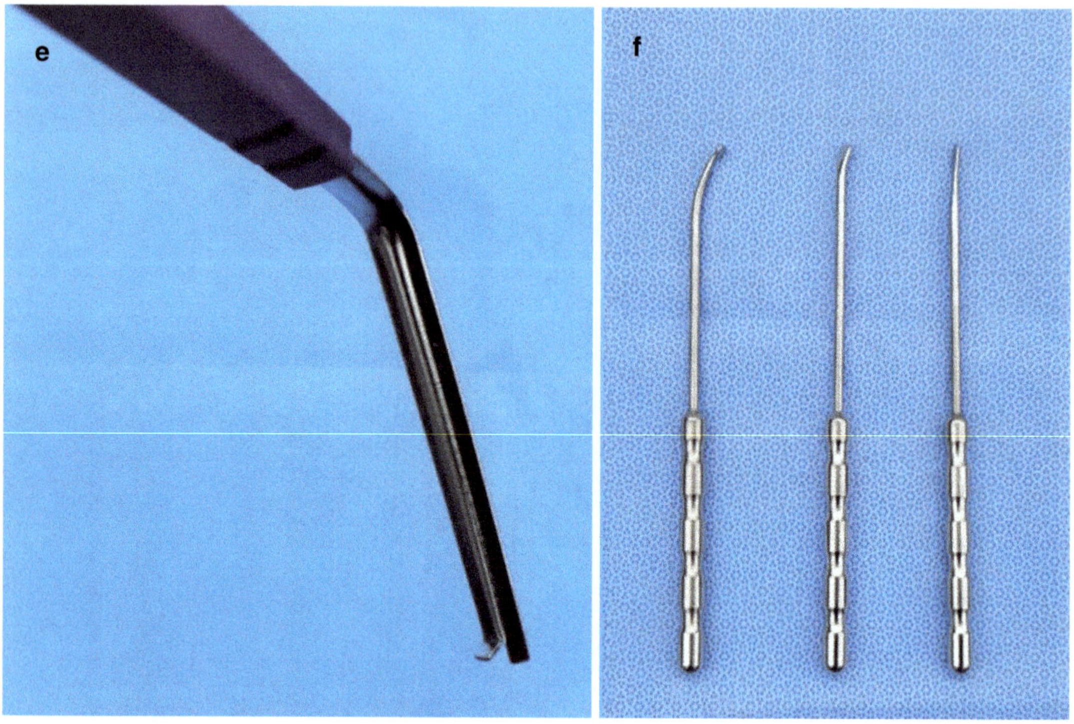

Fig. 12.1 (continued)

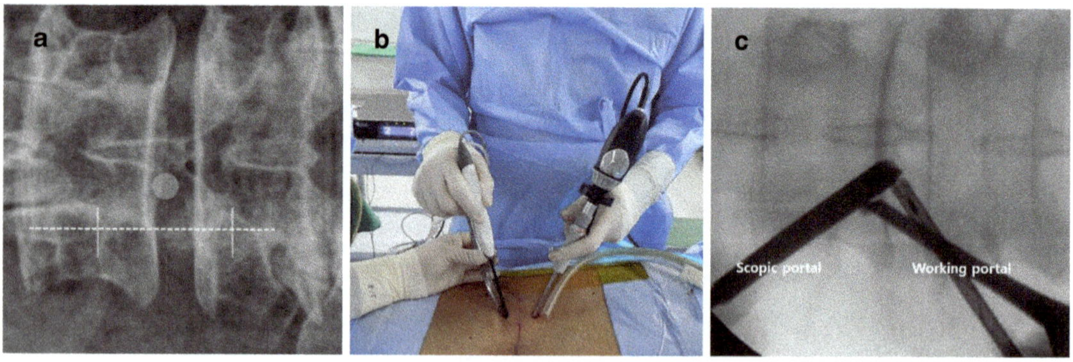

Fig. 12.2 Skin incision and docking point on the fluoroscopic anteroposterior view. The docking point (white circle) is the lower part of the cranial lamina. Two skin incisions (white line) are made about 3 cm apart, with the center being the lower part of the cranial lamina at the midline of the proximal and distal pedicles (dotted line) (**a**). The positioning of the endoscope and surgical instruments with semi-tubular retractor through each portal. A photo in the surgical field (**b**), fluoroscopic view (**c**)

surgical instruments with semi-tubular retractor is crucial to visualize the surgical field and to manipulate the instruments with less motion and vision limitation (Fig. 12.2b, c). Using the muscle detacher, the surgeon is able to feel the base of the spinous process as well as the cranial lamina and the facet joint.

12.5.2 Initial Working Space and Bone Working (Fig. 12.3 and Video 12.1)

After positioning the endoscope and the semi-tubular retractor through each portal, the initial working space is made under endoscopic guid-

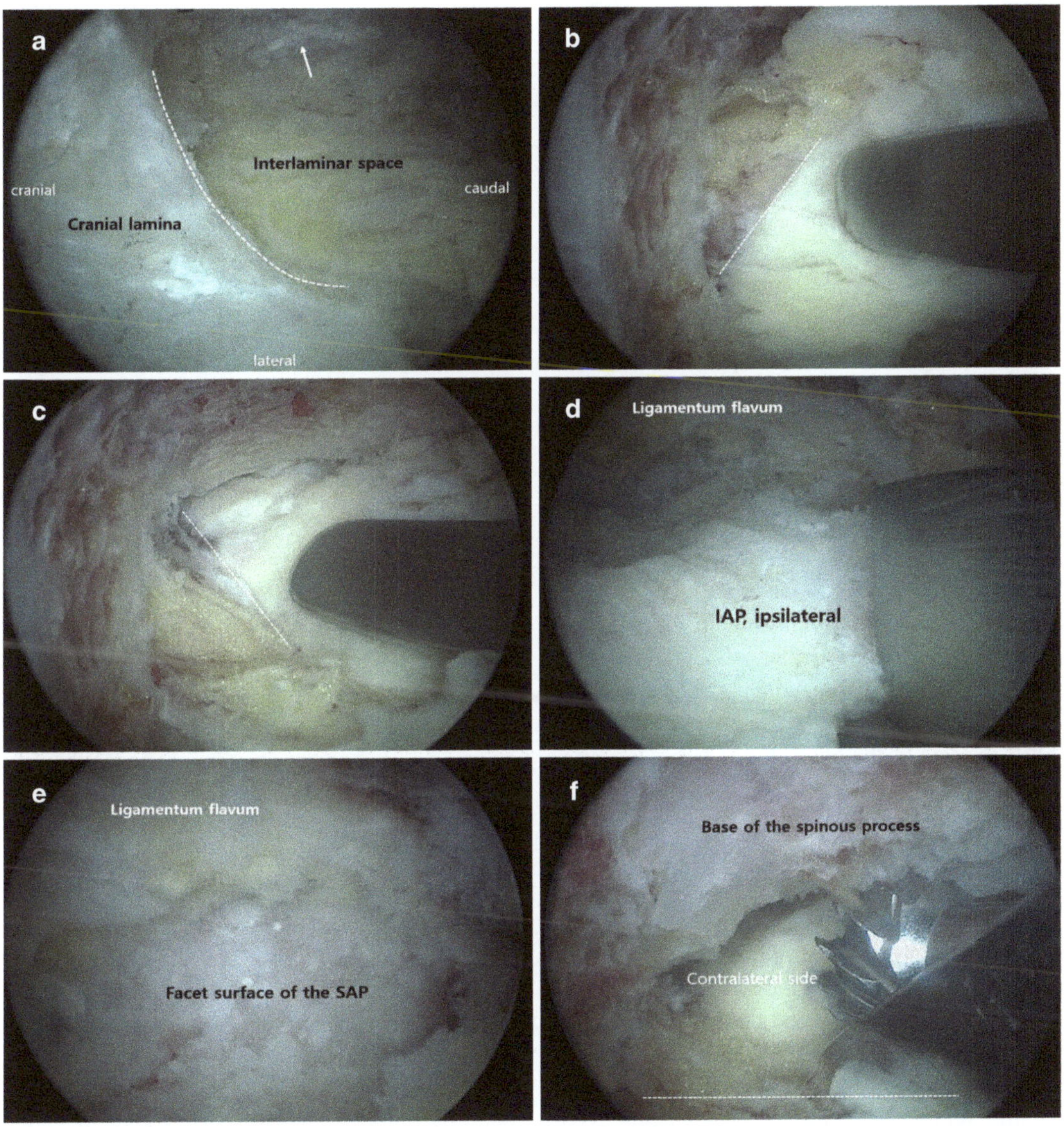

Fig. 12.3 Serial sequence endoscopic images of the bone working. The surgical anatomy is first noticed in the inferior edge of the cranial lamina and the interlaminar space (**a**). Anatomical landmark for cranial bone working. The dotted line indicates cranial end of the ligamentum flavum of ipsilateral side (**b**) and contralateral side (**c**). Removal of inferior articular process by osteotome (**d**) and identification of the articular surfaces of superior articular process (**e**). Removal of the base of the spinous process for contralateral decompression. The dotted line indicates midline (**f**). Removal of inferior articular process by osteotome at contralateral side (**g**)

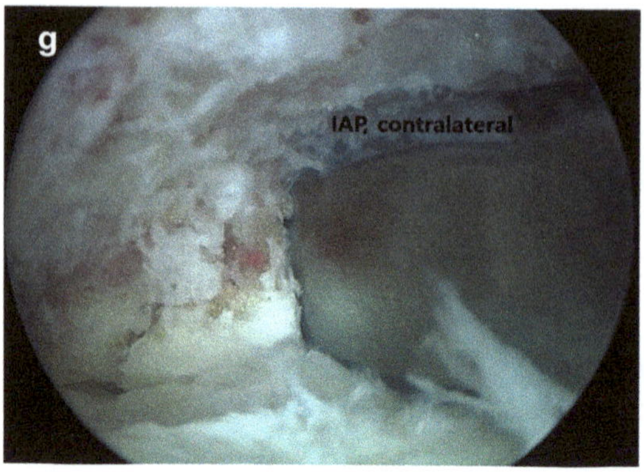

Fig. 12.3 (continued)

ance. Once soft tissue overlying the cranial lamina is coagulated using RF probe, the inferior edge of the cranial lamina and the interlaminar space is identified (Fig. 12.3a). At this point, ipsilateral laminotomy can be performed by using round cutting burr or Kerrison punch. It is preferable not to use a burr, but rather to use Kerrison punch or osteotome to collect the auto bone for bone grafting. Typically, the ligamentum flavum (LF) is left as a protector to avoid neural injury or dural tear until bone working is finished. Laminotomy of the cranial lamina should be performed until exposure of cranial end of the LF (Fig. 12.3b, c). After finishing ipsilateral laminotomy, the inferior articular process (IAP) of the upper vertebra is removed by multiple osteotomies to save the autograft material (Fig. 12.3d, e). If the size of the bone chip is large, it may be difficult to remove through working portal or may cause paraspinal muscle injury. After satisfactory bone working is performed at the ipsilateral side, the bone working is done toward the contralateral side.

A contralateral decompression can be performed through sublaminar approach; the base of the spinous process and contralateral lamina are removed utilizing a round cutting burr or osteotome (Fig. 12.3f). It is important to sufficiently remove the base of spinous process to obtain working space because the base of the spinous process interrupts the manipulation of the endoscope and the surgical instruments. The contralateral facectectomy through sublaminar approach provides release, which helps in reduction of spondylolisthesis and making lordosis (Fig. 12.4a). When the IAP is caudally removed with an osteotome from the tip of IAP, the facet joint surface can be confirmed (Fig. 12.3g). When the facet joint osteophytes are prominent or greater reduction of spondylolisthesis is required, two new portals are created on the contralateral side to perform total removal of IAP (Fig. 12.4b).

12.5.3 Partial Removal of Superior Articular Process and Identification of Disc Space (Fig. 12.5 and Video 12.2)

After removing the superficial layer of ipsilateral LF, the upper portion of the caudal lamina and medial aspect of the superior articular process (SAP) could be identified (Fig. 12.5a, b). The upper portion of the caudal lamina is partially removed with Kerrison punch, continuing along the medial margins of the SAP and detachment of the deep layer of the LF (Fig. 12.5c). The medial aspect of SAP should be removed sufficiently to make space for insertion of the cage. Inadequate resection of SAP could induce retraction-related neurapraxia when the cage is inserted. When the distance from lateral margin of thecal sac to the remaining ledge of the SAP is at least 8 mm, the cage can be safely placed without retraction-related neurapraxia (Fig. 12.5d). Once the deep layer of ipsilateral LF is partially removed, the lateral margin of thecal sac, ipsilateral traversing nerve root, pedicle of lower vertebra, and disc space could be identified (Fig. 12.5e). We do not attempt to fully expose the ipsilateral exiting nerve root before cage insertion because this helps to protect the exiting nerve root from neural injury during cage insertion.

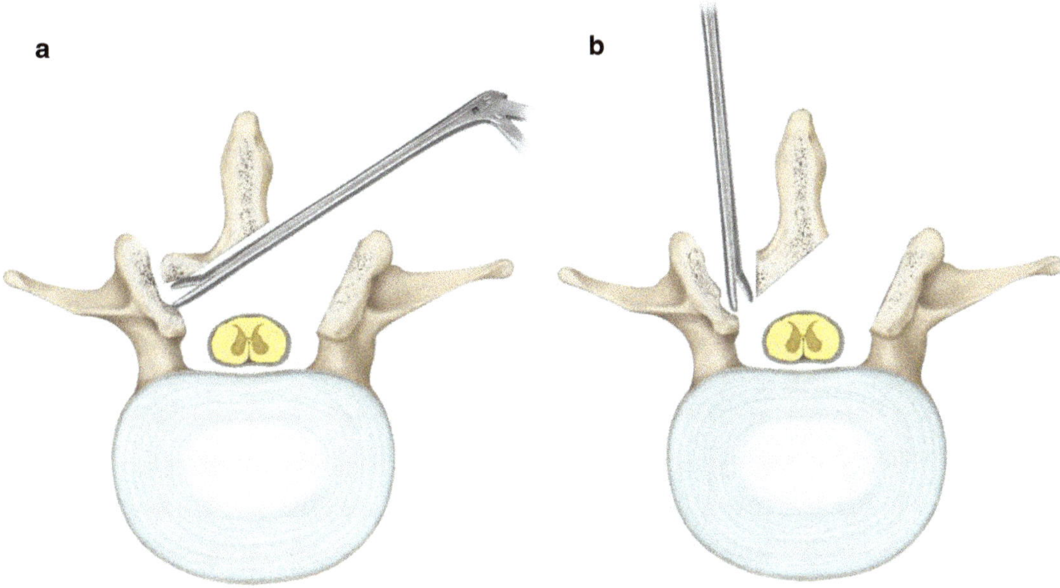

Fig. 12.4 Two types of contralateral facectectomy in lumbar interbody fusion by UBE. Contralateral facectectomy through sublaminar approach (**a**). When the facet joint osteophytes are prominent or greater reduction of spondylolisthesis is required, two new portals are created on the contralateral side to perform total removal of IAP (**b**)

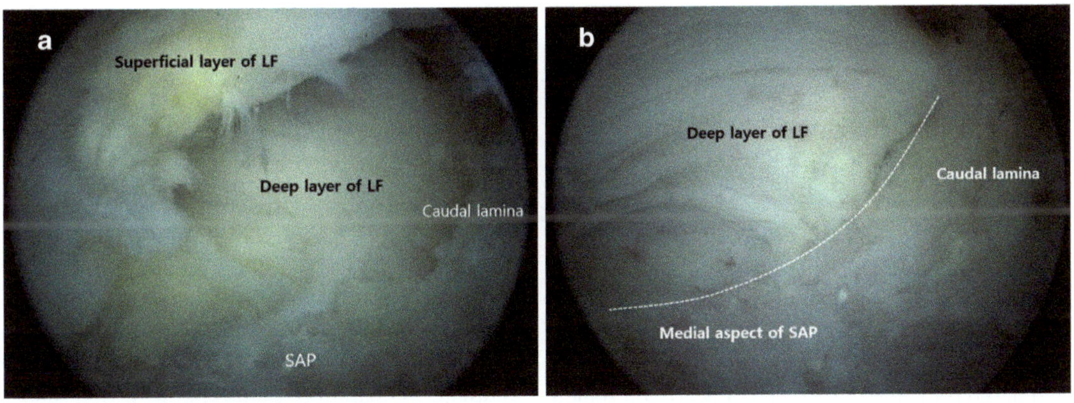

Fig. 12.5 Endoscopic images showing the sequential steps of partial removal of superior articular process and identification of disc space. Detachment of the superficial layer of ligamentum flavum from caudal lamina (**a**). Exposure of the upper portion of the caudal lamina and medial margin of the superior articular process (white dotted curved line) (**b**). The upper portion of the caudal lamina is partially removed with Kerrison punch, continuing along the medial margins of the superior articular process (white dotted curved line) (**c**). When the distance from lateral margin of thecal sac to the remaining ledge of the SAP (double-ended arrow) is at least 8 mm, the cage can be safely placed (**d**). Identification of ipsilateral traversing nerve root, pedicle of lower vertebra, and disc space could be identified (**e**)

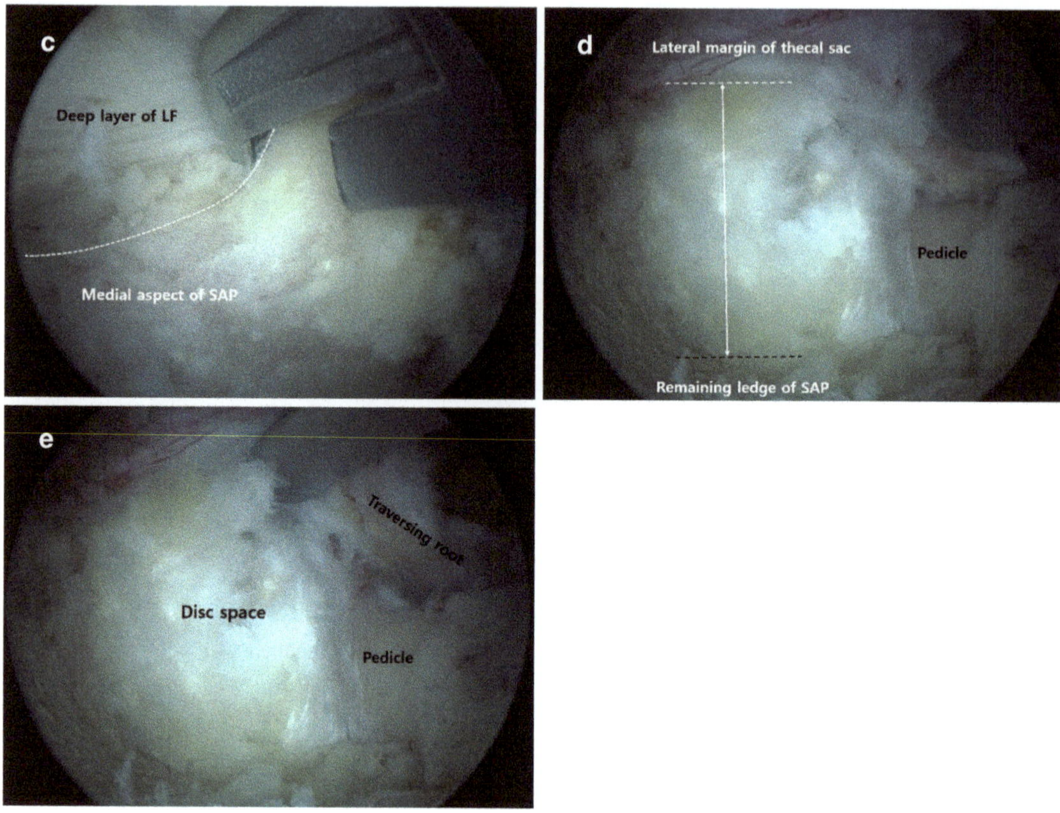

Fig. 12.5 (continued)

12.5.4 Annulotomy and Endplate Preparation (Fig. 12.6 and Video 12.2)

After exposing the ipsilateral disc space, epidural vessels above the annulus are coagulated. Annulotomy can be performed using hook RF probe with attention to protecting the thecal sac and nerve root (Fig. 12.6a). Then, Kerrison punch is used to remove the annulus fibrosus, making the disc space more release (Fig. 12.6b). The nucleus pulposus and cartilaginous endplate are removed using a combination of angled endplate removers and pituitary forceps. Meticulous endplate preparation is crucial for good arthrodesis, and special care should be taken to remove most of the cartilaginous endplate without bony endplate injury, which can prevent the subsidence of the cage into the vertebral body. Detachment of the cartilaginous endplate from the bony endplate can be performed by utilizing a variety of angled endplate removers (Fig. 12.6c). Care should be taken to adequately remove disc material and cartilaginous endplate at the contralateral side, so that the cage is able to be inserted at the contralateral side. With the help of angled endplate removers and curved pituitary forceps, contralateral endplate preparation could be achieved under endoscopic guidance. Using the 30° scope allows more endplate preparation at contralateral side. Generally, about 70%–80% of the disc space could be prepared for fusion with ULIF. In patients with high-grade spondylolisthesis or significant disc narrowing, it may be difficult to perform endplate preparation and cage insertion. In such cases, upper edge of lower vertebral body is removed with an osteotome to obtain a larger entry (Fig. 12.6d). By having a magnified endo-

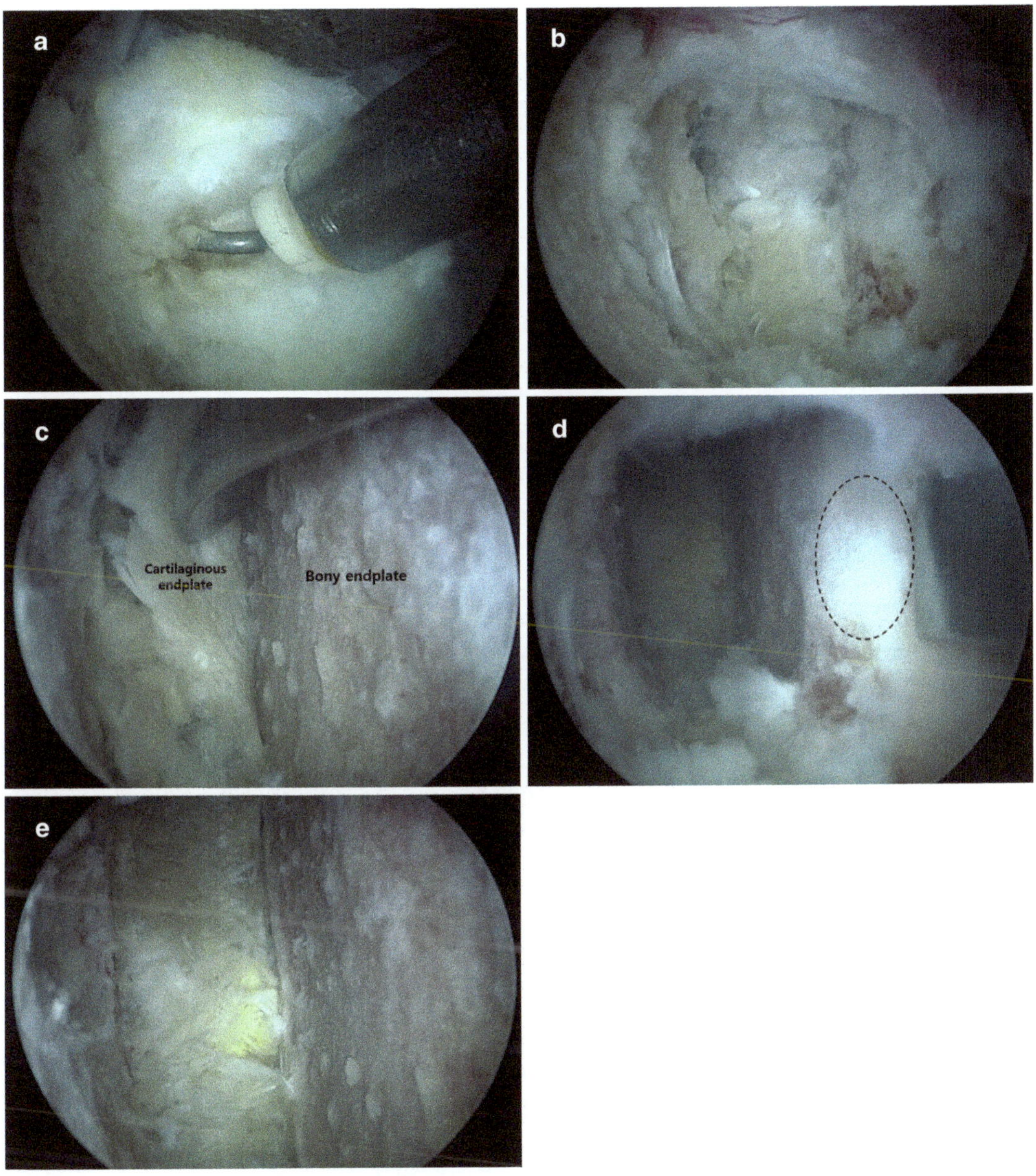

Fig. 12.6 Endoscopic images showing the steps in order of annulotomy and endplate preparation. Annulotomy using hook radiofrequency probe (**a**). Kerrison punch is used to remove the annulus fibrosus, making the disc space more release (**b**). The cartilaginous endplate can be detached from the bony endplate using endplate remover (**c**). Removal of upper edge of lower vertebral body (dotted circle) using an osteotome, which aids in easier cage insertion and prevents exiting root injury (**d**). Confirmation of meticulous endplate preparation (**e**)

scopic view, surgeons can make sure when the meticulous endplate preparation is complete (Fig. 12.6e).

12.5.5 Bone Grafting and Cage Insertion (Fig. 12.7 and Video 12.3)

When placing bone graft or inserting the cage, fluid should be stopped to prevent loss of bone chip by continuous irrigation. After sufficient endplate preparation, insertion of bone graft is performed using specialized bone graft funnel, which is checked on fluoroscopy (Figs. 12.1c and 12.7a, b). Autologous and allogenous bone grafts can be compacted into the anterior portion of the disc space through specialized bone graft funnel. Prior to cage insertion, dilatation of paraspinal muscle can be achieved by using bar dilators to make it easier for insertion of the cage (Figs. 12.1d and 12.7c). Under fluoroscopic guidance during

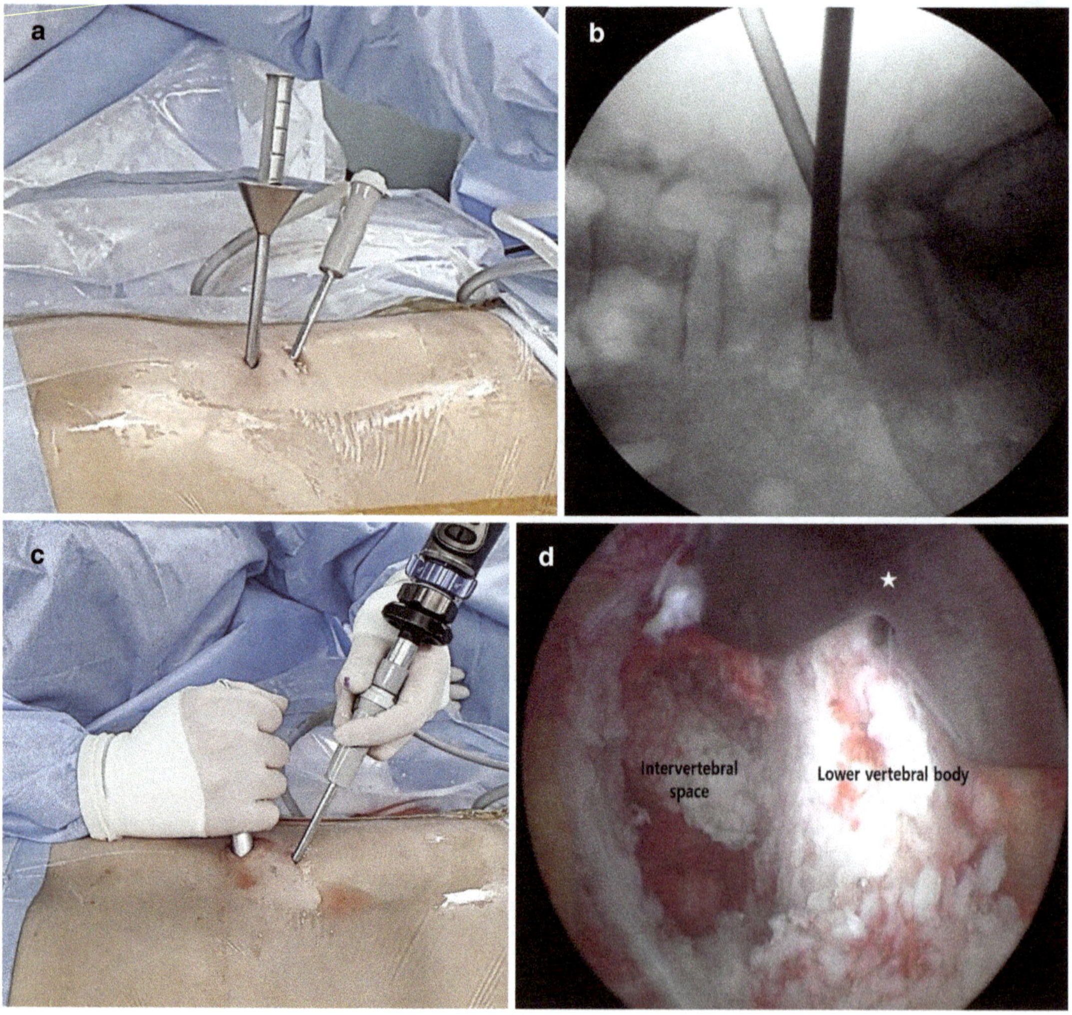

Fig. 12.7 Intraoperative images showing the sequential steps of bone grafting and cage insertion. Bone grafts can be compacted into the anterior portion of the disc space through specialized bone graft funnel. A photo in the surgical field (**a**), Lateral fluoroscopic images (**b**). Prior to cage insertion, dilatation of paraspinal muscle can be achieved by using bar dilators to make it easier for insertion of the cage (**c**). Thecal sac and nerve root can be protected with a specialized root retractor (asterisk) during cage insertion, which is anchored at lower vertebral body edge. Endoscopic view (**d**), Lateral fluoroscopic images (**e**). Serial sequence fluoroscopic images of the insertion of the cage (**f**). Gelfoam is placed to reduce loss of bone graft and bleeding from the bony endplate (**g**)

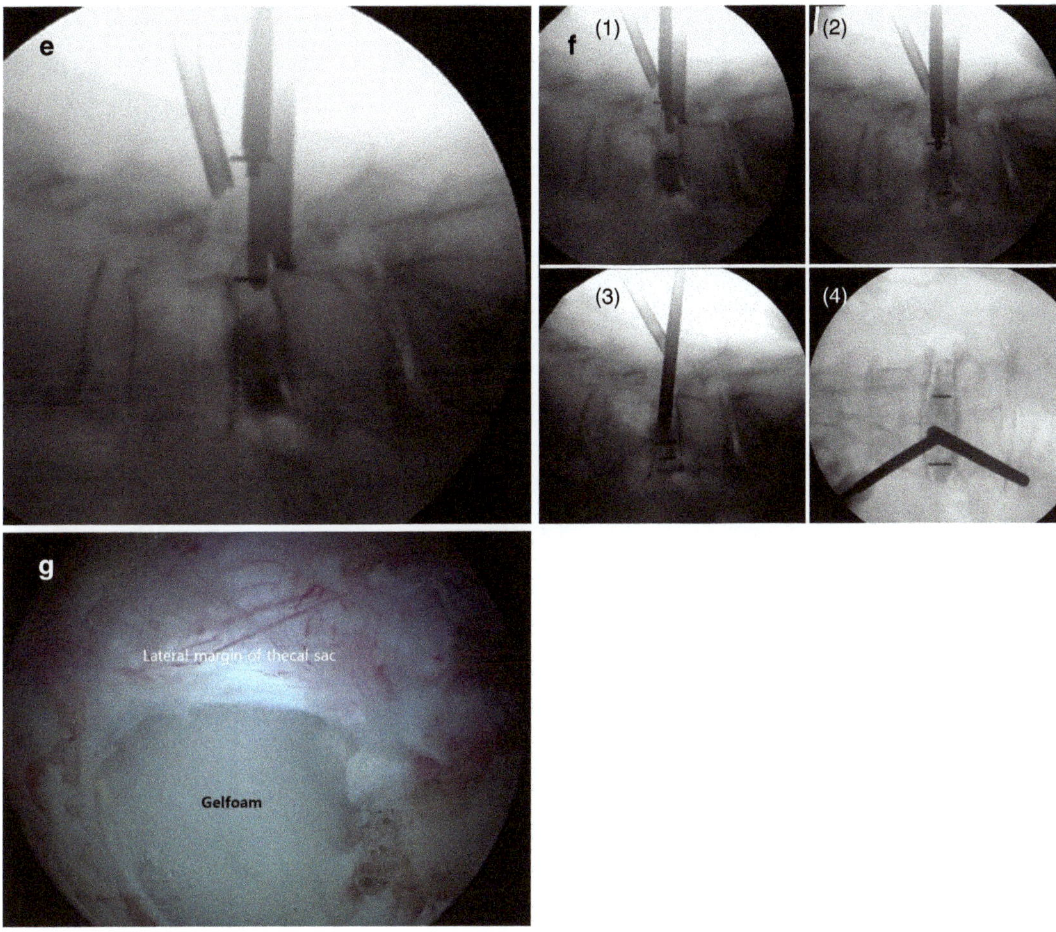

Fig. 12.7 (continued)

cage insertion in ULIF, a blind space is made; thecal sac and nerve root can be protected with a specialized root retractor, anchored at lower vertebral body edge (Figs. 12.1e and 12.7d, e). The cage is then placed transversely using a cage impactor with the aid of fluoroscopy (Fig. 12.7f). Cage should be located between the anterior portion of the disc space on the lateral fluoroscopic image, and centrally place on the anteroposterior fluoroscopic image, which provides segmental lordosis. After insertion of the cage, Gelfoam is applied to the annulotomy site to reduce loss of bone graft and bleeding from the bony endplate (Fig. 12.7g).

12.5.6 Completion of Central and Foraminal Decompression (Fig. 12.8 and Video 12.3)

After finishing the insertion of the cage, the remaining LF is removed to finalize decompression. Once the plane between the dural sac and LF is dissected with freer elevator, the RF probe can be used to detach the LF along the remaining body edge. This technique allows the LF to be removed in an *en bloc* fashion, and minimizes the usage of Kerrison punch, thereby reducing the risk of a dural tear or neural injury. After removing the LF at the contralateral side, we could

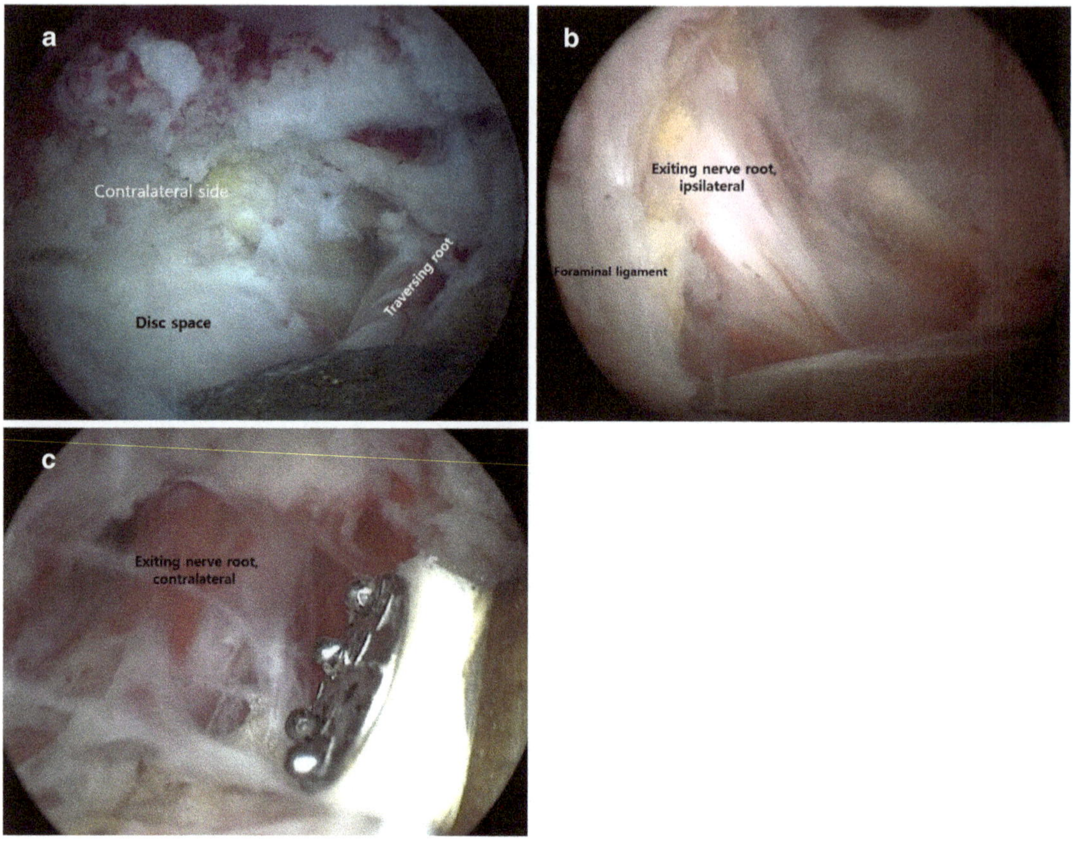

Fig. 12.8 Confirmation of central and foraminal decompression under endoscopic guidance. Contralateral traversing nerve root (**a**), ipsilateral exiting nerve root (**b**), and contralateral exiting nerve root (**c**)

identify the contralateral side disc space and traversing nerve root and then complete the central decompression (Fig. 12.8a).

If direct neural decompression is required in the ipsilateral and contralateral exiting nerve root, it can be done after placing the cage. In the case of an ipsilateral foraminotomy, the exiting nerve root can be identified by removing the foraminal ligament (Fig. 12.8b). Then, palpate the upper vertebral pedicle and remove the inferior aspect of transverse process and the tip of SAP following the exiting nerve root. Decompression of the contralateral exiting nerve root could also be performed using the contralateral sublaminar approach. When the tip of the SAP on contralateral side is removed with a curved osteotome or curved Kerrison punch and then the foraminal ligament is removed, the contralateral exiting nerve root can be identified (Fig. 12.8c). The nerve root and thecal sac can be identified by good pulsation, which is the end point of decompression.

12.5.7 Insertion of Postoperative Drainage and Percutaneous Pedicle Screw Fixation

Jackson–Pratt surgical drain (100 cc) is required after operation to prevent postoperative hematoma. As the drain's line is irritated when the pedicle screw is inserted, Jackson–Pratt surgical drain is inserted through a subcutaneous tunnel created at the medial side of the caudal skin incision. Two ipsilateral incisions are performed for percutaneous pedicle screw insertion. The ULIF is completed with percutaneous pedicle screws.

12.5.8 Postoperative Care

The patient is mobilized with physical activity the first day after the operation. Postoperative standing radiographs and MRI should be checked on the second day after surgery, which will show the placement of the cage and neural decompression in detail. Jackson–Pratt surgical drain is removed 1 or 2 days postoperatively.

12.6 Illustrated Cases

12.6.1 Case 1 (Fig. 12.9)

A 56-year-old female patient complained of pain in both legs and neurological intermittent claudication for 2 years. Simple lateral radiography showed degenerative spondylolisthesis of L4–5 (Fig. 12.9a). Preoperative MRI showed central stenosis with spondylolisthesis at L4–5 level (Fig. 12.9b, c). We performed the ULIF via left-sided approach. Postoperative lateral radiography presented good reduction of spondylolisthesis (Fig. 12.9d). Postoperative MRI T2-weighted images showed improvement in decompressive status of central stenosis (Fig. 12.9e, f). The patient's symptoms significantly resolved after surgery.

12.6.2 Case 2 (Fig. 12.10)

A 71-year-old male patient suffered from right side dominant radicular pain in both legs and

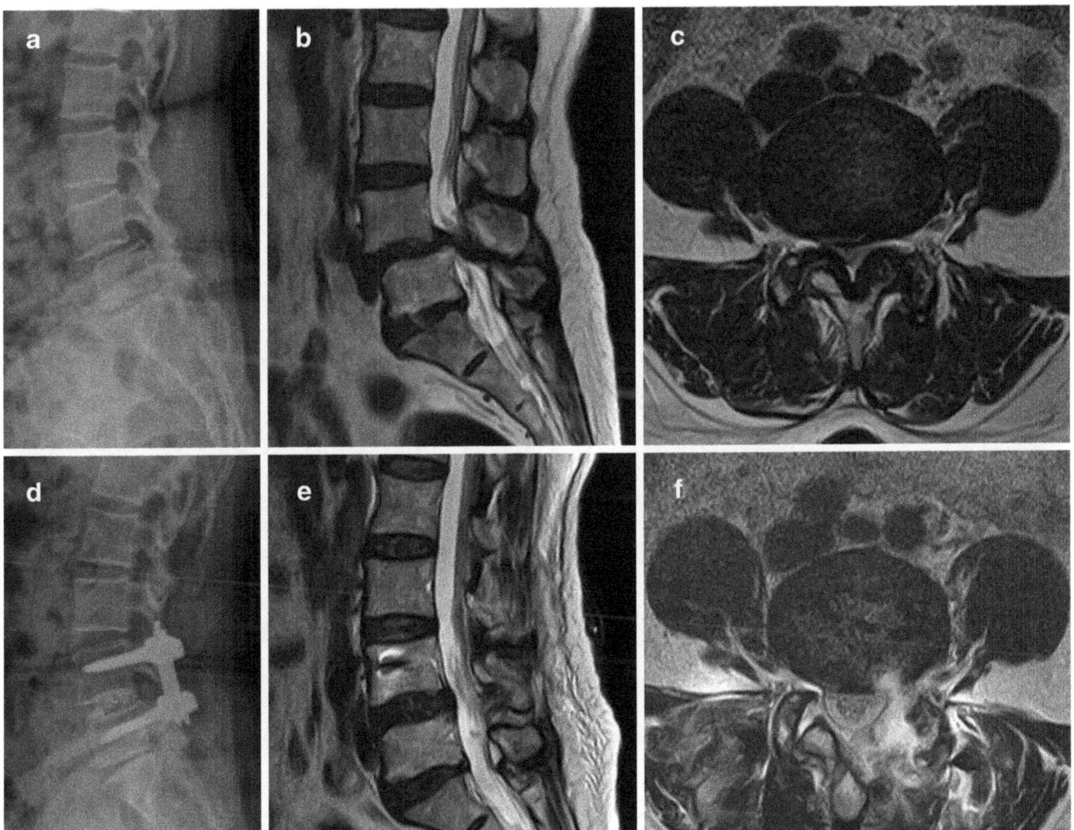

Fig. 12.9 Images of a 56-year-old woman with both buttock and radiating pain. Preoperative lateral radiography showed degenerative spondylolisthesis of L4–5 (**a**). Preoperative MR images show central stenosis with spondylolisthesis at L4–5 level (sagittal: **b**, axial: **c**). Postoperative lateral radiography and sagittal T2-weighted MRI presented good reduction of spondylolisthesis (**d** and **e**). Postoperative axial T2-weighted MRI show enough decompression with minimal paraspinal muscle damage (**f**)

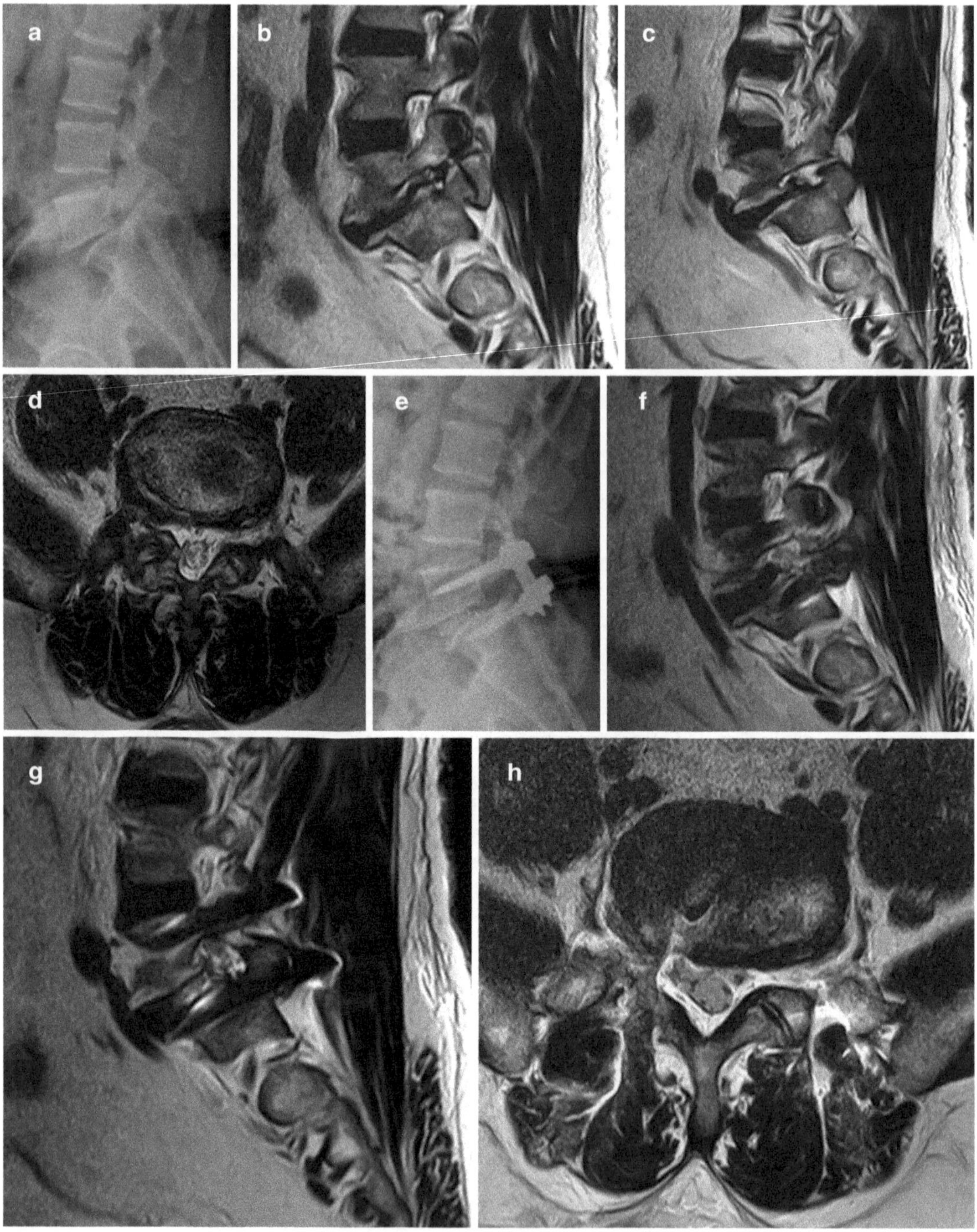

Fig. 12.10 Images of a 71-year-old man with claudication and radicular pain. Preoperative lateral radiography showed isthmic spondylolisthesis of L5-S1 (**a**). Preoperative MR images show bilateral foraminal stenosis on L5-S1 (sagittal: **b** (Right) and **c** (left), axial: **d**). Postoperative lateral radiography presented complete reduction of spondylolisthesis (**e**). Postoperative axial T2-weighted MRI shows well decompression of bilateral foraminal stenosis (sagittal: **f** (right) and **g** (left), axial: **h**)

neurological intermittent claudication for 1 year. Simple lateral radiography showed isthmic spondylolisthesis at L5–S1 (Fig. 12.10a). The patient's preoperative T2-weighted sagittal and axial MRI is shown in Fig. 12.10b–d. There was bilateral foraminal stenosis with isthmic spondylolisthesis at L5–S1. The patient underwent ULIF via right-side approach. Postoperative lateral radiography shows good reduction of spondylolisthesis (Fig. 12.10e). Postoperative MRI confirmed that both exiting roots of L5 were well decompressed (Fig. 12.10f–h). He had a significant reduction in radicular leg pain after surgery.

12.7 Complications and Management

12.7.1 Dural Tear

Most cases of dural tear can be controlled by fibrin collagen patch (TachoComb). Since most of them are not large enough to suture directly dural tears can be repaired by the application of a fibrin collagen patch (TachoComb) and bed rest for 5 to 7 days. Nonetheless, if dural tear is larger than 10 mm, dural defect should be repaired by suture directly under endoscopy or by conversion to microscopic surgery.

12.7.2 Postoperative Hematoma

Bleeding from the removed bone is controlled by applying bone wax. Bleeding from the epidural vessels can be coagulated using a hook RF probe. Hemostatic agents, such as soluble hemostatic gauze (WoundClot) or Gelfoam, are useful to control bleeding from hidden bleeding focus. After insertion of the cage, Gelfoam is applied to the annulotomy site to reduce bleeding from the bony endplate. Jackson–Pratt surgical drain (100 cc) is required after operation to prevent postoperative hematoma for 1 or 2 days. If there are neurological symptoms due to postoperative hematoma, hematoma can be removed by UBE using previous portals.

12.7.3 Fluid-Induced Complications

Headache, neck stiffness, seizure, and retroperitoneal fluid collection are some of the fluid-related complications; therefore caution is important for fluid output as UBE is a fluid medium surgery, and so the fluid-induced complications can be prevented by utilizing a semi-tubular retractor (Fig. 12.1a).

12.7.4 Cage Subsidence/Retropulsion

When placing the cages, injury of the bony endplate can cause cage subsidence. This complication can be avoided with careful endplate preparation under endoscopic guidance, especially in osteoporosis patients. Using a freer elevator or endplate remover rather than using a currette for endplate preparation may reduce endplate injury. The risk of cage retropulsion is reduced by placing the cage transversely without endplate injury, as well as by performing compression of the pedicle screws while locking the screws.

12.7.5 Neural Injury

Prevention is the best way to avoid neural injury. It is recommended not to use sharp instruments such as curettes or knife. Also, the RF probe should be used with much caution around neural structures. When using RF probe around the neural structures, surgeons should use it against neural structure with low power. The LF is left as a protector to avoid neural injury until bone working is finished. When the distance from lateral margin of thecal sac to the remaining ledge of the SAP is at least 8 mm, the cage can be safely placed without retraction-related neurapraxia. In placing the cage, thecal sac and nerve root can be protected with a specialized root retractor under fluoroscopic guidance, which reduces the possibility of retraction-related neurapraxia.

12.8 Surgical Tips and Pitfalls

1. In general, spine surgeons are familiar with left-side approach, but in case of high lordotic angle of surgical level such as L5–S1 level, or when direct neural decompression of right foraminal stenosis is needed, right-side approach is more suitable.
2. When a contralateral decompression can be performed through sublaminar approach, it is important to sufficiently remove the base of the spinous process to obtain working space because the base of the spinous process obstructs the placement of the endoscope and the surgical instruments.
3. The contralateral facectectomy through sublaminar approach provides release, which helps in reduction of spondylolisthesis and making lordosis.
4. When the facet joint osteophytes are prominent or greater reduction of spondylolisthesis is required, two new portals are created on the contralateral side to perform total removal of IAP.
5. As inadequate resection of the medial aspect of SAP can induce neural injury during insertion of the cage, the distance from lateral margin of thecal sac to the remaining ledge of the SAP should be at least 8 mm.
6. When the cage is inserted into the disc space, we do not attempt to fully expose the ipsilateral exiting nerve root because this helps to protect the exiting nerve root.
7. Care should be taken to adequately perform endplate preparation at the contralateral side, so that the cage is able to be inserted from the contralateral side with larger fusion surface area.
8. With the help of angled endplate removers, curved pituitary forceps, and 30° scope, contralateral endplate preparation could be achieved under endoscopic guidance.
9. During endplate preparation, careful attention should be paid not to injure the bony endplate or the anterior longitudinal ligament.
10. In patients with a high-grade spondylolisthesis or significant disc narrowing, removal of upper edge of lower vertebral body using an osteotome aids in easier cage insertion and prevents exiting root injury.
11. It is necessary to avoid continuous irrigation during insertion of bone graft and the cage, in order to prevent bone chip loss.
12. An appropriate cage is inserted under fluoroscopic guidance with a specialized root retractor, which is anchored at lower vertebral body edge, to protect the exposed thecal sac and traversing nerve root.
13. After cage insertion, cage is placed with a cage impactor to ensure it is located in the anterior and central portion of the disc space. To make segmental lordosis, it should be put on the stronger anterior ring apophysis rather than on the soft central cancellous portion.
14. Gelfoam is applied to the annulotomy site to reduce loss of bone chip and bleeding from the bony endplate.

References

1. Gejo R, Matsui H, Kawaguchi Y, Ishihara H, Tsuji H. Serial changes in trunk muscle performance after posterior lumbar surgery. Spine (Phila Pa 1976). 1999;24(10):1023–8.
2. Lee KH, Yue WM, Yeo W, Soeharno H, Tan SB. Clinical and radiological outcomes of open versus minimally invasive transforaminal lumbar interbody fusion. Eur Spine J. 2012;21(11):2265–70.
3. Park MK, Park SA, Son SK, Park WW, Choi SH. Clinical and radiological outcomes of unilateral biportal endoscopic lumbar interbody fusion (ULIF) compared with conventional posterior lumbar interbody fusion (PLIF): 1-year follow-up. Neurosurg Rev. 2019;42(3):753–61.
4. Heo DH, Park CK. Clinical results of percutaneous biportal endoscopic lumbar interbody fusion with application of enhanced recovery after surgery. Neurosurg Focus. 2019;46(4):E18.
5. Kim JE, Yoo HS, Choi DJ, Park EJ, Jee SM. Comparison of minimal invasive versus biportal endoscopic transforaminal lumbar interbody fusion for single-level lumbar disease. Clin Spine Surg. 2021;34(2):E64–71.
6. Kang MS, You KH, Choi JY, Heo DH, Chung HJ, Park HJ. Minimally invasive transforaminal lumbar interbody fusion using the biportal endoscopic techniques versus microscopic tubular technique. Spine J. 2021;21(12):2066–77.
7. Heo DH, Hong YH, Lee DC, Chung HJ, Park CK. Technique of biportal endoscopic transforaminal lumbar interbody fusion. Neurospine. 2020;17(Suppl 1):S129–S37.

13 Unilateral Biportal Endoscopic Transforaminal Lumbar Interbody Fusion, Modified Techniques

Dong Hwa Heo, Young Ho Hong, Jin Hwa Eum, and Hungtae Chung

13.1 Introduction

Various types of endoscopic lumbar interbody fusion surgery have been attempted for the treatment of lumbar degenerative disease [1–5]. Among them, biportal endoscopic lumbar interbody fusion approaches have advantages such as the ability to perform direct neural decompression as in open surgery, a lower incidence of neural injury, the insertion of a conventional transforaminal lumbar interbody fusion (TLIF) cage, and endoscopic endplate preparation [1, 3]. Unilateral biportal endoscopic (UBE) fusion surgery has the benefits of endoscopic spine surgery, as well as those of minimally invasive lumbar fusion surgery [5, 6].

Supplementary Information The online version contains supplementary material available at [https://doi.org/10.1007/978-981-16-8201-8_13].

D. H. Heo
Neurosurgery, Endoscopic Spine Surgery Center, Seoul Bumin Hospital, Seoul, South Korea

Y. H. Hong (✉)
Neurosurgery, Spine Center, Barunsesang Hospital, Bundang, South Korea

J. H. Eum
Neurosurgery, Spine Center, Burjeel Royal Hospital, Al Ain, Abu Dhabi, UAE

H. Chung
Orthopedics, Endoscopic Spine Surgery Center, Seoul Bumin Hospital, Seoul, South Korea

Recently, modified UBE TLIF techniques were introduced and tried. The first was modified far-lateral UBE TLIF using large-sized cages like lateral lumbar interbody fusion cages [2]. The other was the two-cage insertion technique [5]. The goals of these two modified UBE TLIF techniques are the prevention of cage subsidence and the enhancement of interbody fusion [2, 5]. We described the details of these modified UBE TLIF surgical techniques.

13.2 Indications and Contraindications

The indications and contraindications of these UBE fusion techniques are the same as those for minimally invasive TLIF using tubular retractor systems [3]. We have usually recommended these modified UBE TLIF techniques for one or two-level diseases. We suggested that multilevel disease may be a relative contraindication for endoscopic lumbar interbody fusion surgery including the UBE approach [3, 5].

- Indications: spondylolisthesis, spondylolysis, recurrent disc herniation, and central and foraminal stenosis.
- Contraindications: infection, deformity, and congenital anomaly.

D. H. Heo et al. (eds.), *Unilateral Biportal Endoscopic Spine Surgery*,
https://doi.org/10.1007/978-981-16-8201-8_13

13.3 Special Instruments

We used the usual UBE tool kit set and UBE endoscopic systems. Radiofrequency (RF) probes and their console system were used [6]. Customized large-sized cages were newly produced (Fig. 13.1a). Recently, we used new large-sized cages instead of the usual TLIF cages. The size and shape of the customized large-sized cage were similar to those of oblique lumbar interbody fusion cages. A customized cage guide was very useful for the safe insertion of a large-sized cage

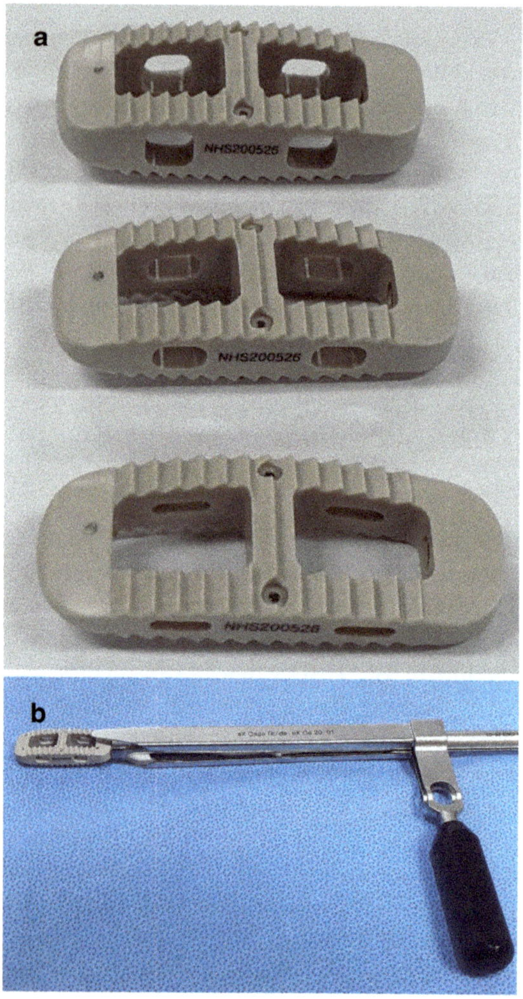

Fig. 13.1 Newly produced cages for far-lateral modified UBE TLIF. The size of the cage was similar to that of OLIF cages (**a**) A customized cage guide for modified far-lateral UBE TLIF (**b**). This cage guide was used for the insertion of a large-sized cage

(Fig. 13.1b). Customized endplate dissectors and angled curettes were useful for endplate preparation.

In the two-cage insertion technique, we usually used posterior lumbar interbody fusion (PLIF) cages.

13.4 Anesthesia and Position

We prefer general endotracheal anesthesia in patients in the prone position. Epidural anesthesia with intravenous sedation was another anesthesia option for single-level UBE interbody fusion procedures in selective cases. Both a Jackson table and Wilson table were available for these UBE fusion techniques.

13.5 Surgical Steps

13.5.1 Modified Far-lateral TLIF Using UBE (Extreme Lateral TLIF, Video 13.1)

Two ipsilateral skin incisions were made on the lateral border of the pedicles to make two portals (Fig. 13.2). The left-side approach was preferred by right-handed surgeons. Two portals (endoscopic portal and working portal) were needed for this technique (Fig. 13.3a). The endoscopic portal was only used for the endoscopy and the working portal was used for the surgical instruments. Serial dilators were inserted for the caudal working portal, and a working sheath was inserted after serial dilation (Fig. 13.3b). An additional cranial skin incision was made, and an endoscopy trocar was inserted (endoscopic portal). The laminar and facet joint were dissected and exposed by radiofrequency (RF). Ipsilateral laminotomy and total facetectomy were performed using a drill, osteotome, and Kerrison punches. If there was central or lateral recess stenosis, we removed the bilateral ligamentum flavum (Fig. 13.4a, b). If the patient had foraminal stenosis and exiting nerve root indentation, we decompressed the exiting nerve root by removing the foraminal ligament. We measured the

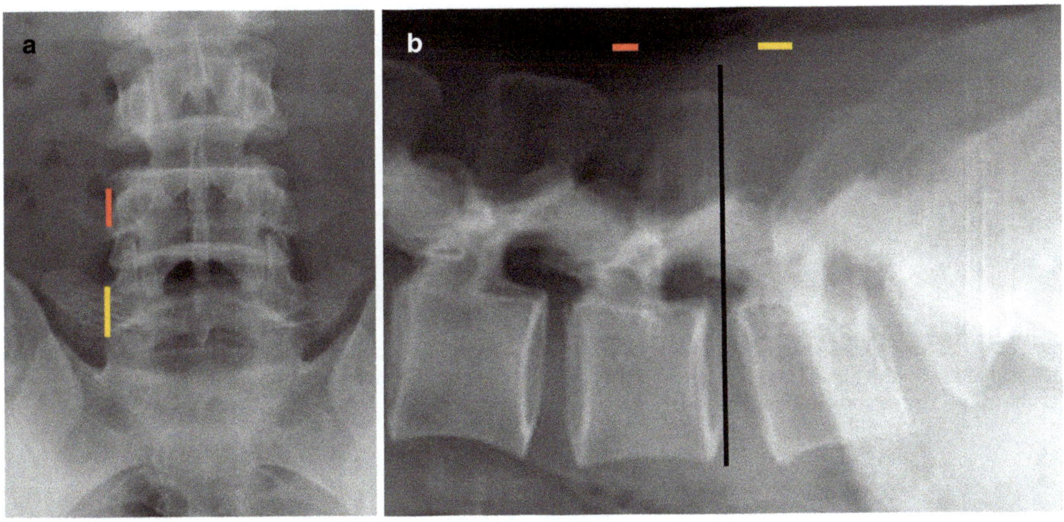

Fig. 13.2 Two skin incision points for two portals (**a**). In a left-side approach, a cranial port (red line) was made for the endoscopic portal and a caudal port (yellow line) was made for the working portal (**b**). Usually, two skin incisions were made at the lateral border of the pedicles (**a**)

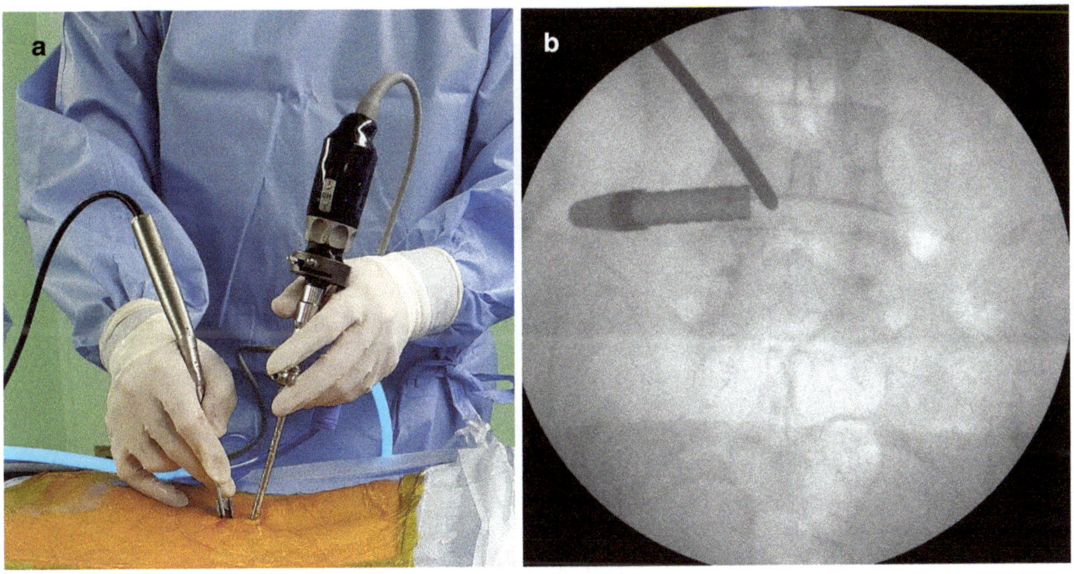

Fig. 13.3 An overview of UBE TLIF surgery (**a**). Intraoperative C-arm fluoroscopic view after making two portals (**b**)

distance between the traversing and exiting nerve roots (Fig. 13.4c). If this distance was greater than 16 mm, a large-sized cage could be safely inserted without nerve root injury. After decompression, a total discectomy was done using a shaver and pituitary forceps. The cartilaginous endplate was separated from the osseous endplate using dissectors and curettes (Fig. 13.5a). Contralateral disc materials and the cartilaginous endplate were removed by angled curettes and angled pituitary forceps (Fig. 13.5).

After endplate preparation was complete (Fig. 13.5b), a large-sized cage was inserted. Sometimes, we made an additional far-lateral portal for the insertion of a large-sized cage [2]. The dura was medially retracted using a dura

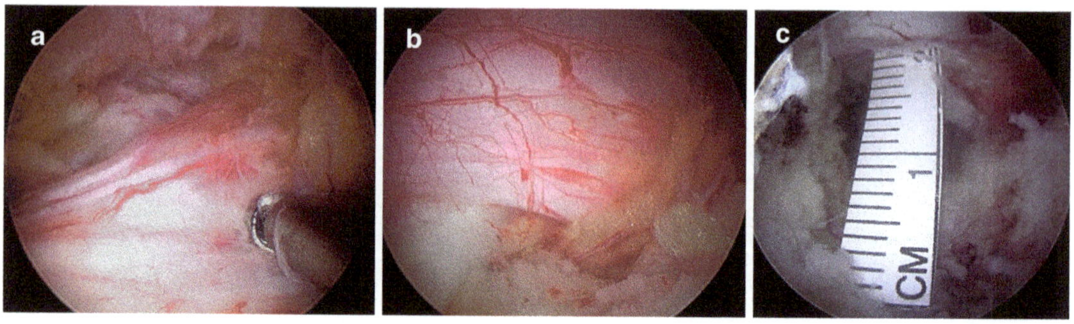

Fig. 13.4 Intraoperative endoscopic images of decompression of the central canal and facetectomy. The contralateral (**a**) and ipsilateral (**b**) traversing nerve roots were completely decompressed. Measurement of the distance between the exiting and traversing nerve roots (**c**)

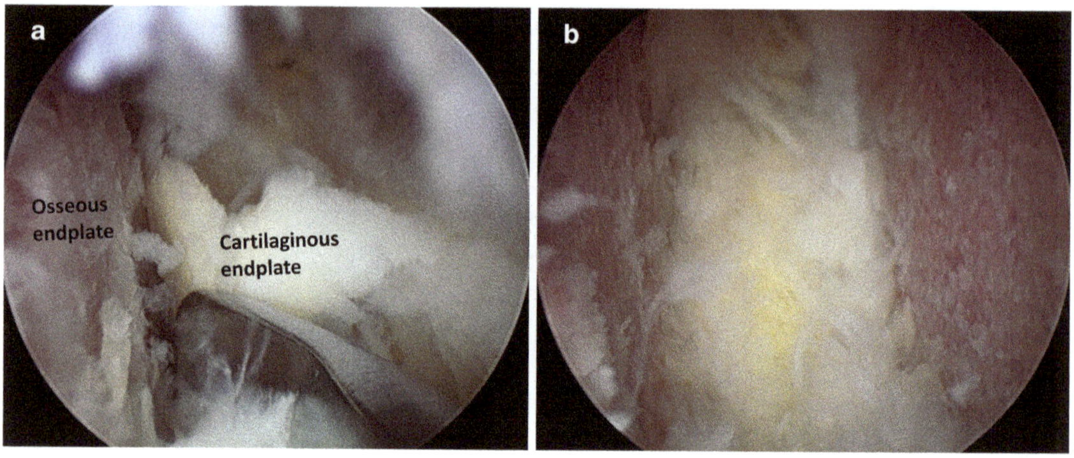

Fig. 13.5 Intraoperative endoscopic views of endplate preparation. The cartilaginous endplate was separated from the osseous endplate using a curette and dissectors (**a**). Complete endplate preparation was performed without osseous endplate injury (**b**)

retractor and a customized cage guide was inserted into the disc space (Fig. 13.6). Finally, we put in a large-sized cage with fusion material packing under C-arm fluoroscopic monitoring (Fig. 13.6). A sagittally oriented cage should be rotated transversely (coronal orientation of cage) for stability and segmental lordosis. We used cage impactors for transverse repositioning under C-arm monitoring (Figs. 13.7 and 13.8). An epidural drainage catheter was inserted and placed to prevent postoperative epidural hematoma. We also inserted bilateral percutaneous pedicle screws.

13.5.2 Modified UBE TLIF Two-cage Insertion Technique (Video 13.2)

The overall procedures were the same as those for routine UBE TLIF or modified far-lateral UBE TLIF. From making the skin incision to making two portals to endplate preparation, this technique was the same as for routine UBE TLIF. This technique used two short PLIF cages instead of TLIF cages. Due to the small size of PLIF cages, we could put in two cages safely and easily.

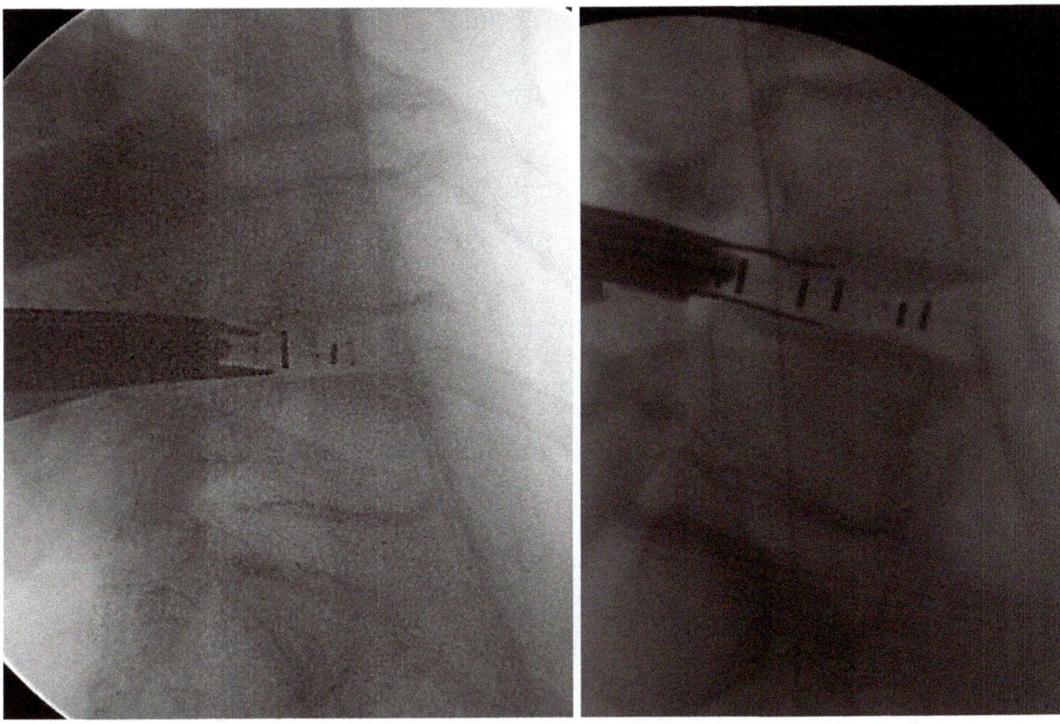

Fig. 13.6 A customized cage guide was used for a large-sized cage insertion

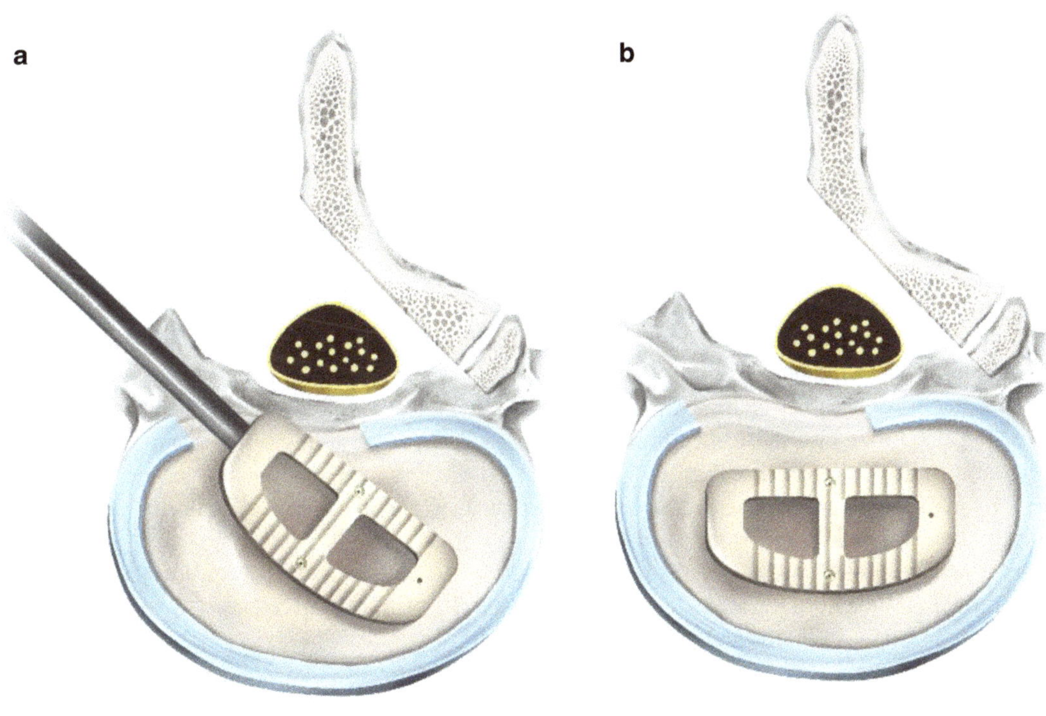

Fig. 13.7 First, a large-sized cage was inserted obliquely (**a**), then it was repositioned transversely using a cage impactor (**b**)

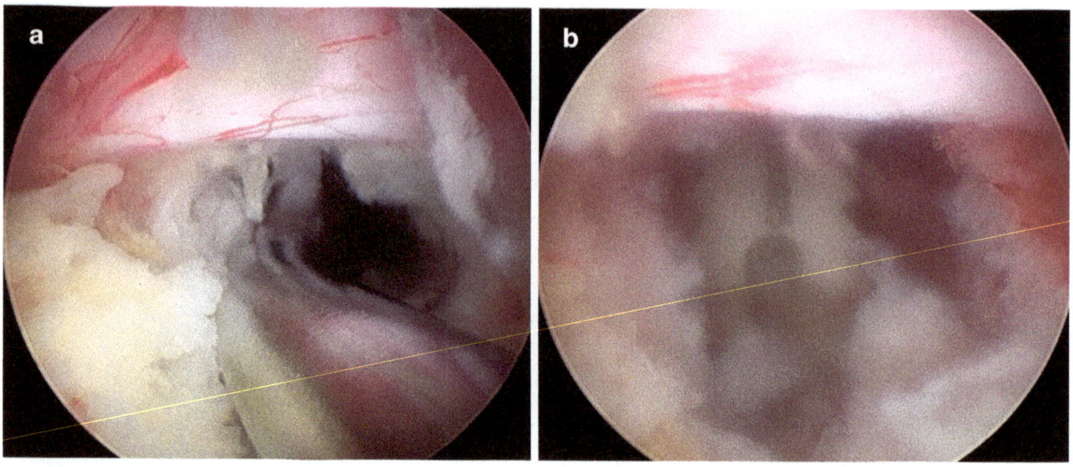

Fig. 13.8 The cage was repositioned transversely using a cage impactor (**a**). The endoscopic image shows the transverse position of a large cage (**b**)

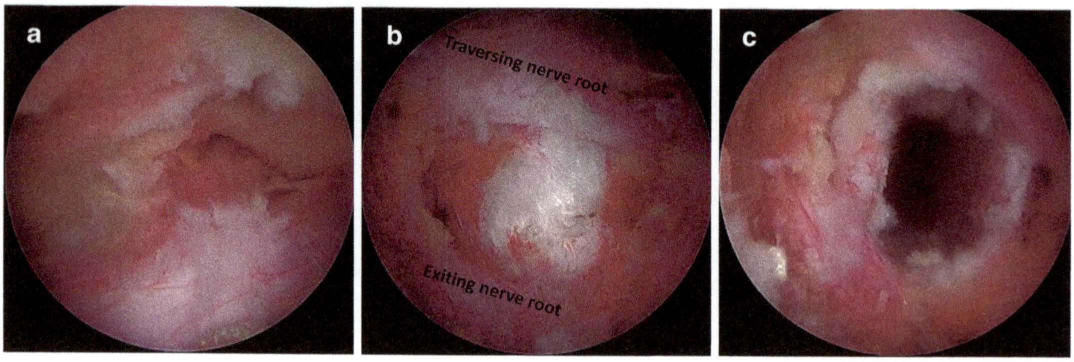

Fig. 13.9 Intraoperative endoscopic images of complete neural decompression and discectomy. The contralateral traversing nerve root (**a**), ipsilateral traversing, and exiting nerve root (**b**) were decompressed. Total discectomy was also performed (**c**)

Before inserting two cages, we performed complete neural decompression including the contralateral traversing nerve root, ipsilateral traversing nerve root, and ipsilateral exiting nerve root (Fig. 13.9). We also performed total discectomy and endplate preparation (Fig. 13.9).

Two PLIF cages were inserted through one side of the unilateral laminotomy and facetectomy area (Figs. 13.10 and 13.11). After medial dura retraction by a dura retractor, the first PLIF cage was inserted medially and contralaterally (Figs. 13.10a and 13.11a). Sometimes, we used a cage pusher for cage insertion more medially. A second PLIF cage was put into the interbody in the space next to the first cage (Fig. 13.10b). Fusion materials such as bone chips were put into the gap space between the two cages (Fig. 13.10c). Two cages were safely inserted under magnified endoscopic view (Figs. 13.10 and 13.11).

After two-cage insertion, we performed percutaneous pedicle screw fixation.

13.6 Case Reports

1. **Case 1:** A 64-year-old female patient complained of severe bilateral leg pain with neurological intermittent claudication.

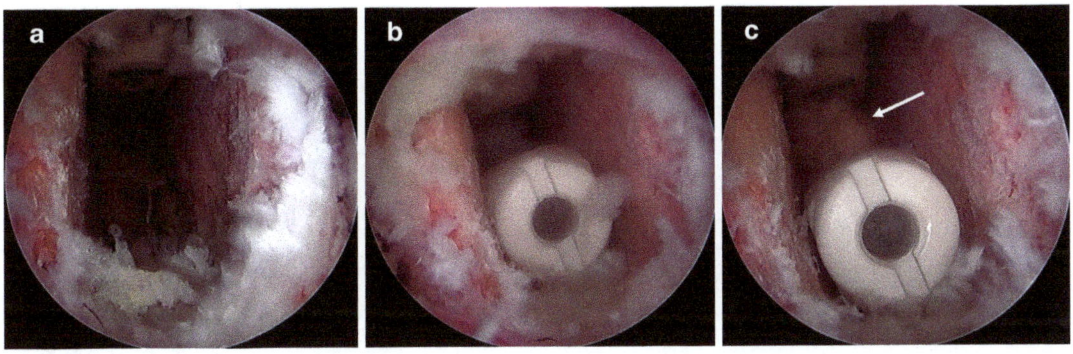

Fig. 13.10 Two PLIF cages were inserted through the left side only. The first cage was inserted medially (**a**). And a second cage was inserted (**b**). Additional fusion materials were put into the gap between the two cages (**c**) (white arrow)

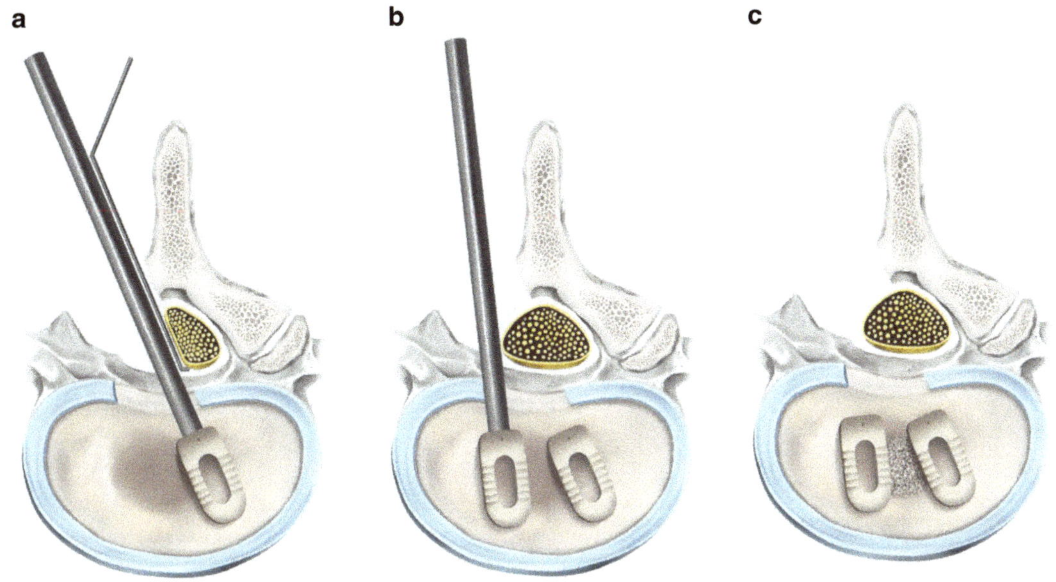

Fig. 13.11 Schematic illustration of the two-cage insertion technique. (**a**) First cage insertion. (**b**) Second cage insertion. (**c**) Final view of two cages insertion

The preoperative X-ray showed degenerative spondylolisthesis of L4–5. Preoperative magnetic resonance imaging (MRI) revealed spondylolisthesis with central stenosis at L4–5. We performed a modified far-lateral UBE TLIF using a large-sized cage at L4–5 (Fig. 13.12 and Video 13.1). After surgery, preoperative spondylolisthesis was completely resolved, and central stenosis was decompressed, and a large-sized cage as in OLIF was placed in the L4–5 interbody area. The preoperative symptoms were significantly improved postoperatively.

2. **Case 2:** A 65-year-old male patient presented with radicular pain and tingling sensations in both legs.

The patient also complained of severe back pain. The preoperative X-ray and MRI images showed spondylolisthesis at L4–5 (Fig. 13.13). Central stenosis with foraminal stenosis was also detected. We performed UBE TLIF using the two-cage insertion technique via a left-side approach (Video 13.2). The postoperative X-ray images showed the reduction of spondylolisthesis and the

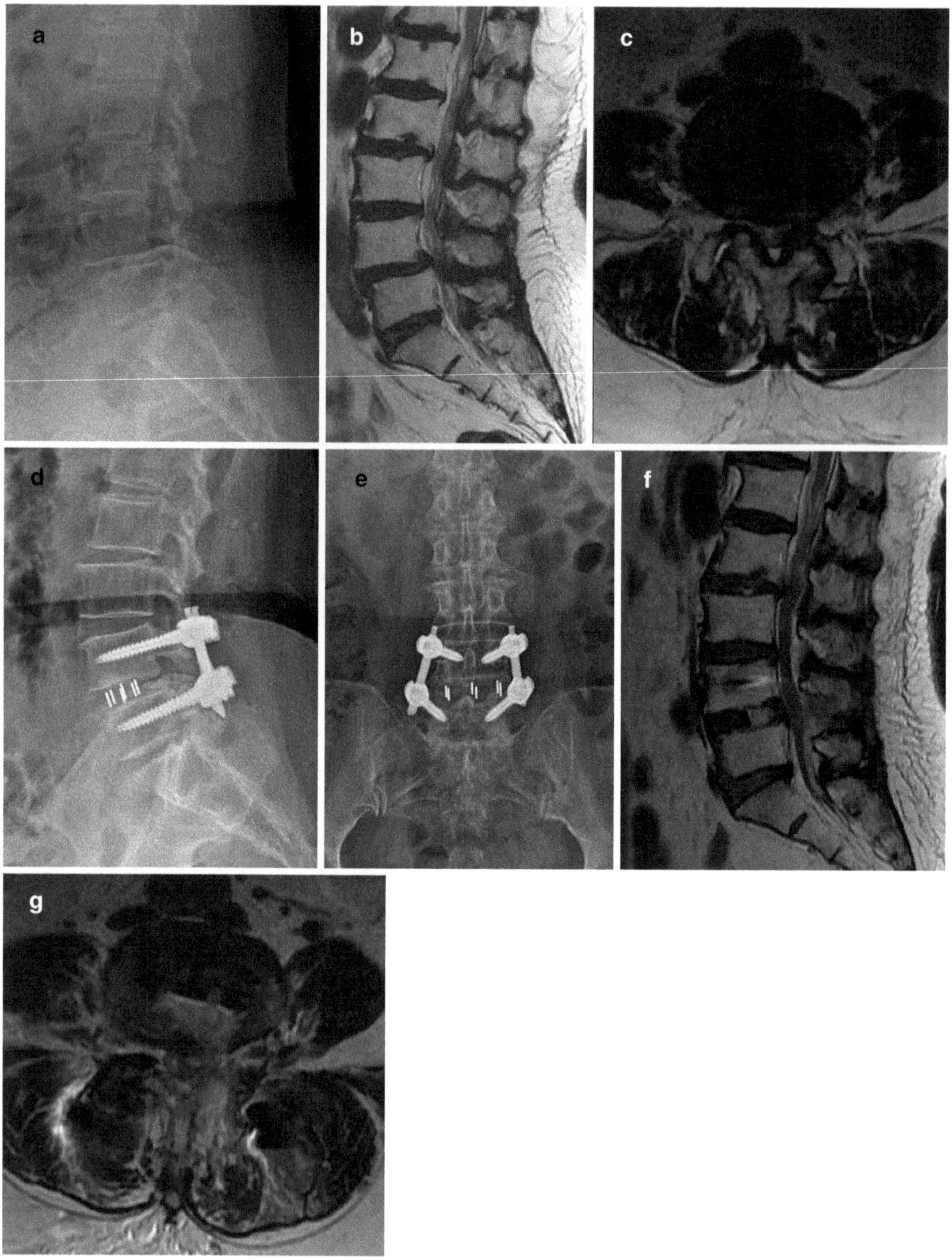

Fig. 13.12 Radiographic images of a 64-year-old female patient. The preoperative X-ray showed degenerative spondylolisthesis of L4–5 (**a**). The MRI images showed spondylolisthesis with severe stenosis of L4–5 (**b** and **c**). This patient underwent a modified far-lateral UBE TLIF at L4–5 (**d** and **e**). The postoperative X-ray and MRI images revealed the complete reduction of spondylolisthesis and decompression of the central canal at L4–5 (**f** and **g**)

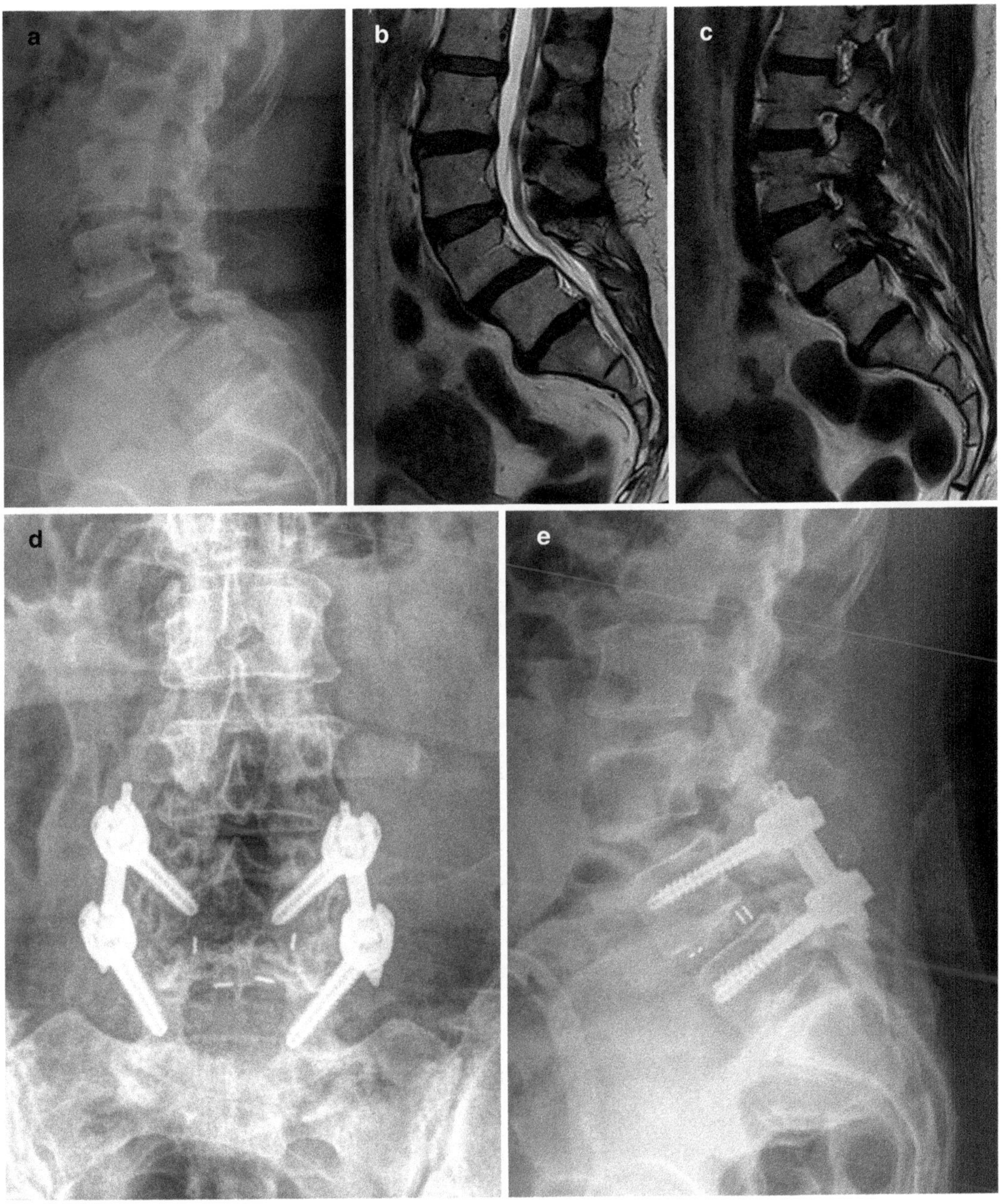

Fig. 13.13 X-ray and MRI images of a 65-year-old male patient. The preoperative X-ray and MRI images showed the spondylolisthesis, foraminal stenosis, and central stenosis of L4–5 (**a**, **b**, and **c**). We performed UBE-TLIF with the two-cage insertion technique via a left-side approach (**d** and **e**). The postoperative X-ray revealed the reduction of spondylolisthesis and two cages inserted at L4–5 (**d** and **e**). The postoperative MRI images showed the resolution of central and foraminal stenosis and the complete reduction of spondylolisthesis at L4–5 (**f**, **g**, and **h**)

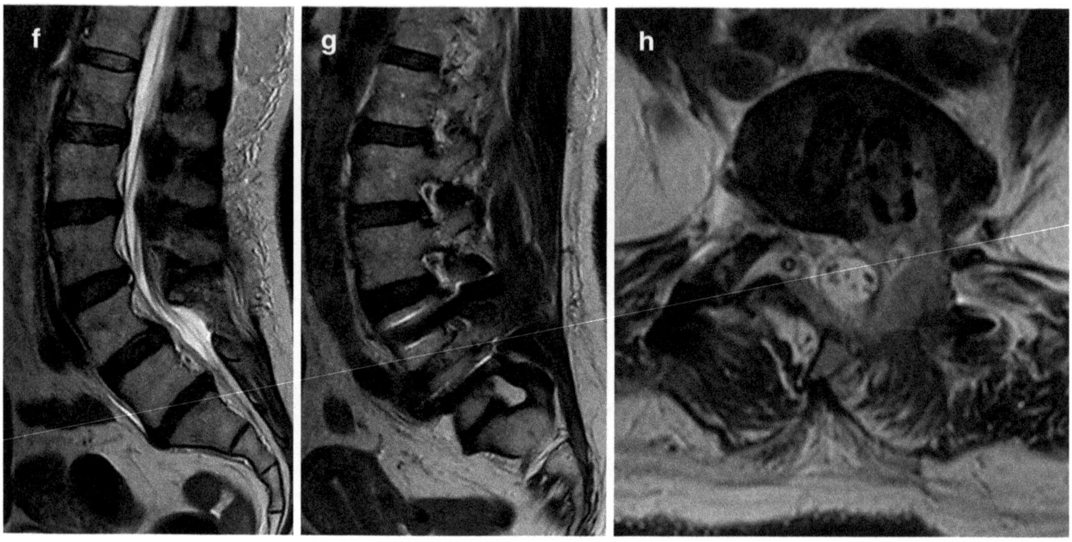

Fig. 13.13 (continued)

insertion of two cages at the L4–5 area (Fig. 13.13). The postoperative MRI images revealed the complete decompression of central and foraminal stenosis. Two PLIF cages were placed at the interbody space of L4–5 (Fig. 13.13). After surgery, pain and tingling sensations in the legs disappeared.

13.7 Complications and Management

The complications of these modified UBE TLIF techniques were similar to those of minimally invasive TLIF using a tubular retractor and were usually minor.

1. Dural tear: A small durotomy area can be repaired by Tachosil or non-penetrating vascular clips [7].
2. Postoperative epidural hematoma: Meticulous bleeding control was important. A drainage catheter was routinely inserted to prevent postoperative epidural hematoma.
3. Neural injury: When we put cages into the disc space, there was a possibility of neural tissue injury. A dura retractor and cage guide were important to prevent neural tissue injury during cage insertion.

13.8 Surgical Tips and Pitfalls

13.8.1 Modified Far-lateral UBE TLIF (Extreme Lateral UBE TLIF)

It is very important to preoperatively measure the distance between the exiting and traversing nerve roots using preoperative axial MRI. If this distance was more than 16 mm, a large-sized cage could be safely inserted without neural injury. This distance is relatively wide in the lower lumbar area including the L4–5 and L5-S1 levels. If the distance between the exiting and traversing nerve roots was narrow (less than 15 mm), we put in routine TLIF cages or two PLIF cages instead of a large-sized cage.

We strongly recommend using a specialized cage guide during cage insertion. C-arm monitoring was important during cage insertion.

13.8.2 Two-cage Insertion Technique

This two-cage UBE TLIF insertion technique used routine PLIF cages. Any PLIF cages can be used in this fusion technique. The first cage should be put in deeply and contralaterally. If the first cage is inserted ipsilaterally, a cage impactor should be used to push the cage to the opposite side. When inserting the second cage, care should be taken not to push the first cage deeply. If there is still space in the disc space after inserting both cages, we inserted fusion materials such as a bone chip into the disc space or in the gap between the two cages. When the cage was inserted, we preferred to use C-arm fluoroscopic monitoring.

References

1. Heo DH, Park CK. Clinical results of percutaneous biportal endoscopic lumbar interbody fusion with application of enhanced recovery after surgery. Neurosurg Focus. 2019;46(4):E18.
2. Heo DH, Eum JH, Jo JY, Chung H. Modified far lateral endoscopic transforaminal lumbar interbody fusion using a biportal endoscopic approach: technical report and preliminary results. Acta Neurochir. 2021;163(4):1205–9.
3. Heo DH, Lee DC, Kim HS, Park CK, Chung H. Clinical results and complications of endoscopic lumbar interbody fusion for lumbar degenerative disease: a meta-analysis. World Neurosurg. 2021;145:396–404.
4. Kang MS, You KH, Choi JY, Heo DH, Chung HJ, Park HJ. Minimally invasive transforaminal lumbar interbody fusion using the biportal endoscopic techniques versus microscopic tubular technique. Spine J. 2021;21(12):2066–77.
5. Heo DH, Hong YH, Lee DC, Chung HJ, Park CK. Technique of biportal endoscopic transforaminal lumbar interbody fusion. Neurospine. 2020;17(Suppl 1):S129–s37.
6. Hwa Eum J, Hwa Heo D, Son SK, Park CK. Percutaneous biportal endoscopic decompression for lumbar spinal stenosis: a technical note and preliminary clinical results. J Neurosurg Spine. 2016;24(4):602–7.
7. Heo DH, Ha JS, Lee DC, Kim HS, Chung HJ. Repair of incidental durotomy using sutureless nonpenetrating clips via biportal endoscopic surgery. Global Spine J. 2020.:2192568220956606; https://doi.org/10.1177/2192568220956606.

Lumbar Interbody Fusion Extension for Symptomatic Adjacent Segment Disease by Unilateral Biportal Endoscopic Approach

14

Ji Soo Ha, Dong Hwa Heo, Kang Hyon Sung, Yong Sang Kim, and Dae Hyun Kim

14.1 Introduction

In an aging society, the overall rates of lumbar or lumbosacral fusion surgery for a variety of spinal pathologies, including degenerative conditions, have exponentially increased [1–3]. Accordingly, the pathological status of adjacent segmental degeneration after lumbar interbody fusion also increases due to acceleration of mechanical stress and unstabilized motion rising on the adjacent segment after surgery [1, 3]. Adjacent segmental disease (ASD) may manifest as spinal stenosis, spondylolisthesis, segmental instability, disc degeneration, and facet arthropathy [1–3]. Conventional lumbar fusion extension surgery (FES) has been considered as a treatment option for symptomatic ASD after lumbar interbody fusion surgery. However, extensive muscle dissection and revision of the previously operated area are significant challenges that can occur with FES. Lumbar interbody fusion using a unilateral biportal endoscopic (UBE) approach has recently been used to treat lumbar degenerative disease [4–6]. However, to our knowledge, the UBE approach to FES has not previously been reported as a treatment option for symptomatic ASD after lumbar interbody fusion surgery.

Lumbar interbody fusion surgery using UBE has the advantage of reducing damage to normal structures [7, 8]. Therefore, using UBE in FES may reduce muscle damage and size of skin incisions. Here, we introduce and describe the UBE approach to performing FES. We include descriptions of two patient cases.

J. S. Ha
Neurosurgery, Spine Center, Seojaigon Linker Hospital, Seoul, South Korea

D. H. Heo (✉)
Neurosurgery, Endoscopic Spine Surgery Center, Seoul Bumin Hospital, Seoul, South Korea

K. H. Sung
Neurosurgery, Spine Center, Samsung Barun Hospital, Seoul, South Korea

Y. S. Kim
Neurosurgery, Jinju Barun Hospital, Jinju, South Korea

D. H. Kim
Neurosurgery, Spine Center, Daegu Catholic University, Daegu, South Korea

14.2 Indication and Contraindication

Briefly, indications of UBE FES are the same as those of conventional FES for symptomatic ASD. However, the difficulty of this technique depends on how laborious it is to remove the previously inserted pedicle screws and rods by endoscopy.

D. H. Heo et al. (eds.), *Unilateral Biportal Endoscopic Spine Surgery*,
https://doi.org/10.1007/978-981-16-8201-8_14

Indications
- Adjacent lumbar stenosis
- Adjacent lumbar instability
- Instrument failure due to fractured screws and rods

Contraindications
- Junctional vertebral fracture
- Infection
- Junctional kyphosis
- Deformity correction surgery

14.3 Anesthesia and Positions

The prone position under general endotracheal anesthesia is recommended. However, for experts, limited epidural anesthesia with sedation may be used for short segments or hardware revision only.

14.4 Special Preparations Before Surgery

Because previously placed pedicle screws or rods must be removed, surgical records should be reviewed to determine the exact type of surgical instruments required. It is necessary to prepare the appropriate surgical instruments required to remove the previously applied hardware, such as a pedicle screwdriver and cap driver.

Furthermore, dynamic X-ray images and three-dimensional computed tomography scans must be performed before surgery to confirm the states of existing pedicle screws and rods. This allows us to note issues such as screw loosening and posterolateral fusion bone mass around the rods and screws.

14.5 Surgical Steps in Cases of L4-5 Interbody Fusion with Rod Extension at L4-L5-S1

14.5.1 Interbody Cage Insertion for ASD

The first step is to implement an endoscopic transforaminal lumbar interbody fusion (TLIF) for adjacent levels that need to be extended before removing the previously inserted pedicle screws and rods. The portal is designed under C-arm fluoroscopy, similar to the well-known UBE TLIF technique [5, 6, 9]. We make three 1.5 cm length ipsilateral skin incisions vertically or transversely on the pedicles or screw heads of the ASD level and previous fusion level (Fig. 14.1). In the case of left-sided approaches for upper-level ASD, the left cranial hole acts as the endoscopic viewing portal, and the right caudal hole acts as the working portal. After making two small skin and fascia incisions, we insert serial dilators and dissectors to make two portals. If it feels like we are touching the dorsal surface of the lamina, periosteal dissection is achieved gently after confirming the location using a C-arm fluoroscope. Finally, endoscopic irrigation systems are used, and the irrigation fluids are drained from viewing the endoscopic portal to the working portal. Irrigation water naturally forms a water chamber above the lamina, which facilitates bleeding control and provides clear surgical field visibility, creating a space for endoscopic interbody fusion. We first perform unilateral laminectomy for bilateral decompression and facetectomy through a highly magnified endoscopic view [5, 6, 9]. Endplate preparation can be achieved safely with confidence by inserting the endoscope directly into the intervertebral space. Finally, a long, straight cage is inserted after dural retraction under fluoroscopic guidance [6, 9]. This technique is very similar to the UBE TLIF procedures.

14.5.2 Previously Inserted "Set Pedicle Screws" Removal

Skin incisions (1–1.5 cm) are made according to the lateral margin of the pedicle. These incisions are used as conduits for removing pre-inserted screws or inserting new percutaneous pedicle screws. If there are skin incisions already made for interbody fusion extension, they can be used to remove or insert screws. To remove the previously inserted screw, we insert the working portal and the viewing portal together through one skin incision directly above the target screw to be

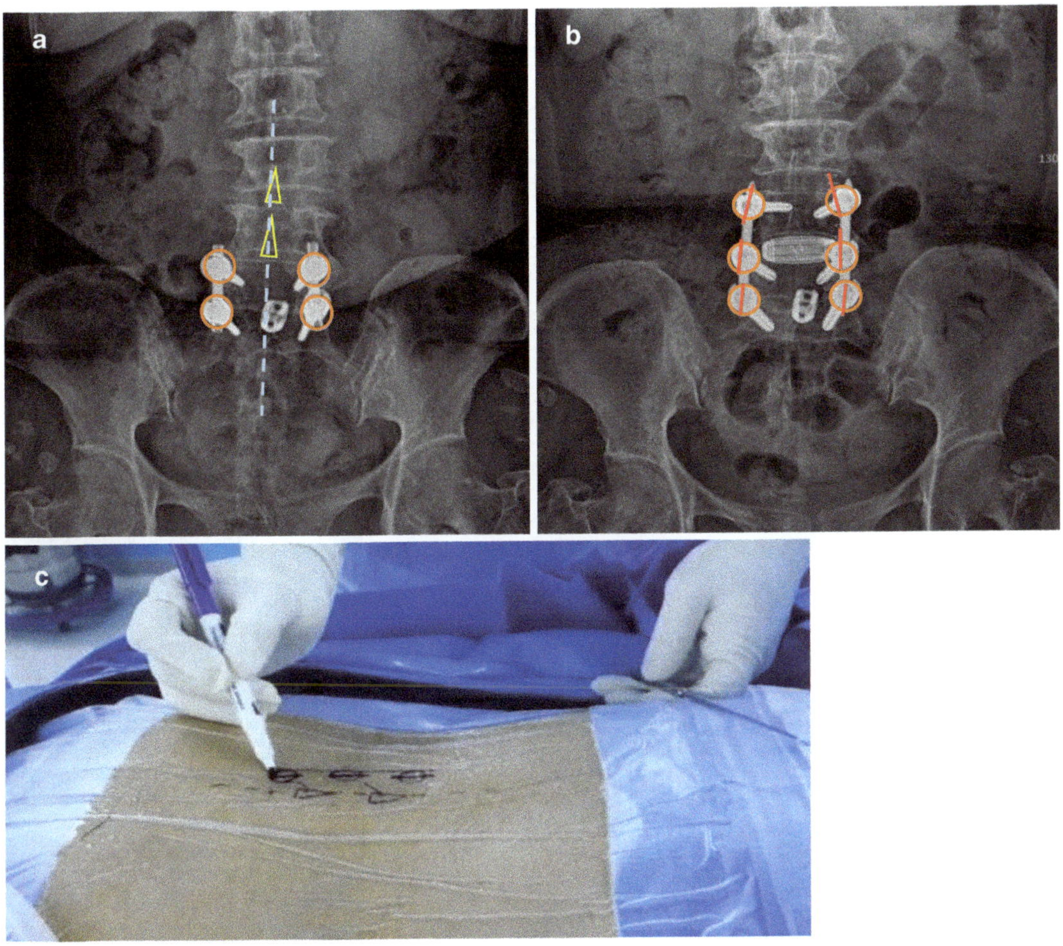

Fig. 14.1 Surgical markings over the pedicle screw heads (circles). Three skin incisions are made vertically on midline of each pedicle (**a, b**, and **c**). The authors prefer vertical skin incisions. These skin incisions are used for endoscopic portals and the working portal. In addition, the skin incision points are also used for the removal of old screws as well as insertion of new percutaneous pedicle screws

removed (Fig. 14.2a). Because the UBE endoscope is approximately 4 mm in diameter, there is enough space to work with two portals at once. We perform muscle dissection using radiofrequency coagulation/ablation and to find the head of the screw. The exposed set screw can be checked after peeling off the adhesion covering the head. Next, the viewing portal is pulled out and inserted through a new incision made for insertion of the nearest pedicle screw. As a result, the working and viewing portals can be inserted into each portal to reduce the burden of using the instrument. If it is possible to find the set screw through the resettled endoscope, it is removed using the set screw remover through the working portal.

14.5.3 Previously Inserted "Rods" Removal

If all the set screws of the previously inserted ipsilateral pedicle screws are removed, we expose the rod around the head. It is not necessary to expose the whole rod because the rod will be naturally pulled out through the skin wound due to its shape instead of removing it in the direction to the top (Fig. 14.2b). If only the rod around the head is exposed sufficiently, the curved curate is placed on the ventral side of the rod, and the rod is lifted slightly through the lever principle. After holding the end part of the exposed rods with a rod holder, we pull out the rods gently toward the incision.

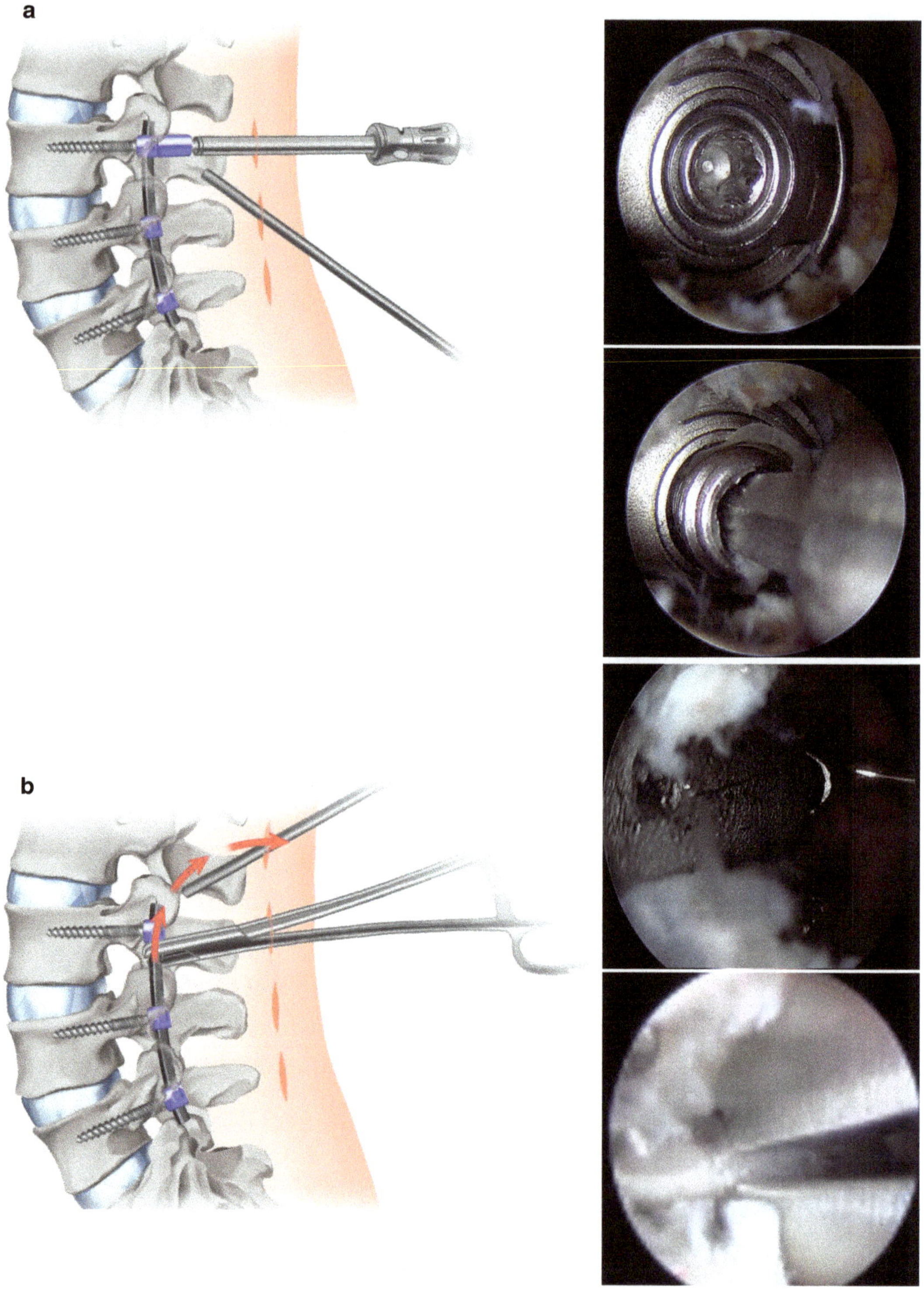

Fig. 14.2 Schematic illustrations and actual endoscopic view photos. (**a**) After exposing the pedicle screw head, the cap driver is inserted into the cap under an endoscopic view. Finally, the caps are removed from the pedicle screw head. (**b**) The rods are removed using a rod holder. We gently remove the rod by pushing it toward the cranial wound. (**c**) After removal of caps and rods, pedicle screws are removed under endoscopic view

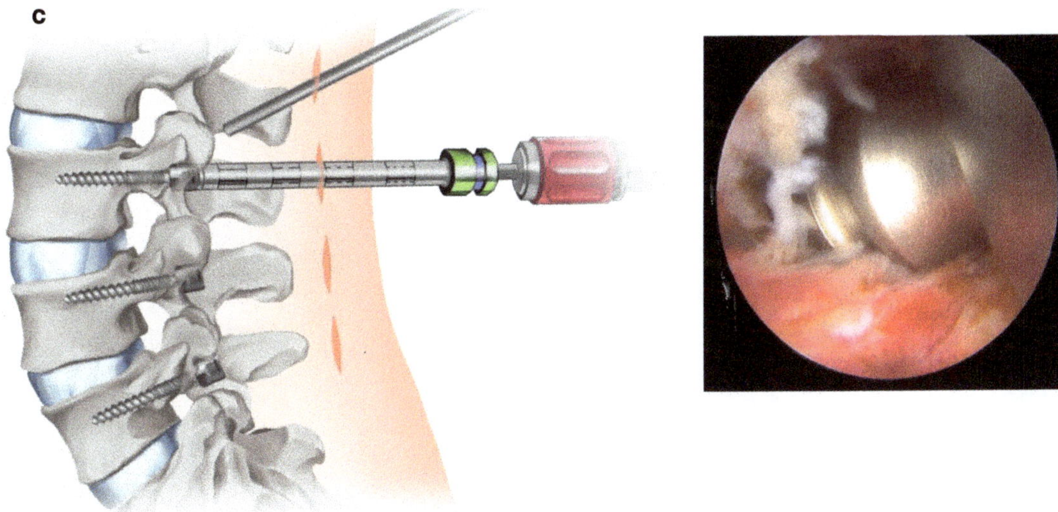

Fig. 14.2 (continued)

14.5.4 Previously Inserted "Pedicle Screws" Removal

After removing the rods, we insert the endoscope into the skin incision point of the adjacent area. We confirm the location of the pedicle screw head using an endoscopic view. Finally, we attach a screwdriver to the screw head under endoscopic guidance. We then remove the pedicle screws (Fig. 14.2c).

14.5.5 Insert New Pedicle Screws and Rods Using Percutaneous Pedicle Screw Systems

After removing the old screw, the entrance of the screw insert hole can be checked directly through the endoscope. We insert guide wires into the pedicle screw holes for the new pedicle screw insertion (Fig. 14.3). The above-mentioned actions are repeated to remove all old screws and replace them with guide wires for new pedicle screws. The subsequent process does not differ from the usual method of using the percutaneous pedicle screw system.

14.6 Complications and Management

In terms of lumbar interbody cage insertion and fusion on the level of ASD, complications of UBE FES techniques were similar to fusion surgeries using the unilateral biportal technique [4–7]. In cases of old hardware retained from previous surgeries, it may be difficult to remove the hardware under endoscopic assistance because the screw and head system may be complicated. In such cases, it is inevitable to switch to open surgery.

14.7 Illustrated Cases

1. Case 1: A 57-year-old male complained of severe buttock pain with intermittent neurological claudication. Twelve years ago, he underwent conventional fusion surgery at L3–4-5. Preoperative magnetic resonance imaging (MRI) showed ASD with foraminal stenosis at L2–3 and L5-S1. We performed UBE FES from L2–3 to L5-S1 (Fig. 14.4). The patient was discharged 7 days after the operation with complete resolution of the symptomatic ASD.

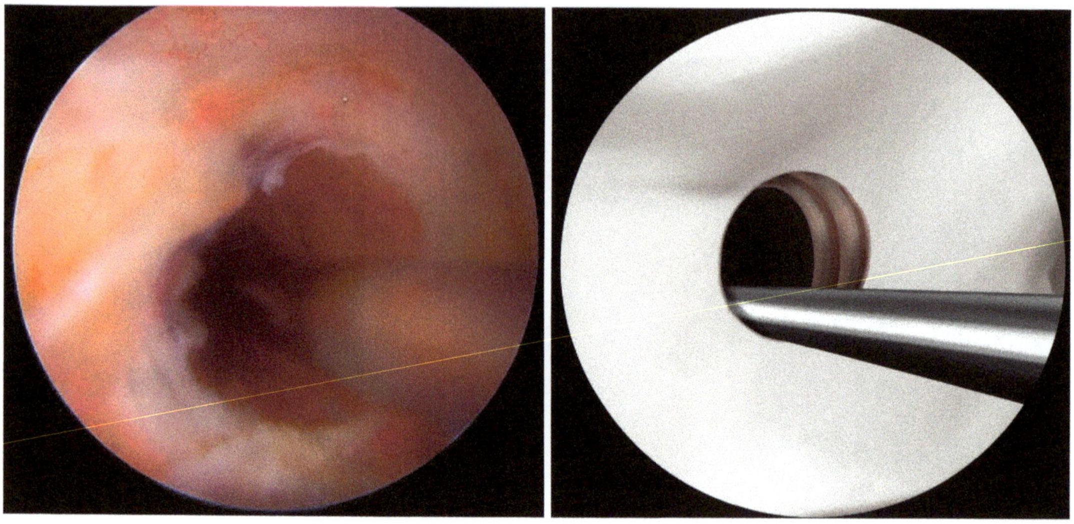

Fig. 14.3 Using guide wire makes it easier to replace percutaneous pedicle screws. After removal of previously inserted screws, guide wires are inserted in the pedicle holes for insertion of new percutaneous pedicle screws

2. Case 2: A 66-year-old female who underwent fusion surgery eleven years ago at the L5-S1 level presented with severe back pain and radicular pain in both legs. She also complained of intermittent neurological claudication. Preoperative X-ray and MRI showed aggravated spondylolisthesis at L4–5. We performed an upper-level extension using UBE FES techniques to resolve ASD. Postoperative X-ray images showed a perfect reduction in spondylolisthesis (Fig. 14.5). Postoperative MRI revealed complete decompression of the foraminal stenosis. After surgery, the pain and tingling sensation of the legs disappeared.

14.8 Discussion

Variable traditional open-based interbody fusion techniques are effective treatment options for adjacent spinal diseases after fusion surgery. Unfortunately, these techniques are often accompanied by troublesome problems including a wide range of muscle damage, a large amount of bleeding, and damage to adjacent joints.

UBE-assisted FES can minimize muscle injury (Fig. 14.6). In this technique, extensive muscle dissection is unnecessary because the screws and rods are removed by exposing only the periphery of the screw head.

Furthermore, cerebral spinal fluid (CSF) leakage from the laminectomy area may occur with conventional open FES [1–3]. Revision dissection of the previous laminectomy area may also cause dural damage and CSF leakage. However, in the case of UBE fusion extension, dissection is only around the ASD level; therefore, the possibility of CSF leakage is very low (Fig. 14.7).

In order to perform this surgery successfully, there are a few things to keep in mind. Skin incisions should be made over the pedicles under C-arm fluoroscopic monitoring. Previously inserted old screws should be replaced with percutaneous pedicle screws (Fig. 14.8). An adjacent skin incision point is used for the endoscopic portal, and a direct skin incision point over the pedicle screw is used as the working portal. Guidewire insertion into the pedicle screw holes is very useful for changing the percutaneous pedicle screws.

In addition, there are supplemental benefits to this approach. Our patients did not require transfusion due to low bleeding during surgery, and drainage systems were not required for operative sites where percutaneous pedicle screw fixation was performed or in segments where we performed interbody fusion. According to previous reports, patients with diabetes healed well with-

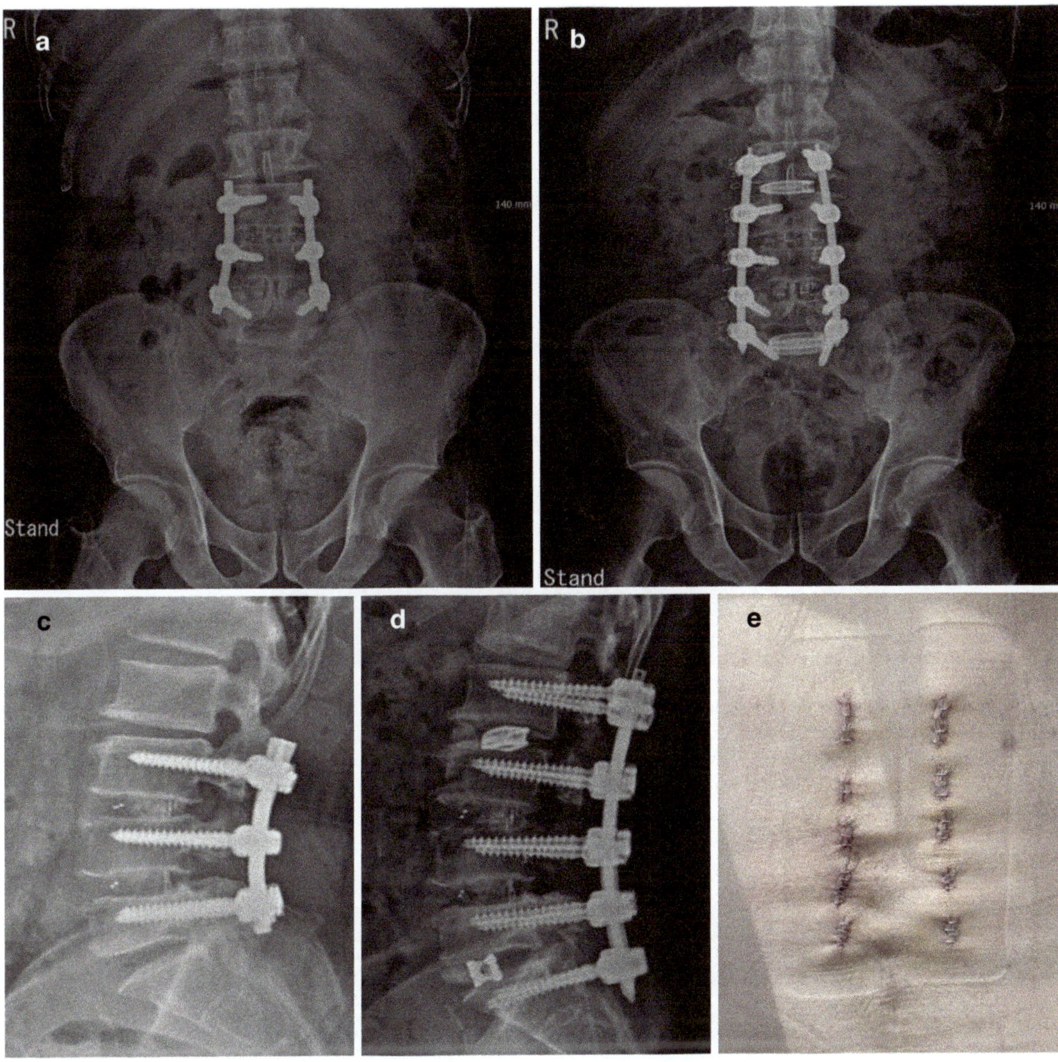

Fig. 14.4 Radiographic images of a 57-year-old male with symptomatic adjacent segmental disease (ASD). Pre and postoperative X-rays show that coronal balance is completely achieved on L2 to S1 after unilateral biportal endoscopic (UBE) fusion extension surgery (FES) (**a, b**). Postoperative X-ray images reveal complete reduction of ASD levels and successful restoration of lumbar curvature (**c, d**). Overview picture of wound shows minimal skin incisions (**e**)

out any major problems due to the small wound, and no patient developed an operative site infection [2, 3].

The concept of enhanced recovery after surgery (ERAS) has been an important focus in the spine surgical field. The ERAS program can accelerate early recovery and prevent postoperative complications [5]. UBE FES may be important for ERAS in major spine surgery because this endoscopic-assisted minimally invasive fusion extension technique might be a safe and effective treatment option for lumbar interbody fusion extension and posterior pedicle screw revision with less morbidity than conventional open surgery [1, 3].

In conclusion, UBE fusion extension techniques may provide a feasible alternative for managing symptomatic ASD with indisputable advantages of reduced muscle damage, blood loss, complications, and length of hospital stay.

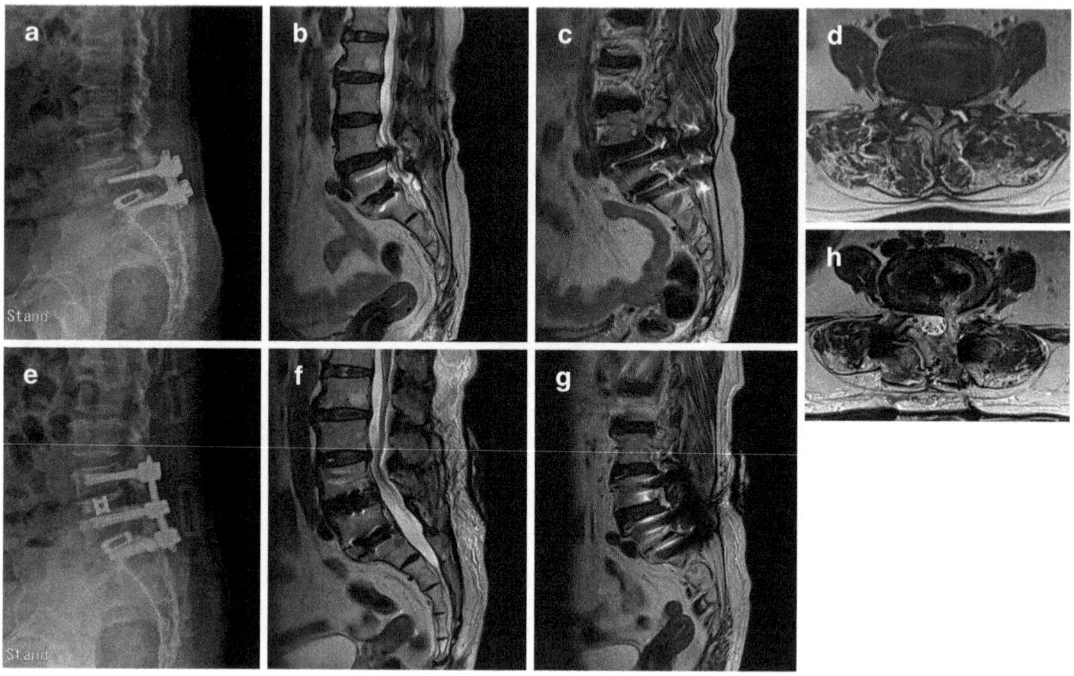

Fig. 14.5 X-ray and magnetic resonance imaging (MRI) of a 66-year-old female. Preoperative X-ray and MRI show the spondylolisthesis, foraminal stenosis, and central stenosis of L4–5 (**a**, **b**, **c**, and **d**). We performed unilateral biportal endoscopic (UBE) fusion extension surgery (FES) (**d** and **e**). Postoperative X-ray reveals the reduction of spondylolisthesis of L4–5 (**d** and **e**). Postoperative MRI reveals the resolution of lumbar central and foraminal stenosis at L4–5 (**e**, **f**, **g** and **h**)

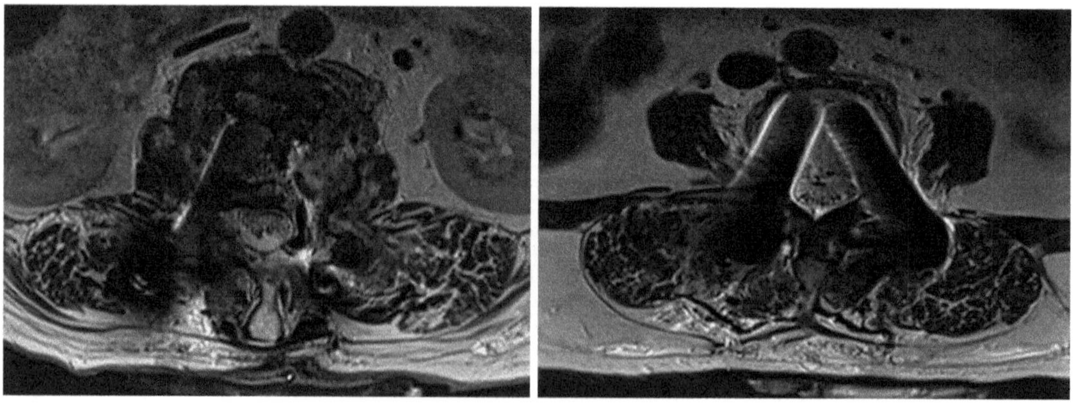

Fig. 14.6 Postoperative magnetic resonance imaging (MRI) reveals minimal muscle damage

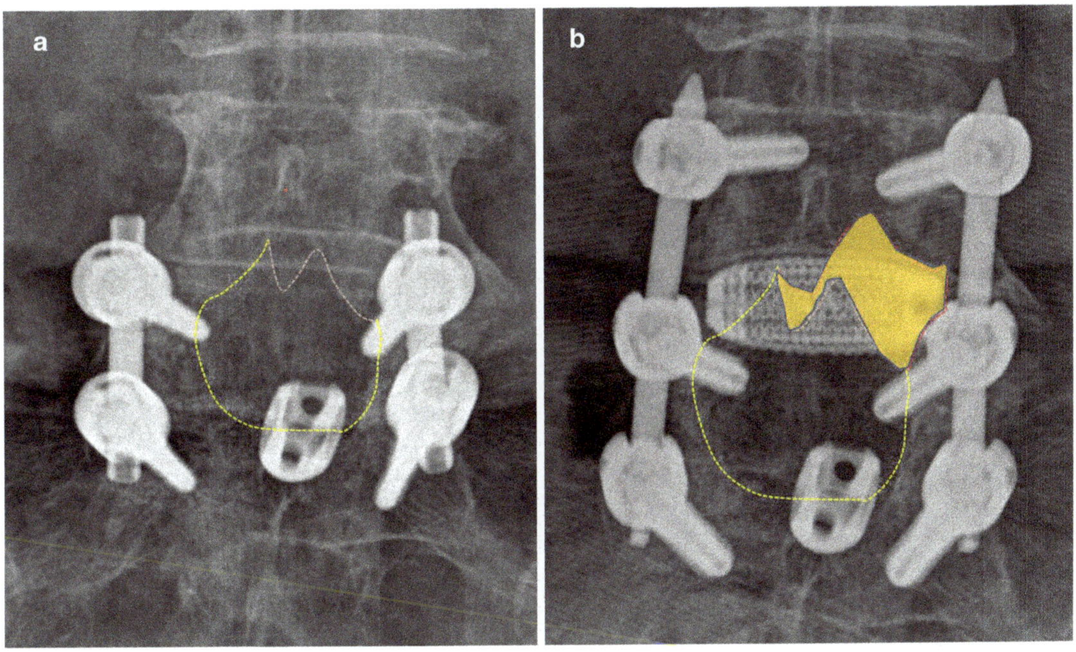

Fig. 14.7 X-ray and magnetic resonance imaging (MRI) of a 73-year-old female. Preoperative X-ray shows subtotal laminectomy at L5-S1 for previous fusion surgery (**a**). There was a high possibility of dura injury during revision dissection. In cases of unilateral biportal endoscopic (UBE) fusion extension surgery (FES), we dissect only the lamina of the adjacent segmental disease (ASD) level and not the previous laminectomy area. Therefore, the incidence of dura tear during dissection may be very low compared to conventional open FES. Yellow-colored schematic drawing of new laminectomy area for UBE FES on postoperative X-ray reveals no need to revise or re-adjust the levels in the previously operated areas (**b**)

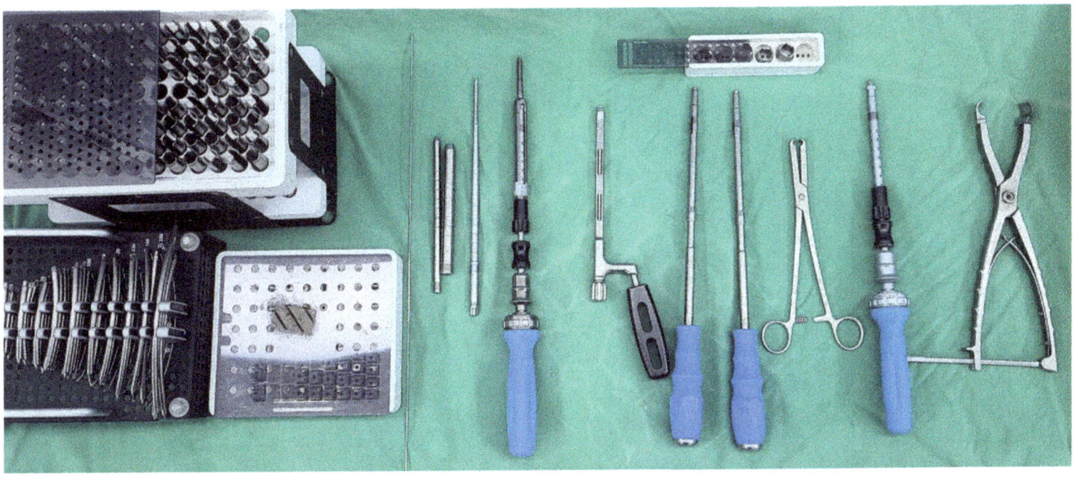

Fig. 14.8 There is no difference in the instruments used in the unilateral biportal endoscopic (UBE) fusion extension surgery (FES) technique compared to conventional FES via percutaneous pedicle screw systems

References

1. Shasti M, Koenig SJ, Nash AB, Bahrami S, Jauregui JJ, O'Hara NN, et al. Biomechanical evaluation of lumbar lateral interbody fusion for the treatment of adjacent segment disease. Spine J. 2019;19(3):545–51.
2. Adogwa O, Parker SL, Shau DN, Mendenhall SK, Devin CJ, Cheng JS, et al. Cost per quality-adjusted life year gained of laminectomy and extension of instrumented fusion for adjacent-segment disease: defining the value of surgical intervention. J Neurosurg Spine. 2012;16(2):141–6.
3. Ryu DS, Park JY, Kuh SU, Chin DK, Kim KS, Cho YE, et al. Surgical outcomes after segmental limited surgery for adjacent segment disease: the consequences of makeshift surgery. World Neurosurg. 2018;110:e258–e65.
4. Ahn Y, Youn MS, Heo DH. Endoscopic transforaminal lumbar interbody fusion: a comprehensive review. Expert Rev Med Devices. 2019;16(5):373–80.
5. Heo DH, Park CK. Clinical results of percutaneous biportal endoscopic lumbar interbody fusion with application of enhanced recovery after surgery. Neurosurg Focus. 2019;46(4):E18.
6. Park MK, Park SA, Son SK, Park WW, Choi SH. Clinical and radiological outcomes of unilateral biportal endoscopic lumbar interbody fusion (ULIF) compared with conventional posterior lumbar interbody fusion (PLIF): 1-year follow-up. Neurosurg Rev. 2019;42(3):753–61.
7. Heo DH, Hong YH, Lee DC, Chung HJ, Park CK. Technique of biportal endoscopic transforaminal lumbar interbody fusion. Neurospine. 2020;17(Suppl 1):S129–s37.
8. Heo DH, Lee DC, Kim HS, Park CK, Chung H. Clinical results and complications of endoscopic lumbar interbody fusion for lumbar degenerative disease: a meta-analysis. World Neurosurg. 2021;145:396–404.
9. Heo DH, Son SK, Eum JH, Park CK. Fully endoscopic lumbar interbody fusion using a percutaneous unilateral biportal endoscopic technique: technical note and preliminary clinical results. Neurosurg Focus. 2017;43(2):E8.

15 Hybrid Surgery Combining Unilateral Biportal Endoscopy and Lateral Lumbar Interbody Fusion

Min Seok Kang, Hyoung Bok Kim, Dong Hwa Heo, and Hyun Jin Park

15.1 Introduction

Posterior lumbar instrumented fusion surgery for degenerative lumbar disc disease often incurs a risk of paravertebral muscle injury and significant blood loss, and minimally invasive surgical techniques proposed to overcome this challenge have been increasing in popularity over the past decade [1]. Among these, lateral lumbar interbody fusion (LLIF) has been proposed as an alternative to minimally invasive surgical modalities for anterior lumbar interbody fusion, with a specially designed retractor system under a small skin incision allowing a large-footprint interbody cage to be inserted into the intervertebral disc, thus approaching the anterolateral aspects of the intervertebral disc without injury to the paravertebral musculature or intrusion of major blood vessels. LLIF includes oblique lumbar interbody fusion (OLIF; Medtronic Inc., Memphis TN, USA), which is performed via a corridor located anterior to the psoas muscle; direct lumbar interbody fusion (DLIF; Medtronic Inc., Memphis TN, USA); and extreme lateral interbody fusion (XLIF; NuVasive Inc., San Diego, CA, USA), which is performed via psoas muscle penetration. LLIF can correct coronal and sagittal alignment and obtain indirect neural decompression via ligamentotaxis by placing a long lordotic cage on the bilateral cortical epiphyseal ring of the vertebral endplate [2]. In particular, it is potentially useful in multi-segment surgery with deformity correction and can also be applied to some cases of osteoporotic vertebral collapse, which requires anterior column reconstruction [3].

However, LLIF is ineffective in patients with severe central canal stenosis or concomitant ruptured disc herniation. In addition, LLIF is not always indicated for patients with hard stenotic lesions, including endplate or facet articular osteophytes, and ossification of spinal ligaments [4, 5]. In particular, additional surgery may be necessary to yield favorable results under the aforementioned conditions, and combination with unilateral biportal endoscopy (UBE) for direct neural decompression may be an effective collaboration. Although the outcomes of transforaminal lumbar interbody fusion using UBE are reportedly beneficial, most previous studies have focused on single- or two-level fusion, and the exclusion criteria of most published studies included high-grade spondylolisthesis (grade > 2) or coexisting advanced coronal imbalance

M. S. Kang · H. B. Kim
Orthopedic Surgery, Endoscopic Spine Surgery Center, Seoul Bumin Hospital, Seoul, Republic of Korea

D. H. Heo
Neurosurgery, Endoscopic Spine Surgery Center, Seoul Bumin Hospital, Seoul, Republic of Korea

H. J. Park (✉)
Orthopedic Surgery, Kangnam Sacred Heart Hospital, Hallym University College of Medicine, Seoul, Republic of Korea

D. H. Heo et al. (eds.), *Unilateral Biportal Endoscopic Spine Surgery*,
https://doi.org/10.1007/978-981-16-8201-8_15

(Cobb's angle >25°) [6–9]. However, the combination of LLIF and UBE may be clinically important because the radiological advantages of the anterior surgical approach and clinical advantages of UBE are clear.

Herein, the hybrid surgical procedure that combines LLIF and UBE will be described in detail, and relevant cases will be reviewed.

15.2 Indications and Contraindications

Hybrid surgery combining LLIF with UBE is a minimally invasive surgical form of anterior-posterior spine surgery, and it can be applied to a variety of adult spines and in some cases of osteoporotic vertebral collapse.

I. Inclusion criteria:

- Lower back and/or leg radicular pain with neurogenic intermittent claudication and/or progressive neurological deficits
- Neural foraminal stenosis (> moderate base on Wildermuth's grading system)
- Central canal stenosis (> grade 3 based on the Borenstein lumbar central canal stenosis grading system)
- Segmental instability (> 4.5 mm of translation or > 15° of angulation evident on flexion–extension radiographs
- Degenerative lumbar scoliosis
- Flat back deformity with sagittal imbalance (> 5 cm of sagittal vertical axis and > 25° of pelvic tilt)
- Failure of >3 months of conservative treatment
- Osteoporotic vertebral collapse (= Kümmell disease stage 3) with lumbar spinal canal stenosis

II. Exclusion criteria:

- Spinal infection or tumorous condition
- Inflammatory spondylitis
- Acute spinal trauma

15.3 Anesthesia and Position

Once general endotracheal anesthesia was performed and appropriate IV access obtained, each patient initially underwent LLIF. The patient was placed on a bendable surgical table in a right-sided lateral decubitus position under fluoroscopic guidance. (Fig. 15.1a) The flexion of the table is potentially useful in aiding the opening of the space between the 12th rib and iliac crest. Once the desired position was achieved, the patient was secured. Thereafter, the patient was prepped and draped in a sterile fashion.

15.4 Surgical Steps: LLIF

C-arm fluoroscopy was used to confirm the target disc level, which was marked on the skin. A skin incision of approximately 3 cm was made for a single-level fusion, centered on the target segment and parallel to the external oblique muscle, followed by a blunt dissection of the internal oblique muscle fascia and transverse abdominis fascia along the direction of the muscle fibers. For multi-segment fusions, a sliding window technique was used to approach the disc spaces without expansion of the initial incision. After blunt dissection of the retroperitoneal space, the peritoneum and major vessels were mobilized ventrally with posterior retraction of the psoas muscle. Subsequently, the outer annulus of the intervertebral disc was exposed through a corridor between the abdominal aorta and psoas muscle, and a specialized tubular retractor system was applied. (Fig. 15.1b) Neuromonitoring was performed when psoas muscle fibers were exposed. Discectomy was performed sequentially, contralateral annulotomy was performed using the Cobb elevator, and the cartilaginous endplate was carefully removed to expose the subchondral bone so as not to damage the bony endplate. The size of the interbody cage was determined by increasing the size of the trial cage until a snug fit was confirmed. (Fig. 15.1c, d) To prevent over-distraction while inserting the cage, the average height of the adjacent segment's disc

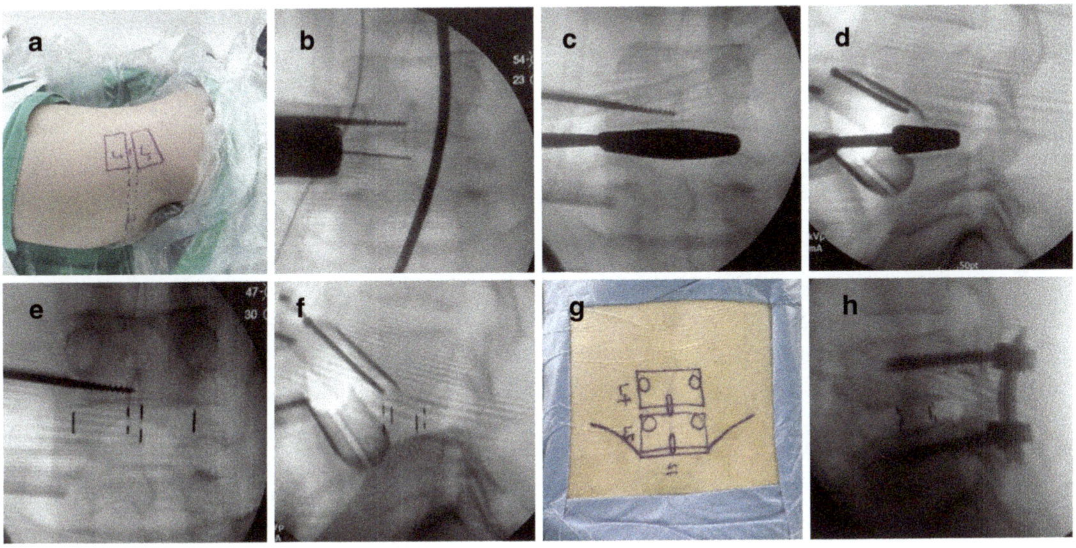

Fig. 15.1 Surgical steps—LLIF via anterior-to-psoas approach. (**a**) Right-sided lateral decubitus position for LLIF. (**b–f**) Step-by-step intraoperative findings of LLIF. The C-arm fluoroscopy confirmed that the implant was in the proper position. (**g**) And then, the patient was placed in the prone position for additional decompression using UBE technique. (**h**) After UBE decompression, percutaneous pedicle screw insertion was performed for posterior fixation

space was measured preoperatively to determine the adequate height of the corresponding level. A properly sized Clydesdale PEEK cage (Medtronic Sofamor Danek Inc., Memphis, TN, USA) was filled with demineralized bone matrix (Grafton; Medtronic, Minneapolis, MN, USA). Cage insertion commenced in the lateral oblique direction, proceeding through the true lateral direction using the rotation maneuver. C-arm fluoroscopy was performed to confirm that the implants and instruments were in their proper positions. (Fig. 15.1e, f).

15.5 Surgical Steps: UBE and Percutaneous Pedicle Screw Fixation

After LLIF, the patient was placed in the prone position and draped in a water-proof, sterile fashion. (Fig. 15.1g) Decompressive laminectomy or lateral foraminotomy was performed using the unilateral biportal endoscopic technique. In a decompressive laminectomy, two separate skin incisions were made above the superior and lower margins of the interlaminar space; usually, the left-side incision serves as a viewing portal, and the right-side incision is used as a working portal. After endoscopic visualization of the interlaminar space, superior and inferior laminotomies were performed on both sides, and complete flavectomy was performed to the greatest possible extent. Adequate neural decompression was confirmed when the ipsilateral traversing nerve root and contralateral exiting and traversing nerve roots were identified with the free movement of these nerve roots, and discectomy was performed where necessary. In the case of lateral foraminotomy, two separate skin incisions were made above the lower margin of the superior transverse process and the upper margin of the inferior transverse process 2 cm outward from the lateral interpedicular line. After obtaining endoscopic visualization of the superior transverse process, isthmus, and superior facet articular process, the Kambin triangle was identified by performing lateral foraminotomy and partial flavectomy. Finally, a lumbar discectomy was performed. After UBE decompression, percutaneous pedicle screw insertion was performed for posterior fixation. (Fig. 15.1h) After saline irrigation of the operative wound, no bleeding focus was confirmed, and wound repair was performed.

15.6 Illustrated Cases

15.6.1 Case 1: LLIF + UBE Decompressive Laminectomy for Adult Scoliosis with Multilevel Spinal Stenosis

A 74-year-old woman complained of severe back and right leg pain as well as gait disturbance 1 month prior. Fifteen years prior, she underwent right-sided hemilaminotomy at L4–5–S1 for lumbar spinal stenosis. However, the back pain did not improve after the operation, and she received intermittent, conservative treatment; however, she complained of progressive claudication and radicular leg pain. On physical examination, right ankle dorsiflexion, plantar flexion, and long-toe dorsiflexion power decreased to grade 3. Preoperative plain radiographs revealed degenerative scoliosis; multilevel, severe disc-space narrowing; and wedge shape deformity of the L4 body. (Fig. 15.2a, b) Further, preoperative magnetic resonance imaging (MRI) exhibited intervertebral disc protrusion at L2–3, moderate-to-severe central canal stenosis at L3–4, and bilateral neural foraminal stenosis at L4–5–S1, with both-facet hypertrophy due to prior right hemilaminotomy. (Fig. 15.2c–h) Although the central canal was decompressed, severe stenosis was observed from the right lateral recess to the foraminal area due to facet hypertrophy. Finally, the patient underwent anterior total discectomy with OLIF at L2–3–4–5–S1 in the right lateral decubitus position. Thereafter, the patient's position was altered to the prone position. For additional posterior decompression, UBE was used. Subsequently, right-side foraminotomy at L4–5–S1 (Fig. 15.2k, l) as well as unilateral laminotomy and bilateral decompression (ULBD) at L3–4 followed. (Fig. 15.2m, n) A percutaneous pedicle screw was inserted at L2–3–4–5–S1. (Fig. 15.2i, j) After the operation, the preoperative symptoms significantly improved.

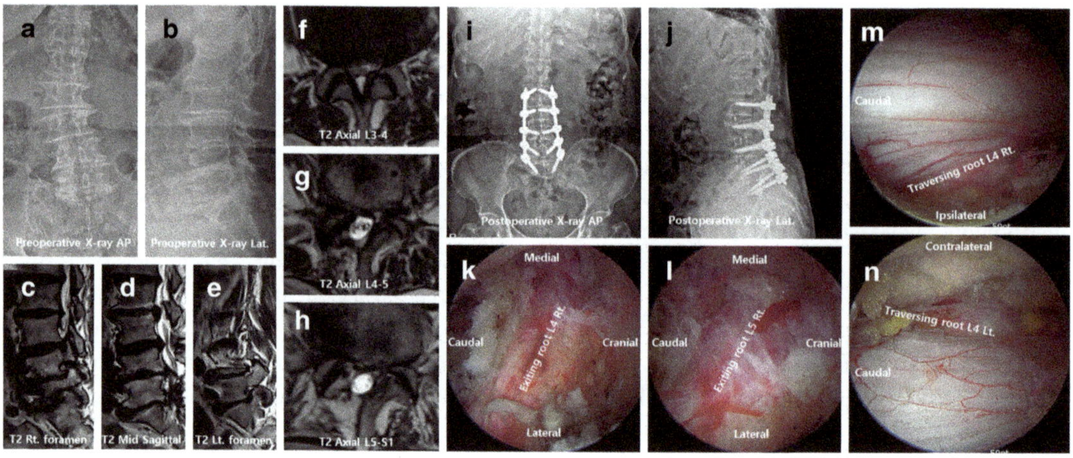

Fig. 15.2 Case of hybrid surgery combining oblique lumbar interbody fusion and selective neural decompression using unilateral biportal endoscopy. (**a, b**) Preoperative plain radiographs and (**c–h**) MRI T2-weighted images. (**i, j**) In postoperative plain radiographs, the coronal Cobb angle was corrected, and lumbar lordosis increased compared to that in preoperative images. (**k, l**) Intraoperative endoscopic findings of far-lateral approach for foraminotomy. Rt. L4 and L5 exiting roots were well decompressed. (**m, n**) Intraoperative endoscopic findings of posterolateral approach for ULBD. Thecal sac and bilateral L4 traversing root were well decompressed

15.6.2 Case 2: LLIF + UBE Foraminotomy for Osteoporotic Vertebral Collapse with Far-lateral Ruptured HNP

A 78-year-old man complained of severe back and left anterior thigh pain as well as gait disturbance 2 months prior. A year before, he underwent anterior lumbar interbody fusion at L4–L5 for lumbar spinal stenosis. However, 2 months prior, he suffered back pain without any special trauma, and he was diagnosed with an L3 vertebral compression fracture in another hospital and received conservative treatment; nevertheless, he complained of progressive deterioration of intermittent claudication and radicular leg pain. On physical examination, the left femoral nerve stretch test was positive, and the left-knee extension power decreased to grade 3. Preoperative plain radiographs revealed L3 osteoporotic vertebral collapse with left side wedging of the vertebral body, post-traumatic retrolisthesis, and anterior lumbar interbody fusion status at L4–L5. (Fig. 15.3a–c) Moreover, preoperative MRI revealed an L3 vertebral burst fracture involving the left neural foramen with L3 retrolisthesis and left far-lateral ruptured herniated nucleus pulposus at L3–4. (Fig. 15.3d–h) Finally, the patient underwent LLIF via psoas muscle penetration, cement-augmented short-segment percutaneous pedicle screw fixation, (Fig. 15.3i, j) and left lateral foraminotomy with lumbar discectomy using the UBE technique. (Fig. 15.3k) After the operation, the preoperative symptoms significantly improved.

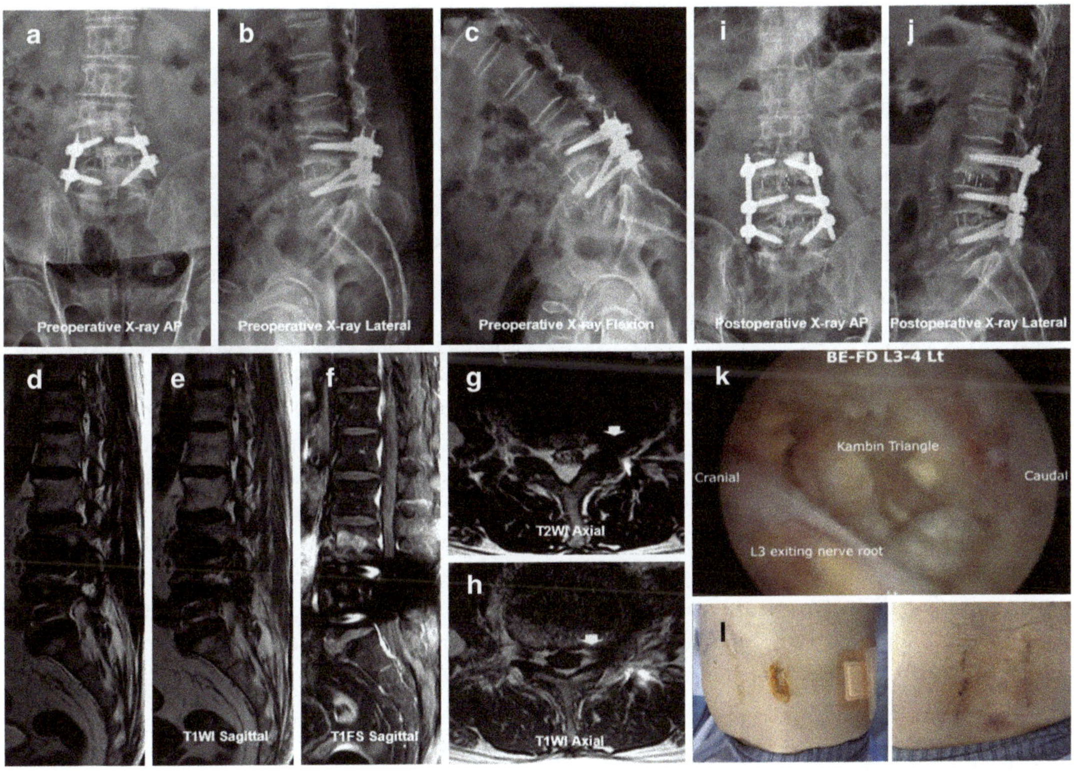

Fig. 15.3 Case of hybrid surgery combining lateral foraminotomy using unilateral biportal endoscopy and lateral lumbar interbody fusion. (**a–c**) Preoperative plain radiographs and (**d–h**) preoperative MRI images. In particular, a white arrow refers to the left far-lateral ruptured herniated nucleus pulposus of L3–4. (**i, j**) In postoperative plain radiographs, traumatic retrolisthesis was corrected compared to that in preoperative images. (**k**) Intraoperative endoscopic findings confirmed that the L3 exiting nerve root was well-decompressed. (**l**) Clinical photographs of operative wounds exhibiting a 3-cm-longitudinal skin incision for lateral lumbar interbody fusion and four skin incisions for percutaneous pedicle screw insertion

15.7 Complications and Their Management

The overall complications associated with hybrid surgery combining LLIF and UBE are consistent with the complications of each surgical technique. The complications associated with UBE have been described in the previous section. The most common post-LLIF complication was incisional pain followed by transitory weakness of the psoas muscle, transient neurological symptoms, segmental-artery lesion, and pseudohernia [10]. Most complications improved by conservative treatment. However, lumbar plexus injury, which occurs after surgery and penetrates the psoas muscle, can be accompanied by permanent motor deficits and dysesthesia. To prevent these complications, it is important to conduct appropriate neurophysiological monitoring while the tubular retractor is being placed, especially at the L4–L5 level. After LLIF via a corridor located anterior to the psoas muscle, painful lower-extremity swelling, paresthesia due to sympathetic trunk injury, and ureter and major vessel injuries were reported. In the case of ureter or major vessel injuries, a specialist is generally consulted for assistance. In particular, it is recommended to cooperate with a vascular surgeon if L5–S1 is included in the surgical range.

15.8 Surgical Tips and Pitfalls

In addition to increasing the volume of the neural foramen, LLIF also stretches the buckled ligamentum flavum and posterior longitudinal ligaments, a process that can partially widen the anteroposterior diameter of the central canal. This phenomenon is called ligamentotaxis, which can make decompressive laminectomy or lateral foraminotomy performance easier; thus, the authors recommend that LLIF be performed first in hybrid surgery. In addition, if sequestrated or subligamentous extruded herniated nucleus pulposus coexist, we recommend that only lesions located above and below the posterior longitudinal ligament should be removed and the posterior longitudinal ligament and annulus fibrosus preserved as much as possible to maintain ligamentotaxis.

LLIF has the advantage of being able to place the large footprint interbody cage on the bilateral cortical epiphyseal ring of the vertebral endplate, thus obtaining indirect neural decompression by ligamentotaxis and correcting coronal and sagittal alignment. However, subsidence of the interbody cage can occur in cases of bony endplate fracture during endplate preparation or implant insertion, processes that potentially cause serious problems, such as pseudoarthrosis and/or loss of indirect neural decompression. For older patients with osteoporosis, it is recommended to minimize the use of disc shavers for endplate preparation, manipulate implants gently, and insert pedicle screws as long as possible to the anterior vertebral cortex, where the interbody cage is located.

LLIF is known to be a typical modality used for lumbar degenerative disc disease; nevertheless, it has recently been attempted as a treatment for post-traumatic lumbar spinal stenosis following osteoporotic vertebral collapse in older patients [3]. This condition is reportedly difficult to treat and requires various reconstructive surgical procedures. Although there is insufficient clinical evidence, short-segment anteroposterior surgery combined with LLIF tailored to the morphology of the collapsed vertebra has reportedly achieved favorable clinical outcomes in terms of sufficient neural decompression, reconstruction of the anterior column, and correction of local alignment. In particular, optional decompressive laminectomy or discectomy using UBE is expected to preserve the stability of the posterior vertebral structure without paravertebral muscle injury, while ensuring improvement of radicular pain through direct neural decompression.

References

1. Meng B, Bunch J, Burton D, Wang J. Lumbar interbody fusion: recent advances in surgical techniques and bone healing strategies. Eur Spine J. 2021;30(1):22.
2. Lee HJ, Park EJ, Ahn JS, Kim SB, Kwon YS, Park YC. Clinical outcomes of biportal endoscopic inter-

laminar decompression with oblique lumbar interbody fusion (OLIF): comparative analysis with TLIF. Brain Sci. 2021;11(5):630.

3. Fukuda K, Katoh H, Takahashi Y, Kitamura K, Ikeda D. Minimally invasive anteroposterior combined surgery using lateral lumbar interbody fusion without corpectomy for treatment of lumbar spinal canal stenosis associated with osteoporotic vertebral collapse. J Neurosurg Spine. 2021:1–9. https://doi.org/10.3171/2020.10.SPINE201293.
4. Heo DH, Kim JS. Clinical and radiological outcomes of spinal endoscopic discectomy-assisted oblique lumbar interbody fusion: preliminary results. Neurosurg Focus. 2017;43(2):E13.
5. Nakashima H, Kanemura T, Satake K, Ishikawa Y, Ouchida J, Segi N, et al. Unplanned second-stage decompression for neurological deterioration caused by central canal stenosis after indirect lumbar decompression surgery. Asian Spine J. 2019;13(4):584.
6. Kang MS, You KH, Choi JY, Heo DH, Chung HJ, Park HJ. Minimally invasive transforaminal lumbar interbody fusion using the biportal endoscopic techniques versus microscopic tubular technique. Spine J. 2021;21(12):2066–77.
7. Park MK, Park SA, Son SK, Park WW, Choi SH. Clinical and radiological outcomes of unilateral biportal endoscopic lumbar interbody fusion (ULIF) compared with conventional posterior lumbar interbody fusion (PLIF): 1-year follow-up. Neurosurg Rev. 2019;42(3):753.
8. Heo DH, Park CK. Clinical results of percutaneous biportal endoscopic lumbar interbody fusion with application of enhanced recovery after surgery. Neurosurg Focus. 2019;46(4):E18.
9. Kim JE, Yoo HS, Choi DJ, Park EJ, Jee SM. Comparison of minimal invasive versus biportal endoscopic transforaminal lumbar interbody fusion for single-level lumbar disease. Clin Spine Surg. 2021;34(2):E64–e71.
10. Quillo-Olvera J, Lin GX, Jo HJ, Kim JS. Complications on minimally invasive oblique lumbar interbody fusion at L2-L5 levels: a review of the literature and surgical strategies. Ann Transl Med. 2018;6(6):101.

Part V

Cervical and Thoracic Lesion

16 Cervical Posterior: Foraminotomy and Discectomy

Kwan-Su David Song, Seung Deok Sun, and Dae Hyun Kim

16.1 Introduction

Cervical radiculopathy is often caused by disc herniation or degenerative change.

Historically, the posterior cervical approach had been performed a long time ago, but there had been some serious problems. For example, the surgical field was too deep. So, there were a lot of muscle tissues that had to be sacrificed to reach the target area. Therefore, even access to small surgical sites also requires long skin incisions and excessive force retraction of the surrounding muscles.

However, with the research and effort of minimally invasive spinal surgery, these disadvantages have been overcome by the use of tubular retractors, such as microendoscopic decompression systems.

Supplementary Information The online version contains supplementary material available at [https://doi.org/10.1007/978-981-16-8201-8_16].

K.-S. D. Song (✉)
Department of Neurosurgery, Him-Plus Hospital, Suncheon-si, Jeollanam-do, Republic of Korea

S. D. Sun
Department of Orthopedic Surgery, Sun's Orthopedics Clinic, Seoul, Republic of Korea

D. H. Kim
Department of Neurosurgery, Daegu Catholic University Medical Center, Daegu, Republic of Korea

In addition, with the development of endoscopic spinal instruments and optimal surgical techniques using endoscopes, minimally invasive surgical techniques are being further developed [1, 2].

In this chapter, we describe the surgical procedure of the posterior cervical foraminotomy (PCF) and posterior cervical inclinatory foraminotomy (PCIF) with the UBE system step-by-step, using video and pictures.

16.2 Indications and Contraindications

The indications are unilateral radiculopathy resulting from nerve root compression within the neural foramen, refractory pain to conservative treatments, or progressive neurologic symptoms [3].

The classic indication of the conventional microscopic PCF corresponded to the lesion of the nerve root which was located on the lateral board of the dura. So, the contraindication of PCF was a central lesion.

However, the indication of the endoscopic PCF has expanded to paracentral lesions.

The exclusion criteria are the presence of segmental instability, central disc, and severe kyphotic deformity. Any associated infection, tumor, or fracture in the region of the cervical segment is also considered a contraindication.

D. H. Heo et al. (eds.), *Unilateral Biportal Endoscopic Spine Surgery*,
https://doi.org/10.1007/978-981-16-8201-8_16

In PCIF, the operative indication and contraindication are the same as in PCF. However, the PCIFs are more ideological if the lesion is located in the more distal area and the facet is vulnerable, and there is a risk that during facetectomy, instability may be promoted. On the other hand, it should also be considered that depending on the shape and deviation of the spinous process, there may be relative surgical limitations on the PCIF.

16.3 Equipment

(A) **Bur** (Fig. 16.1a, b)
3.5 mm diamond bur (ELNA 4 Aesculap, B Braun Germany),
3 mm bendable diamond burs (All care, Korea).
(B) **Scope retractor** (Fig. 16.1c)

16.4 Anesthesia and Position

The patient's position and anesthesia for PCF and PCIF are the same.

The surgical position is assumed in a prone position under general anesthesia. The abdomen is relaxed using an H-shape pillow to avoid increased abdominal pressure. A facial gel pad is used to protect the eyeballs and chin from direct high contact pressure. (Fig. 16.2a).

The neck must be flexed, while the upper back must be slanted down. This helps maintain good venous return and reduces bleeding during surgery. Therefore, creating this posture is a very important point for this operation. Usually, lateral fluoroscopy can be viewed up to the C5–6 level, but C6–7 and below that level can be obscured by soft tissue in the shoulder. So even though a cervical traction device is not used, the patient's head must be fixed, and both shoulders must be pulled by plasters (Fig. 16.2b).

Also, one of the most important factors in bleeding control is the patient's blood pressure. The cooperation of an anesthesiologist for hypotensive anesthesia is the most important thing in securing surgical vision. In my personal experience, I think it is appropriate to lower the mean arterial pressure to 80 mmHg.

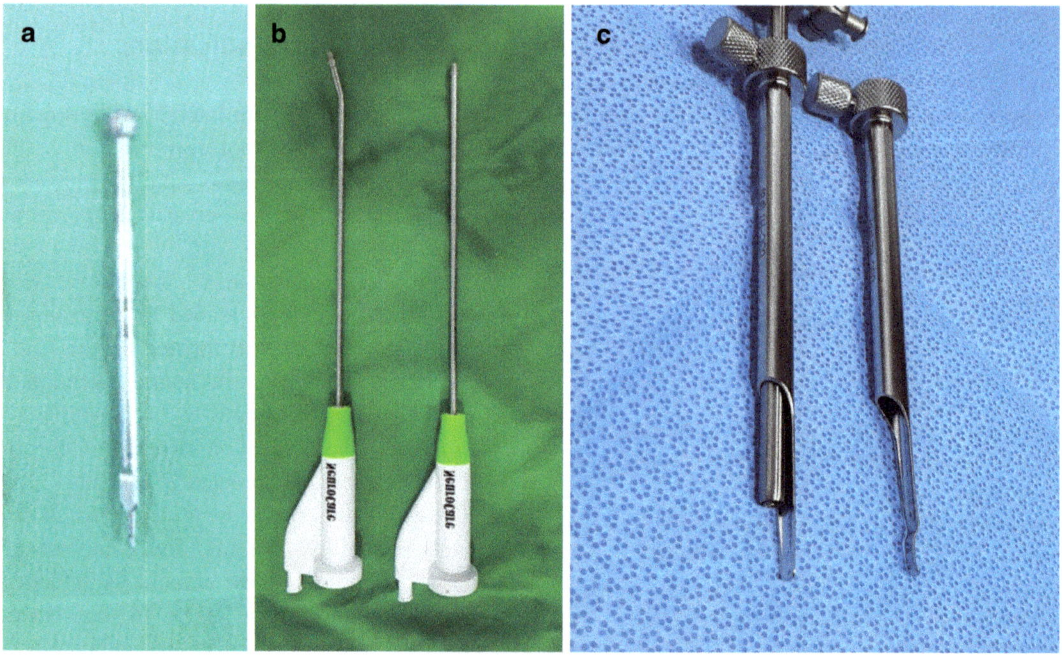

Fig. 16.1 The equipment used in PCF and PCIF. 3.5 mm spherical diamond bur (**a**), 3.0 mm conical diameter bendable diamond burs (**b**), Scope retractor (**c**)

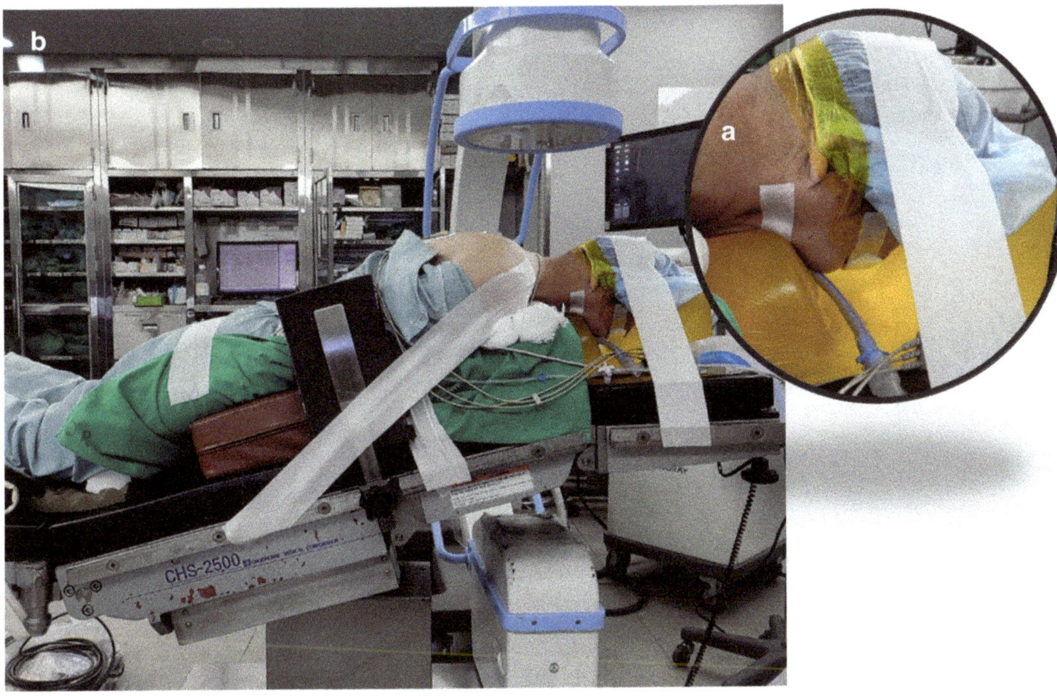

Fig. 16.2 Patient's operative position. The eye-ball must be protected by a gel facial pad (**a**). Neck and bilateral shoulders must be fixed with plaster, without headrest. The upper back must be slanted down, because of good venous return (**b**)

16.5 Surgical Steps

PCIF is a surgical procedure in which the PCF and the operator are located differently. Therefore, the location of the portal is different, and the inclinatory angle approaching the target point during surgery is different [4].

However other surgical techniques of the steps, which include bone work, flavectomy, and nerve root decompression, are the same.

Therefore, PCF and PCIF are described separately for making portals that have significant differences. In addition, instead of explaining the main surgical techniques for PCF, we explain the detailed surgical techniques for PCIF.

16.6 Posterior Cervical Foraminotomy (Videos 16.1, 16.2, and 16.3)

16.6.1 Skin Marking and Incision

After the antiseptic is draped, the surgeon stands on the same side as the lesion. To make 2 portals, 2 skin incisions of 0.5 cm length are made vertically on the pedicle under the guidance of C-arm fluoroscopy. Each skin incision for the portal is made at the upper and lower pedicle related to the target level. The distance between these 2 portals is about 2 cm (Fig. 16.3a).

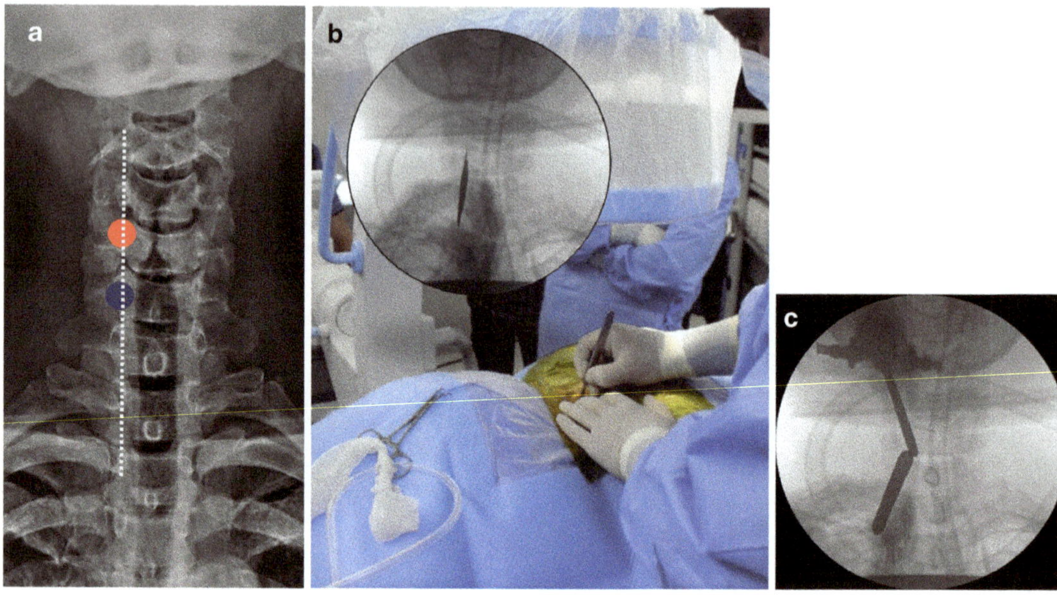

Fig. 16.3 The skin incision points of PCF are marked on the upper and lower pedicles around the target level. Two skin incisions for the scope portal (Red circle) and the working portal (Blue circle) are illustrated in the figure. White dotted line means the medial margin of pedicle (**a**). The skin incision is recommended under the fluoroscopic image guide (**b**). After skin incision, the right triangulation scopes and instruments can be checked on the target points (**c**)

The interval of scope portal and working portal need to be located some distance apart. If the distance is too close, the surgical procedure would be difficult, due to a conflict between scopes and instruments. Conversely, if the distance between the two is too great, it is difficult for endoscopes and instruments to handle within the target point.

After making two portals, a #10 blade is used to make a deeper incision into the fascia until it touches the bone, with the guidance of C-arm fluoroscopy. The use of a wide blade is much safer, because it is less likely to penetrate through the inter-lamina, and when this is done, it is much faster to clear the remnant muscle around the lamina (Fig. 16.3b).

Serial dilators are used to dissect the neck muscle and acquire operative space. After inserting the cannula, a 0° endoscope is inserted through the viewing portal.

In the author's case, the saline irrigation system is applied as a natural drainage system, but in the case of surgery using the pump system, a pressure of about 30 mmHg can be safely maintained, without affecting the rise of intracranial pressure [5]. Surgical instruments are inserted through the working portal.

After triangulation with the endoscope and instrument on the margin of the superior laminar, inferior laminar, and medial point of the facet joint (V-point) (Fig. 16.3c), remove the remnant soft tissue around the V-point, and control the minor bleeding with a radiofrequency (RF) probe to clean the surgical field [6].

16.6.2 Laminectomy and Flavectomy

Using a 3.5 mm diamond bur, a partial laminectomy–facetectomy is performed beginning at the V-point (Fig. 16.4a). The inferolateral portion of the upper lamina is drilled out in the craniolateral direction with the 3.5 mm spherical diamond bur, until the ligament flavum is detached from the site (Fig. 16.4b) (Video 16.1).

The superolateral part of the lower lamina is drilled out in the caudolateral direction until the

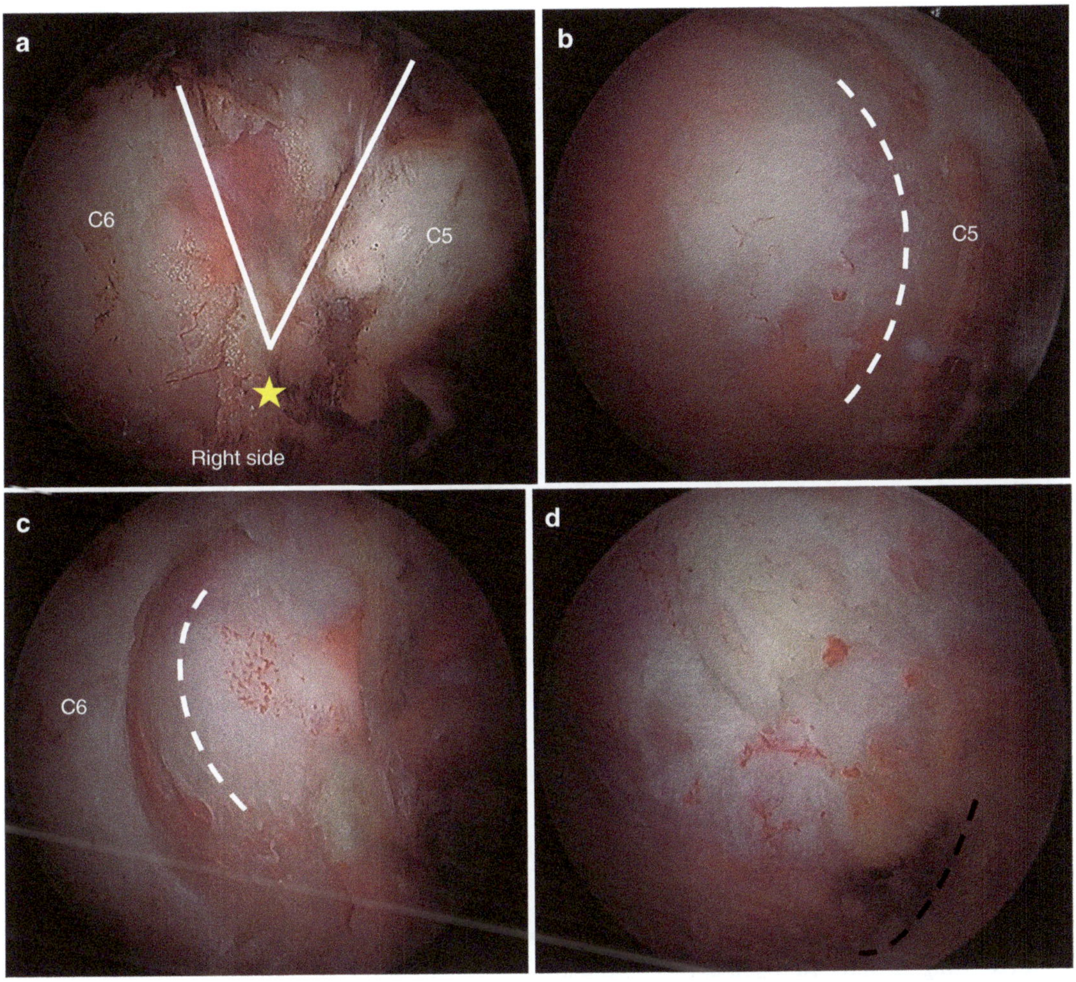

Fig. 16.4 Intraoperative endoscopic images showing the V-point (Yellow asterisk) of the right C5–6 level (**a**). Drilling out the lower margin of the upper lamina in the cranial direction can expose the point at which the ligament flavum is detached (White dashed line). This area is the end-point of the upper lamina bone work (**b**). When the upper margin of the lower lamina is drilled out in the caudal direction, the bone becomes very thin like an eggshell that penetrates into the silhouette of the dura. This area is the end-point of the lower laminectomy (White dashed line) (**c**). When drilling the medial aspect of the facet joint (Black dashed line), be careful not to damage more than 50%. It is safer to work without removing the ligament flavum (**d**)

bone is thin like an eggshell, so the dura is visible inside (Fig. 16.4c).

The bur is then directed toward the lateral side along the inner surface of the facet joint for foraminotomy. The medial one-third to one-half of the facet is progressively removed (Fig. 16.4d). Depending on the size and location of the herniation and surgical level, the hole of foraminotomy can be extended toward the lateral or craniocaudal side.

If more than 50% of the facet joints are damaged, there is a risk of instability, so less than 50% must be removed, until the lateral margin of the ligament flavum appears [7, 8].

It is recommended that the ligament flavum be preserved until the bone work is completely finished, because during bone drilling work, the ligament flavum acts as a protector of the neural structure.

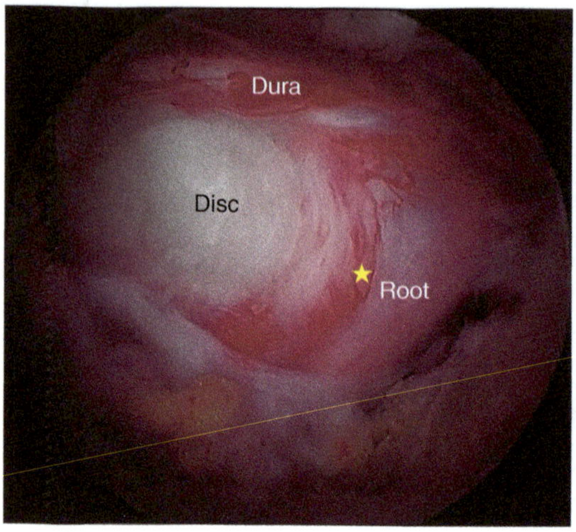

Fig. 16.5 One good way to distinguish between the nerve root and dura is to check the direction of the capillary vessel of the nerve root (Yellow asterisk). This is because they also drive the vessel along the nerve root

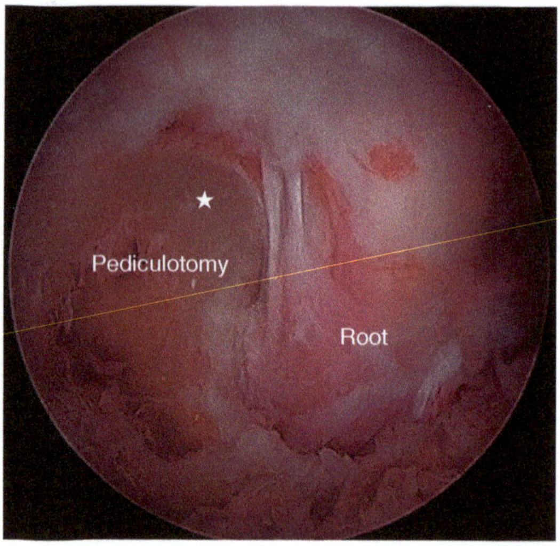

Fig. 16.6 If there is insufficient space for decompression of the nerve root, or for manipulation of the nerve root, it may be necessary to secure space through pediculotomy (Asterisk)

16.6.3 Nerve Root Decompression

After flavectomy and hemostasis, the medial border of the pedicle should be identified first. The purpose is to establish the surgical anatomy of dura and nerve root. Also, checking the pathway of a capillary vessel of the dura can be a good tip for finding the exiting nerve root (Fig. 16.5).

The exiting nerve root is identified and decompressed using 1 mm Kerrison's punches and curettes. These are useful for foraminotomy without compression of neural tissue during nerve root compression (Video 16.2).

If there is a protruded disc particle around the nerve root, it can be gently retracted superiorly to carefully incise and remove the disc herniation. Because disc herniation is usually developed at the axillar portion of the nerve root. If there is less workspace to remove the disc, the pediculotomy can provide more space around the nerve root, making it easier to manipulate the nerve root (Fig. 16.6). The scope retractor is useful for this work. The surgeon must be careful during this procedure to avoid iatrogenic spinal cord injury (Video 16.3).

After nerve root decompression, a ball-tip type hook is then used to palpate the lateral margin of the pedicle to ensure adequate foraminal decompression through the neural foramen.

16.7 Posterior Cervical Inclinatory Foraminotomy (Videos 16.4 and 16.5)

16.7.1 Skin Marking and Incision

The surgeon stands on the opposite side of the lesion. To make 2 portals, under the guidance of C-arm fluoroscopy, 2 skin incisions of 0.5 cm long are made vertically along the medial margin of the spinous process (Fig. 16.7a). Sometimes, 18-gauge needles are useful for finding a proper inclinatory angle and target levels before the skin incision (Fig. 16.7b). Each skin incision for the portal is made at the upper and lower cervical spinous process related to the target. The distance between these 2 portals is about 2–3 cm. After triangulation with the endoscope and instrument on the V-point, the ideal inclinatory angle for surgery is about 20 degrees to 25 degrees (Fig. 16.8a–c).

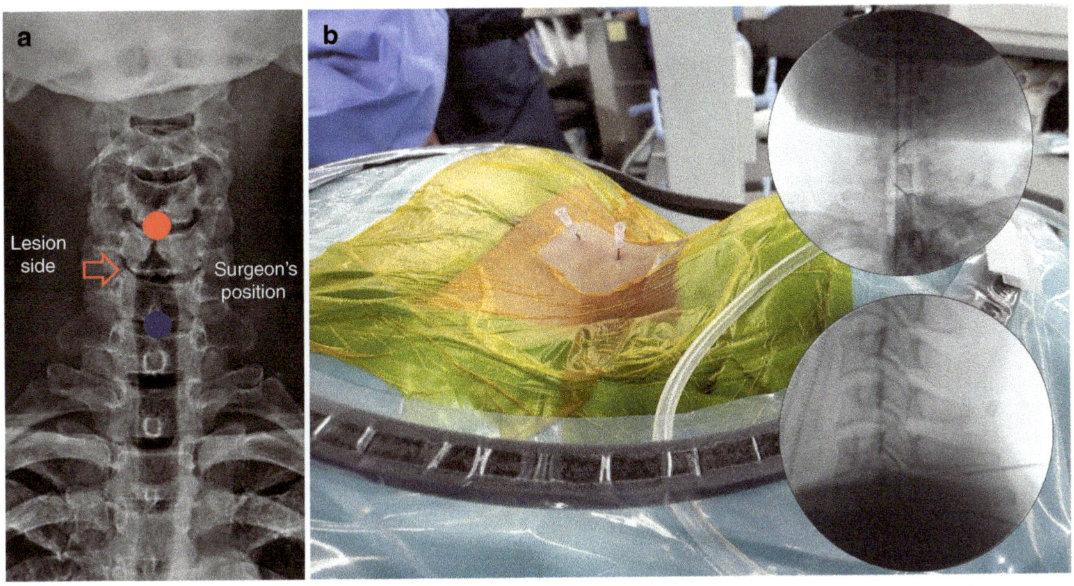

Fig. 16.7 The skin incision points of PCIF are marked on the upper and lower spinous process around the target level. Two skin incisions for the scope portal (Blue circle) and the working portal (Red circle) are illustrated in the figure. A red open arrow means target lesion (**a**). The skin entry points for two portals and needle targeting before skin incision is shown. Needle targeting toward the V-point of the lesion site to determine the two skin entry points and approach angle is shown by the C-arm fluoroscopic image (**b**)

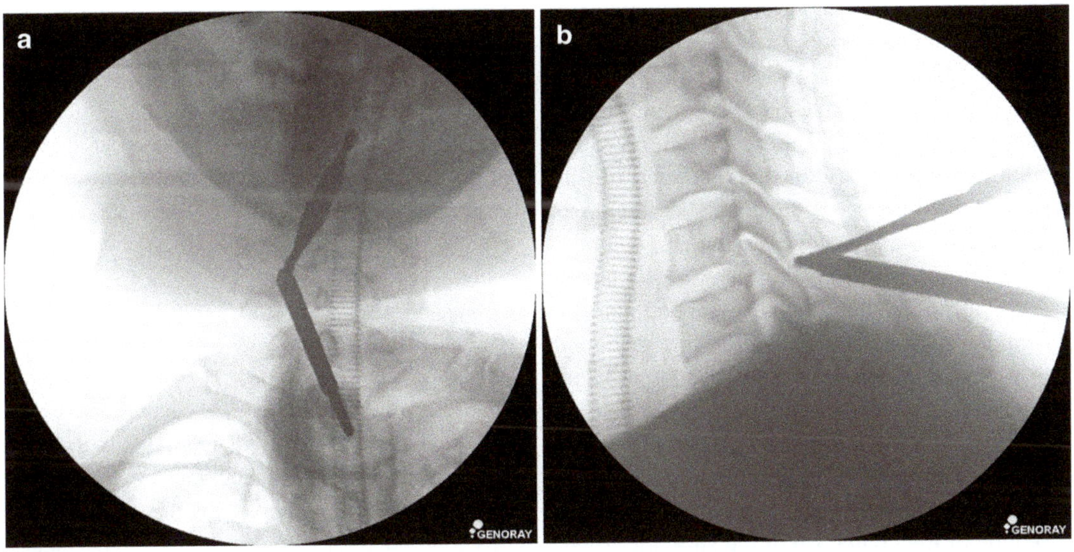

Fig. 16.8 Triangulation with endoscope and instruments. Triangulation of endoscope and instruments is done at the docking point (V-point) under the C-arm fluoroscopic views (**a, b**). The proper inclinatory operative angle is about 20 degrees to 25 degrees. The schematic shows the surgical trajectory of PCIF and endoscopic surgical view (Blue square) of the PCIF approached from right to left side (**c**)

c

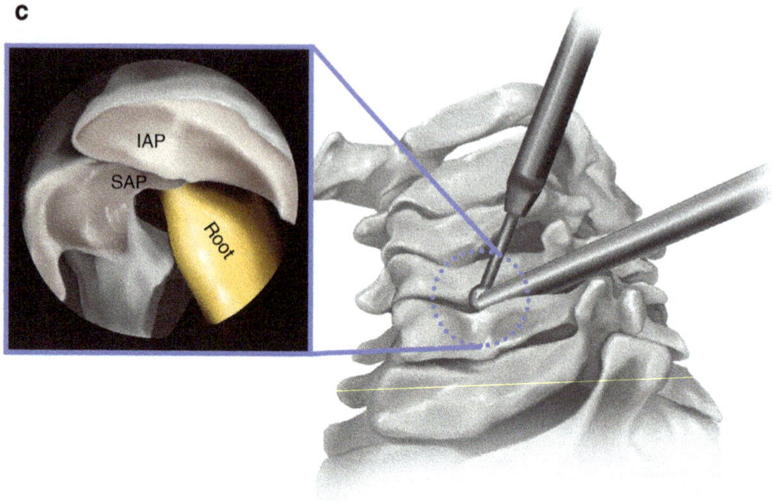

Fig. 16.8 (continued)

16.7.2 Foraminotomy and Flavectomy

The inferolateral portion of the upper lamina and the superolateral part of the lower lamina are drilled out as in the PCF (Video 16.4).

The ligament flavum can be a protector of the neural structure during drilling for laminectomy. Drilling around the V-point is continued till the caudocranial margin of the ligament flavum is exposed. The Surgeon could assume the shape of the nerve root through a thin layer at the lateral margin of the ligament flavum. The boundary of decompression is extended to the further lateral part of the foramen by using a bendable 3 mm diamond bur.

After circumferential drilling along the passage of the nerve root, additional decompression for the distal portion of the nerve root is done by resection of the cranial tip of the superior articular process with the 1 mm Kerrison's punch or small curette (Video 16.4).

After sufficient bony decompression, the ligament flavum is removed at last. While removing the ligament flavum, bleeding control is performed. Immediate hemostasis around the nerve root origin is done by using the small RF probe, because the venous plexus is abundant around the nerve root origin area, and sometimes it makes troublesome intraoperative bleeding. When hemostasis is carried out using an RF probe, the RF tip is located under the vessel, lifted up from contact with the nerve root. Then it can prevent neural damage.

Sufficient foraminal decompression is confirmed by passing a ball tip probe through the foraminal canal without any resistance (Fig. 16.9).

16.7.3 Discectomy

Annulotomy is implemented using an Indian knife or ball tip type small RF. At this time, be careful of nerve root damage. Discectomy is conducted by using the hook and the pituitary forceps, after adequate foraminotomy and perineural adhesiolysis (Video 16.5). Scope retractor is used for the acquisition of enough space for discectomy or removal of the bony spur with nerve root protection (Video 16.5).

After PCF or PCIF, a surgical drain is inserted, and kept for 24 h, until spontaneous bleeding is controlled. The wound is closed with subcutaneous

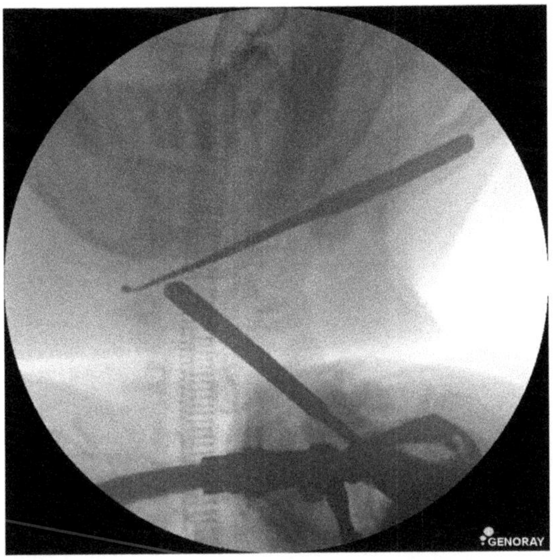

Fig. 16.9 Sufficient decompression in the foraminal area is verified by passing the ball tip probe through the foraminal canal

suture and skin tape. After surgery, patients are advised to wear a neck collar for a week.

16.8 Illustrated Cases

16.8.1 Case 1: PCF C5–6 Right

A 38-year-old female patient had right shoulder and scapular pain and numbness of the right upper extremity about four months ago. In the neurologic examination, Spurling's test was positive, and there was right-side motor weakness (grade 4) in elbow flexion with the right C6 dermatome paresthesia. The Visual Analogue Scale (VAS) of the right shoulder was 8. Preoperative Magnetic resonance imaging (MRI), and computed tomography (CT) showed right-side herniated disc on C5–6 level (Fig. 16.10a–c).

The PCF with discectomy was performed under general anesthesia. After sufficient foraminotomy, the extruded disc was identified in the axillary area of the right C6 nerve root, which was removed (Fig. 16.10d, e). Pulsation of the nerve root was all recovered. Postoperative images showed the ideal foraminal decompression and removal of the disc with minimal facet joint and muscle damage (Fig. 16.10f–i). The pain and weakness of the patient improved. The VAS of the right shoulder was changed from 8 to 1. The VAS of neck pain was about 1 after the operation. The motor weakness was recovered to normal immediately after the operation.

16.8.2 Case 2: PCIF C3–4, C4–5 Right

A 60-year-old male patient visited the hospital due to chronic occipital neuralgia with the right shoulder and scapular pain area that occurred 11 months ago. In the neurologic examination, Spurling's test was positive, and there was the right C4, 5 dermatome paresthesia without motor weakness. The VAS of headache and right shoulder were 6 and 7, respectively. Preoperative MRI and CT documented right-side foraminal stenosis at the C3–4, C4–5 levels (Fig. 16.11a–d).

The PCIF was performed under general anesthesia. After sufficient nerve roots decompression, the pulsation of nerve roots was all recovered (Fig. 16.11e, f). Postoperative images showed the ideal two-level foraminal decompression with minimal facet violations (Fig. 16.11g–k). The patient's headache and shoulder pain improved. The VAS of headache and shoulder were changed to 0 and 1, respectively.

16.8.3 Case 3: PCIF C5–6 Left

A 59-year-old male patient suffered from acute left scapular and shoulder pain with weakness. The symptoms occurred 7 days ago. In the neurologic examination, Spurling's test was positive, and there was left-side motor weakness (grade 4) in elbow flexion with the left C6 dermatome paresthesia. The VAS of the left shoulder was 9. Selective root block was effective only for 2 days. Preoperative MRI and CT documented left-side foraminal stenosis at the C5–6 level (Fig. 16.12a–c).

The PCIF was performed under general anesthesia. In the surgical findings, a severe adhesive fibrotic band was formed between the left C6 nerve root and the left C5 pedicle medial aspect, which was entrapping the nerve root, and hinder-

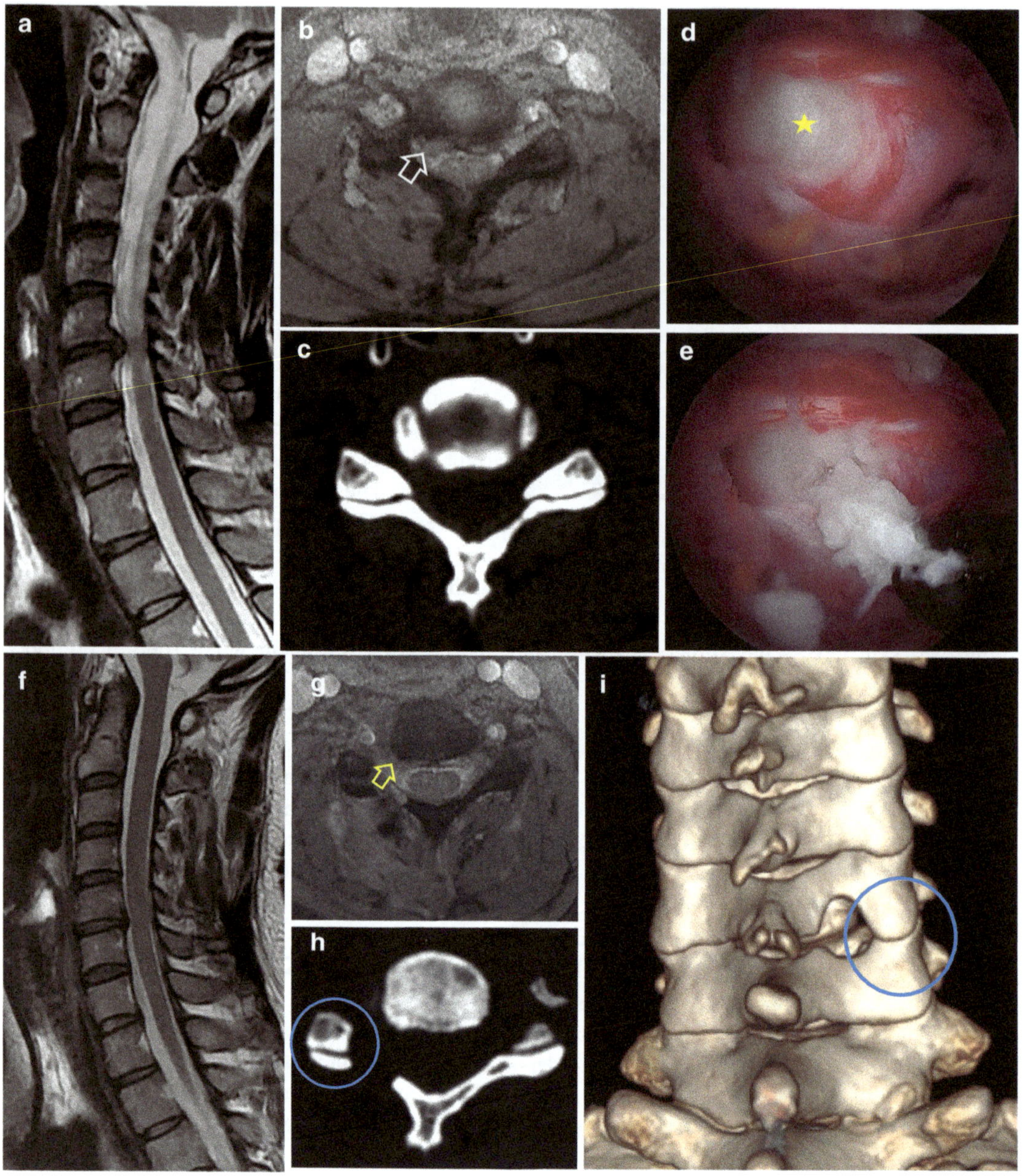

Fig. 16.10 The Case of PCF and discectomy at the C5–6 level. The preoperative T2 sagittal MR image shows the herniated disc at C5–6 level (**a**). The preoperative T2 axial MR image (**b**) and CT axial scan (**c**) show the herniated disc on the right side C5–6 level without facet hypertrophy (White open arrow). An intraoperative endoscopic image shows the extruded disc (Yellow asterisk) at the axillary portion of the right C6 nerve root (**d**). After annulotomy, the disc particle is pushed out (**e**). The postoperative T2 sagittal and axial MR image (**f, g**) show the sufficient removal of the disc at the C5–6 level (Yellow open arrow). The CT axial scan (**h**) and the three-dimensional reconstructive CT scan (**i**) show minimal damage to the facet joint (Blue circles)

ing the normal pathway of the nerve root (Fig. 16.12d). After sufficient nerve root decompression, the pulsation of nerve root was all recovered. Postoperative images showed sufficient left C5–6 foraminal decompression with minimal facet joint injury (Fig. 16.12e–h). The patient's pain and weakness improved. The VAS of the shoulder was changed to 9 and 1, respectively. The motor grade was recovered to normal immediately after the operation.

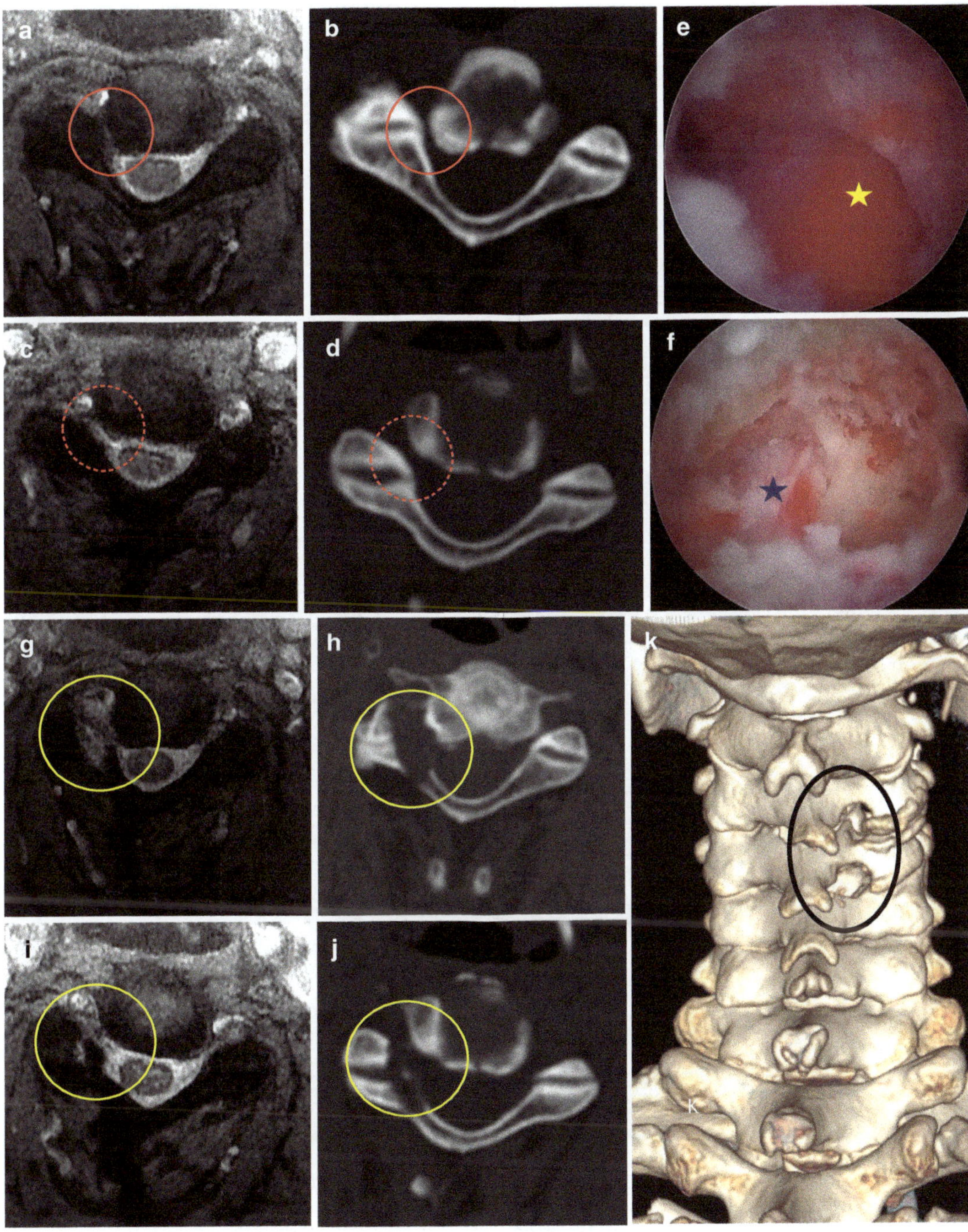

Fig. 16.11 The Case of PCIF at the right C3–4, C4–5 levels. The preoperative T2 axial MR image (**a**) and CT axial scan (**b**) show the foraminal stenosis on the right side C3–4 level with facet hypertrophy (Red circles). The preoperative T2 axial MR image (**c**) and CT axial scan (**d**) show the foraminal stenosis on the right side C4–5 level without facet hypertrophy (Red dashed circles). An intra-operative endoscopic image shows the engorged right C4 nerve root (Yellow asterisk) and C5 nerve root (Blue asterisk) after decompression (**e, f**). The postoperative T2 axial MR image (**g**) and CT axial scan (**h**) show sufficient foraminal decompression of the C3–4 right foramen (Yellow circles). Also, the postoperative T2 axial MR image (**i**) and CT axial scan (**j**) show the foraminal decompression of the C4–5 level on the right side (Yellow dashed circles). The 3-dimensional reconstructive CT scan shows the foraminotomy site, which is located on the more medial side. So the dorsal surface of the facet joint (Black dashed circle) is more preserved (**k**)

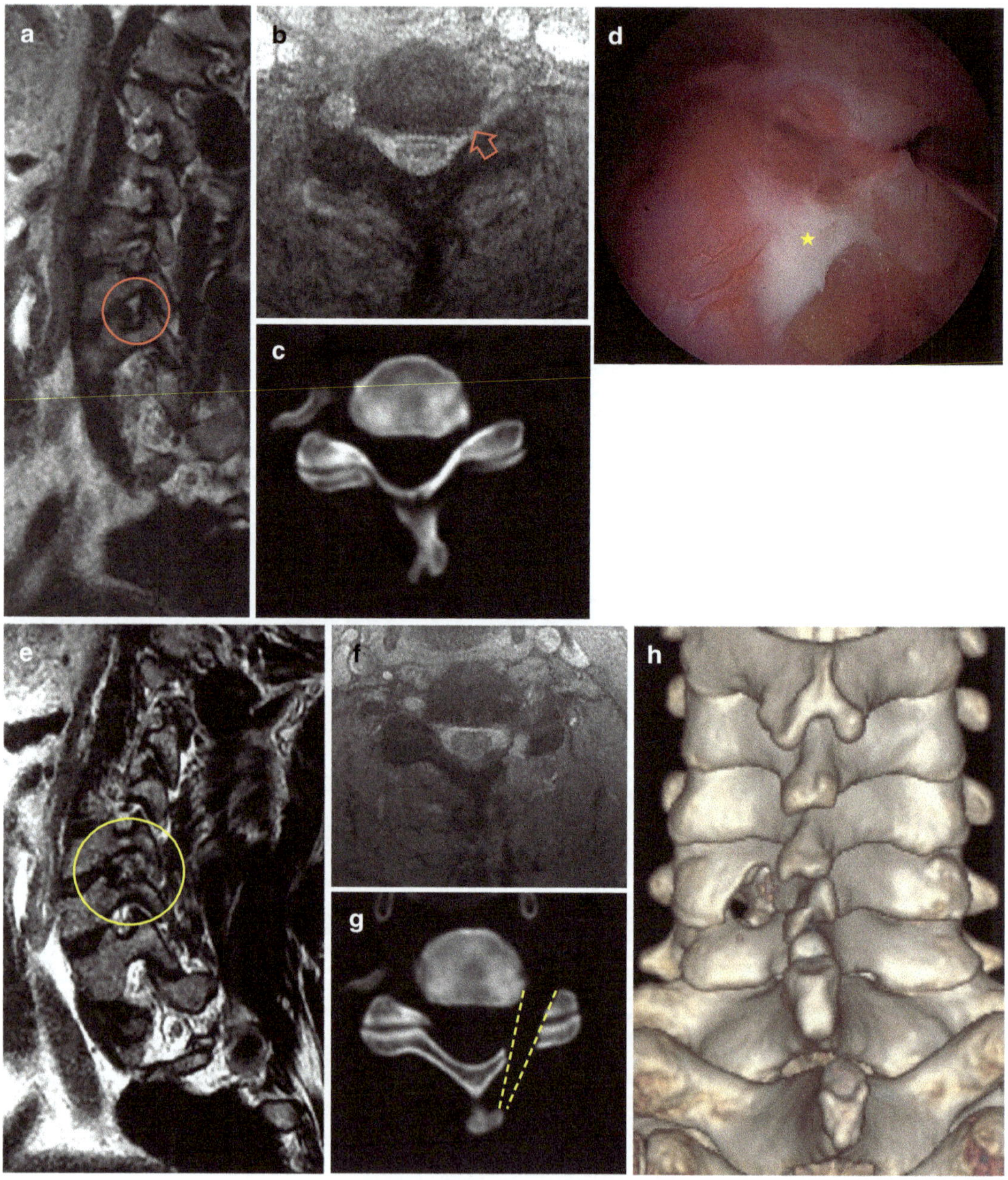

Fig. 16.12 The Case of PCIF at the left C5–6 level. The preoperative T2 left para-sagittal MR image shows the foraminal stenosis C5–6 level (Red circle) (**a**). The preoperative T2 axial MR image (**b**) and CT axial scan (**c**) show the foraminal stenosis on the left C5–6 level without facet hypertrophy (Red open arrow). An intraoperative endoscopic image shows the severe adhesion between the left C6 nerve root and the medial aspect of the C5 pedicle. The adhesive fibrotic band (Yellow asterisk) is cut by a small RF, and the nerve root is released (**d**). The postoperative T2 left para-sagittal MR image (**e**) and axial MR image (**f**) and CT axial scan (**g**) show the cutting surface of the facet joint with inclinatory angle (Yellow dashed lines) and the sufficiently widened left C5–6 foramen (Yellow circle). The three-dimensional reconstructive CT scan (**h**) shows the foraminotomy site, which is located on the more medial side

16.9 Complications and Their Management

16.9.1 Bleeding

The most important reason to ensure clear surgical vision is to minimize the technical complications that can occur during surgery. To do this, the bleeding that occurs during surgery must be controlled.

The most important key to the posterior cervical approach is the position of the patient. By slanting down the upper back, the venous return can be reduced. The use of this method can greatly reduce the amount of bleeding that occurs during surgery.

We also recommend the use of a diamond bur to reduce the bone bleeding that occurs during laminectomy. It also works as a drill to stop the bleeding. Bone wax is useful to stop bleeding also.

The main cause of bleeding after flavectomy is epidural blood vessels covering the dura. A small RF device can stop the bleeding by stopping this vessel.

16.9.2 Dura Tear

The dural tear during cervical spine surgery is less common than during lumbar spine surgery, and the incidence is reported to be about 3% [9]. Nevertheless, the dural tear remains one of the complications that spine surgeons do not want to meet during surgery.

In particular, UBE allows the surgical field to be viewed at high magnification, and the saline from continuous pressure irrigation enables slight compression of the dura during procedures. Therefore, it can be difficult to find cerebrospinal fluid leakage. A significant dural tear should be repaired directly by converting to microscopic surgery; however, severe dura tear occurs rarely in PCF or PCIF.

Most of the dura tears in PCF and PCIF occur in drill work after flavectomy. Drill work after removing the ligament flavum should be performed very carefully. In particular, dust that occurs during drill work in endoscopic surgery obscures vision. There is also the possibility that the surrounding tissue can be moved by the saline flow, and the ligament flavum that can protect the nervous structure has been removed, so the possibility of a drill causing neural tissue injury should be kept in mind (Fig. 16.13).

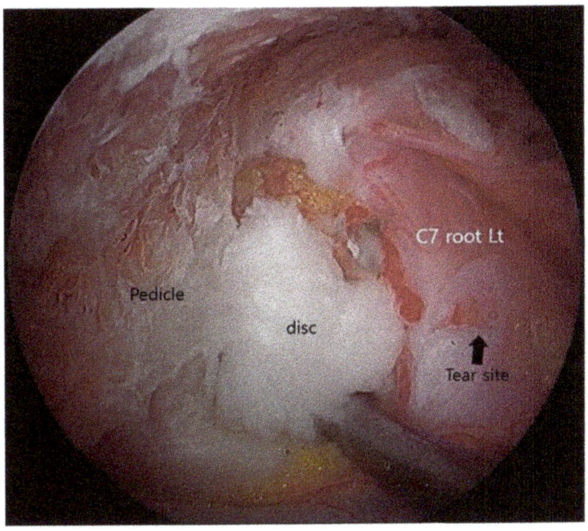

Fig. 16.13 An intraoperative endoscopic image shows the small dura tear (Black arrow) on the proximal left C7 nerve root. This was developed by drilling after flavectomy

Most of the small dural tear can be resolved with the application of sealant materials and placing the patient on bed rest.

16.10 Surgical Tips and Pitfalls

First, it is important to make sure of finding the V-point of the level the surgeon wants to operate on before drilling. In particular, it should be noted that the position of the V-point can always change, depending on the degree of neck flexion in the patient's surgical position.

Second, laminectomy using drill should be done until the attachment of the ligament flavum is exposed. It is easy to remove the ligament flavum at once. Removing the ligament flavum piecemeal is more likely to result in neural injury due to punches.

Third, hemostasis of the epidural vessel must be done right away. Venous plexus around the nerve root is very abundant, and if bleeding cannot be stopped there, the surgical endoscopic vision will be interrupted, and surgery will no longer be possible.

Fourth, PCIF is an operation performed at a narrow, inclinatory angle. Therefore, the use of surgical instruments, such as Kerrison's punches and burs, may be difficult. So, other devices, such as small curettes and chisels, should be prepared for use.

Fifth, the same is true for all surgeries, but the surgical anatomy, the pathway of the nerve root, the locational relationship between the ruptured disc and the nerve root, and the direction facet joint aspect must be known before surgery. Because disc rupture is often located in the axillar portion of the nerve root, the nerve root retraction is usually done in the cranial direction. This requires an appropriate scope position and instrument position. PCF and PCIF have different portal locations for the same lesion, so simulate the location of the preoperative lesion to find the best approach.

References

1. Park JH, Jun SG, Jung JT, Lee SJ. Posterior percutaneous endoscopic cervical foraminotomy and diskectomy with unilateral biportal endoscopy. Orthopedics. 2017;40(5):e779–e83.
2. Kim HS, Wu PH, Lee YJ, Kim DH, Kim JY, Lee JH, et al. Safe route for cervical approach: partial pediculotomy, partial vertebrotomy approach for posterior endoscopic cervical foraminotomy and discectomy. World Neurosurg. 2020;140:e273–e82.
3. Leheta F, Kazner E, Kollmannsberger A. Therapy of cervical nerve root compression syndromes. Indication, technic and results of foraminotomy. Fortschr Med. 1973;91(17):725–31.
4. Song KS, Lee CW. The biportal endoscopic posterior cervical inclinatory foraminotomy for cervical radiculopathy: technical report and preliminary results. Neurospine. 2020;17(Suppl 1):S145–S53.
5. Kang MS, Park HJ, Hwang JH, Kim JE, Choi DJ, Chung HJ. Safety evaluation of biportal endoscopic lumbar discectomy: assessment of cervical epidural pressure during surgery. Spine (Phila Pa 1976). 2020;45(20):E1349–E56.
6. Kim CH, Shin KH, Chung CK, Park SB, Kim JH. Changes in cervical sagittal alignment after single-level posterior percutaneous endoscopic cervical diskectomy. Global Spine J. 2015;5(1):31–8.
7. Voo LM, Kumaresan S, Yoganandan N, Pintar FA, Cusick JF. Finite element analysis of cervical facetectomy. Spine (Phila Pa 1976). 1997;22(9):964–9.
8. Zdeblick TA, Zou D, Warden KE, McCabe R, Kunz D, Vanderby R. Cervical stability after foraminotomy. A biomechanical in vitro analysis. J Bone Joint Surg Am. 1992;74(1):22–7.
9. Yoshihara H, Yoneoka D. Incidental dural tear in cervical spine surgery: analysis of a nationwide database. J Spinal Disord Tech. 2015;28(1):19–24.

Unilateral Biportal Endoscopy for Cervical Decompressive Laminectomy

17

Ji Yeon Kim, Jin Hwa Eum, and Choon Keun Park

17.1 Introduction

Cervical myelopathy is caused by degenerative cervical spondylosis, cervical disc protrusion, and cervical ossification of posterior longitudinal ligament (OPLL). Cervical myelopathy usually requires surgical treatments such as decompressive laminectomy, laminoplasty, anterior cervical discectomy and fusion, anterior cervical corpectomy, or anterior-posterior combined approaches rather than minimally invasive approaches or endoscopic spine surgery [1]. However, posterior cervical laminoplasty or laminectomy with instrumentation are extensive surgeries, and have a high possibility of injury of the posterior neck muscles [2], and may have perioperative morbidities and mortality related to extensive surgical procedures.

Supplementary Information The online version contains supplementary material available at [https://doi.org/10.1007/978-981-16-8201-8_17].

J. Y. Kim
Department of Neurosurgery, Spine Center, Wiltse Memorial Hospital, Anyang, South Korea

J. H. Eum (✉)
Department of Neurosurgery, Spine Center, Burjeel Royal Hospital, Al Ain, UAE

C. K. Park
Department of Neurosurgery, Spine Center, Wiltse Memorial Hospital, Suwon, South Korea

Therefore, various minimally invasive surgical methods have been developed to preserve the cervical extensor muscle, such as selective laminectomy and microendoscopic laminoplasty [3–5]. Endoscopic posterior cervical decompression obviates the need for extensor muscle dissection and the disruption of the posterior spinous process-ligament-muscle complex and can prevent post-laminectomy kyphosis. It does not require the sacrifice of a cervical motion segment, thereby lessening the need for additional fusion. Jian et al. [6] reported a case series with 21 patients who had undergone a full-endoscopic posterior cervical unilateral laminectomy for bilateral decompression and observed a favorable clinical outcome with a one-year follow-up, and none of the patients showed increasing kyphosis after surgery or serious complications.

Unilateral biportal endoscopy has been tried and developed to treat cervical radiculopathy caused by foraminal stenosis or foraminal disc herniation through posterior foraminotomy and discectomy [7, 8]. With the development of the instruments such as a scope retractor, working cannula, and a fine endoscopic diamond drill, the biportal endoscopic system can access the bilateral side through the unilateral laminotomy. Therefore, we can perform unilateral laminotomy (laminectomy) with bilateral decompression surgery to treat cervical spondylotic myelopathy with safe and well-designed surgical procedures [9].

D. H. Heo et al. (eds.), *Unilateral Biportal Endoscopic Spine Surgery*,
https://doi.org/10.1007/978-981-16-8201-8_17

17.2 Indications and Contraindications

Biportal endoscopic unilateral laminotomy (laminectomy) with bilateral decompression could be considered for selective patients with one or two levels of cervical stenosis as follows.

- Indication
  - Cervical stenosis due to hypertrophied ligament flavum
  - Cervical stenosis with concomitant foraminal stenosis
  - Cervical stenosis with OPLL involving less than 50% of the spinal canal
- Relative Contraindication
  - Multiple level cervical stenosis involving more than three levels
  - Cervical stenosis with disc herniation
- Contraindication
  - Cervical stenosis with segmental instability
  - Cervical stenosis with OPLL involving more than 50% of the spinal canal
  - Cervical stenosis with prominent disc herniation
  - Cervical stenosis with prominent ossification of ligamentum flavum

In the cases of contraindication, conventional anterior cervical discectomy and fusion (ACDF), or posterior cervical surgery such as laminoplasty or laminectomy could be considered instead of trying posterior endoscopic decompression. ACDF can be proposed when a herniated disc causes persistent pain or symptomatic segmental instability following posterior endoscopic decompression.

17.3 Special Instruments (See Detailed Figures in Chapters for Instruments)

A compressed spinal cord is vulnerable and may be injured with even slight pressure by the instruments. Therefore, several optimized surgical instruments are essential for safe and adequate neural decompression while avoiding spinal cord injury.

1. 3.5-mm and 3.0-mm endoscopic diamond drill for intimate bone drilling along the free end of the ligamentum flavum (LF).
2. Working cannulas to maintain proper outflow of the saline and prevent increasing water pressure to the spinal cord.
3. Scope self-retractor to protect the surrounding structures during drilling.

17.4 Anesthesia and Position

The patient underwent surgery under general anesthesia in the prone position on a radiolucent Wilson frame for posterior surgery equipped with a chest bar. A compression-free sponge device was placed under the face of the patient, and the neck was slightly flexed. The slightly flexed neck position can be maintained using skin tape without skull fixation. It is the same with a surgical position for the posterior endoscopic cervical foraminotomy and discectomy.

17.5 Surgical Steps of Laminectomy with Bilateral Decompression (Video 17.1)

Surgical steps of biportal endoscopic C6 laminectomy with bilateral decompression at the C5-C6-C7 levels through right-sided approach to treat cervical spondylotic myelopathy.

17.5.1 Making Two Portals

Under image intensification, fluoroscopic confirmation of the level is performed with the insertion of spinal needles at the target area. We usually need one pair of portals to decompress the two-level posterior cervical decompression surgery to avoid the crowding between an endoscope and surgical instruments. Two paramedian portals (one pair of portals) were first created over the C5

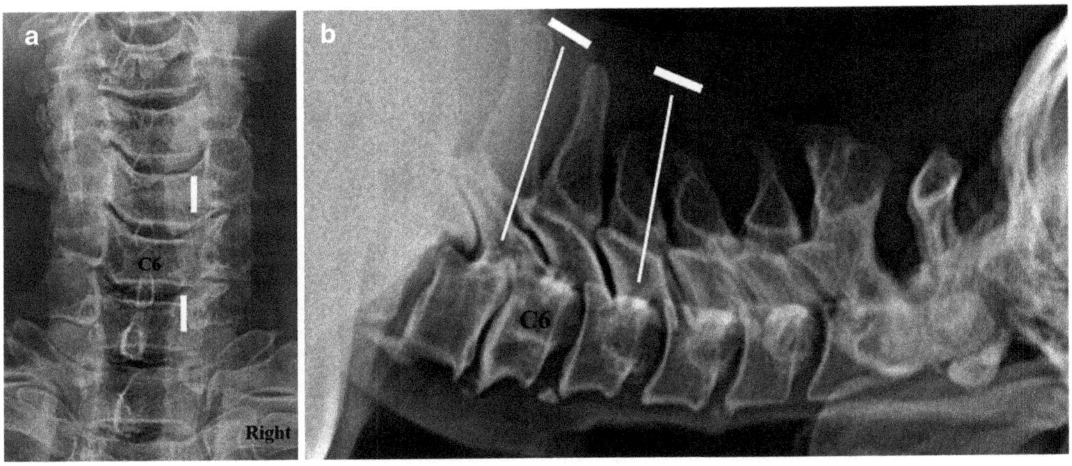

Fig. 17.1 Skin incision points of making two portals for bilateral decompression of the C5-C6-C7 levels. One pair of portals over ipsilateral pedicles at the upper (C5) and lower (C6) involved levels is sufficient to decompress the two adjacent cervical levels. Anteroposterior view (**a**); lateral view (**b**)

and C7 pedicles along the medial pedicle line (approximately 2 cm lateral to the midline) in the anteroposterior view to decompress the C5-C6-C7 levels (Fig. 17.1). Paraspinal muscles in the cervical spinal levels consisted of multiple layers of muscle and facia, blocking the outflow of the infused water. Therefore, sufficient skin incisions of approximately 1.0-cm and longitudinal linear skin incisions (Fig. 17.1) parallel with the muscle fiber direction are critical to keeping proper outflow of the saline. Serial dilators were inserted at the working portal, and then a working cannula was inserted along the serial dilator.

17.5.2 Soft Tissue Dissection and Expose the Targeted Lamina and Interlaminar Area

Incidental instrument insertion into the interlaminar area before clear identification may cause spinal cord injury with penetration of the LF. The position of serial dilators and instruments should be confirmed with an intraoperative X-ray. Furthermore, if the instruments and endoscope are located on the C6 lamina before starting soft tissue dissection, the risk of accidental cord compression injury may be decreased. We should expose the whole part of targeted laminas and interlaminar areas before bone drilling using the radiofrequency (RF) probe (Fig. 17.2a). Initial drilling of the superior part of the lamina (C6) makes easy access to the contralateral side of the adjacent interlaminar area and inferior border of the upper lamina (C5) (Fig. 17.2b).

17.5.3 Ipsilateral Hemilaminectomy and Contralateral Sublaminar Bony Drilling

Ipsilateral outer cortical bone and cancellous bone of the involved lamina (C6) were removed using a fine endoscopic drill while preserving inner cortical bone (Fig. 17.2c). Then, sublaminar bony drilling of the contralateral side was performed until the medial border of the facet joint was exposed while retaining the spinous process and contours of the contralateral outer cortical bone (Fig. 17.2d). After confirming the extent of the remaining inner cortical bone and its boundaries, the inner cortical bone was further drilled along the medial border of the bilateral facet joint (Fig. 17.2e, g), similar to thin paper. Subsequently, thinned parts of the lamina were cut using a fine dissector (Fig. 17.2f, h).

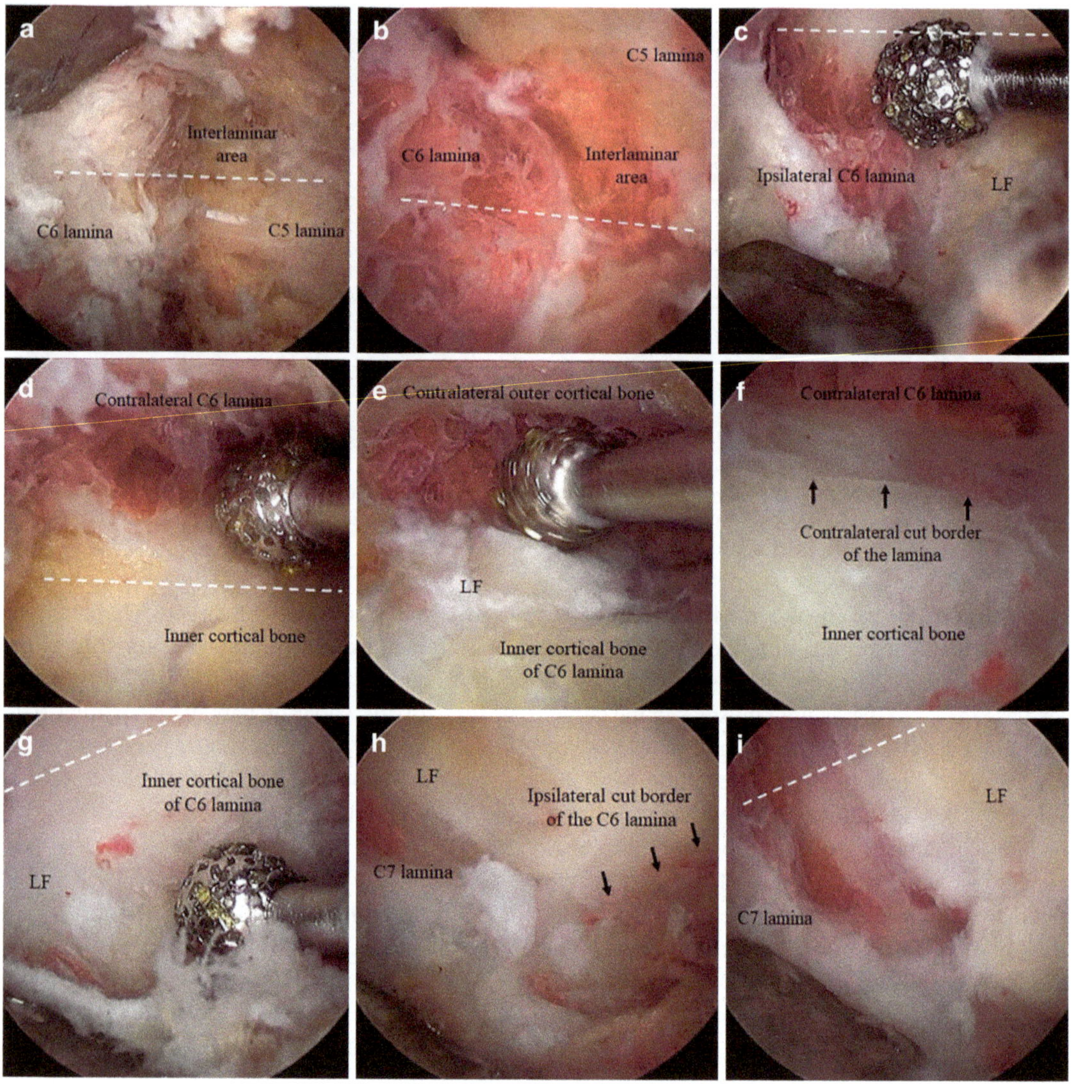

Fig. 17.2 Endoscopic view of surgical steps. Soft-tissue dissection and exposing the targeted lamina and interlaminar area (**a, b**). Ipsilateral hemilaminectomy (**c**) and contralateral sublaminar bony drilling (**d**) while preserving the bilateral inner cortical bone and contralateral outer cortical bone. Remained inner cortical bone was drilled along the medial border of the facet joint, similar to thin paper, at the contralateral side (**e, f**) and ipsilateral side (**g, h**). A partial laminotomy along the inferior border of the C5 lamina (**k**), and superior border of the C7 lamina (**i, j**). Detached ligamentum flavum (LF) from the laminotomy sites using a fine hook and dissectors (**l, m**) and cut the LF along the bilateral medial border of the facet joints (**n**). Removed the secured flap with forceps with en bloc fashion (**p**) after sufficient epidural dissection (**o**). A fully decompressed dural sac was found after hemostasis (**q**) then inserted a drainage catheter (**r**). *LF* ligamentum flavum. White dotted line: midline

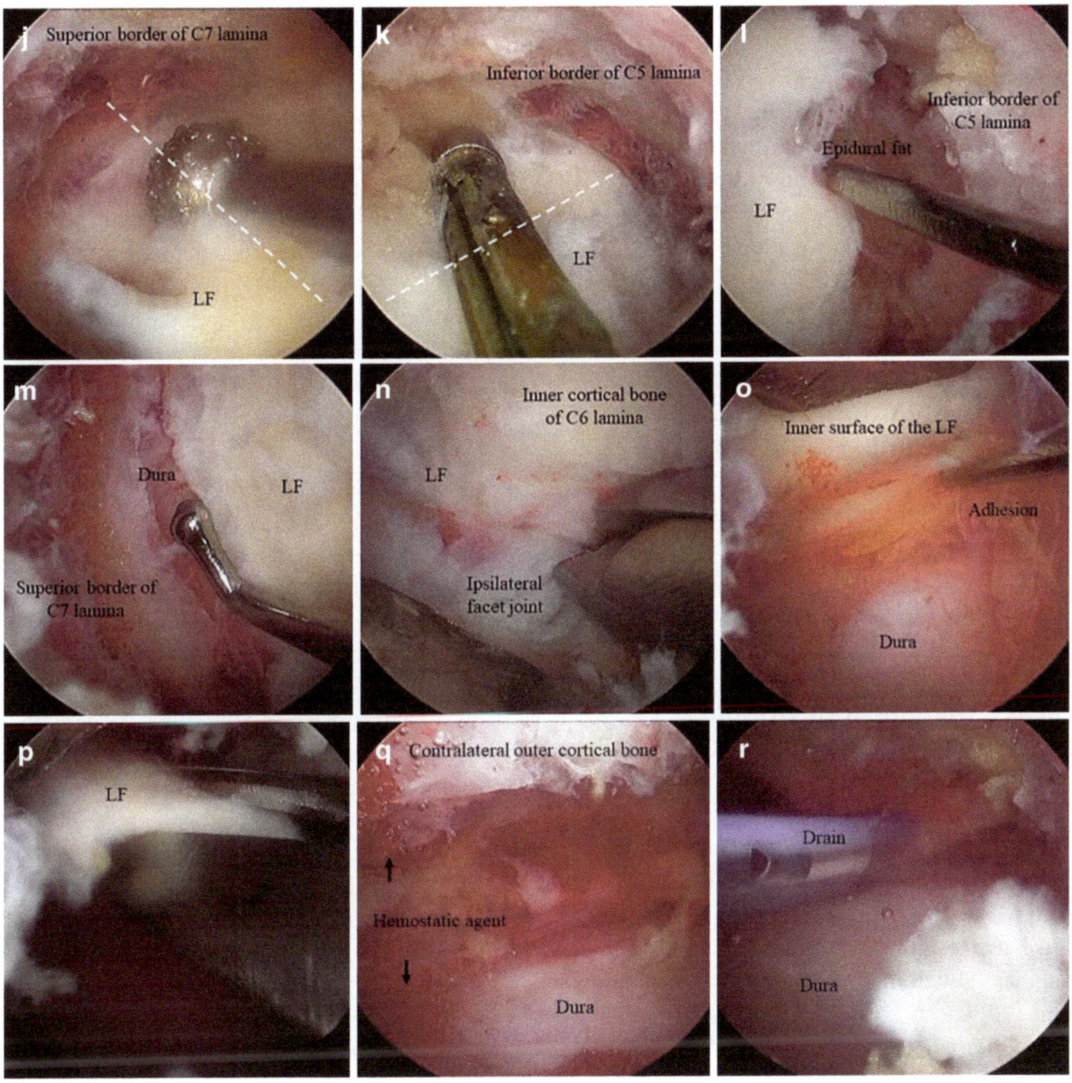

Fig. 17.2 (continued)

17.5.4 Partial Laminotomy to Detach the LF from the Adjacent Laminas

A partial laminotomy was performed along the inferior border of the one level upper (C5) lamina (Fig. 17.2k), and superior border of the one level lower (C7) lamina (Fig. 17.2i, j) using a fine endoscopic drill until the proximal and distal free margin of LF were exposed. Subsequently, we detached LF from the laminotomy sites using a fine hook and dissectors (Fig. 17.2l, m) and cut the LF along the bilateral medial border of the facet joints using 1.0-mm punches (Fig. 17.2n). At this time, the entire flap consisted of the C6 inner cortical bone with an inferiorly and superiorly attached LF was created.

17.5.5 Neural Decompression

The secured flap was lifted from the ipsilateral free edge to expose the epidural space using a scope self-retractor. Sufficient epidural dissection was performed between the lamina and dura without causing irritation of the dura (Fig. 17.2o). Subsequently, en bloc removal of the secured flap was performed using fine forceps (Fig. 17.2p). Epidural bleeding was controlled using the hemostatic agent rather than an radiofrequency (RF) probe (Fig. 17.2q). A drainage catheter was finally inserted to prevent postoperative epidural hematoma (Fig. 17.2r).

17.6 Surgical Steps of Unilateral Laminotomy with Bilateral Decompression (Video 17.2)

Surgical steps of biportal endoscopic unilateral C5 laminotomy with bilateral decompression at the C5-C6 level through left-sided approach to treat cervical spondylotic myelopathy.

17.6.1 Midline Bony Drilling and Expose the Bilateral Interlaminar Area

We first exposed the involved interlaminar area and adjacent upper and lower-level laminas after soft tissue dissection (Fig. 17.3a) then performed ipsilateral laminotomy and drilling of the spinolaminar junction and contralateral sublaminar bone to wholly expose the bilateral interlaminar area (Fig. 17.3b, c).

17.6.2 Partial Laminotomy along the Superior and Inferior Border of the Interlaminar Area

A partial laminotomy was performed along the inferior border of the upper (C5) lamina (Fig. 17.3d), and superior border of the lower (C6) lamina (Fig. 17.3e) using a fine endoscopic drill until the proximal and distal free margin of LF were exposed.

17.6.3 Neural Decompression

We detached LF from the laminotomy sites and ipsilateral medial border of the facet joint using a fine hook and dissectors (Fig. 17.3f, g). Detached flavum was elevated from the ipsilateral border using a dissector. Subsequently, LF was removed with en bloc fashion using fine forceps (Fig. 17.3h). Finally, the compressed dural sac was fully expanded, and the contralateral medial border of the facet joint was found (Fig. 17.3i).

17.7 Illustrated Cases

1. An 88-year-old woman presented with motor weakness of insidious onset and gradual progression in the lower and upper extremities. Preoperative MR and CT images revealed central cervical stenosis at the C5-C6-C7 levels, which compressed the spinal cord secondary to ligamentum flavum hypertrophy with a calcified herniated disc at the C5-C6 level. There was no definite segmental instability on the preoperative X-ray images (Fig. 17.4). We performed the biportal endoscopic C6 laminectomy with bilateral decompression of C5-C6 and C6-C7 levels through the right unilateral approach (Video 17.1). Postoperative MR T2-weighted images showed adequate decompression of dural sac with well-preserved bilateral facet joints. Intraoperative images revealed the fully decompressed dural sac. The extracted specimen is consisted of the C6 inner cortical bone and superiorly and inferiorly attached LF (Fig. 17.4). Myelopathic symptoms were gradually improved after surgery.
2. A 45-year-old man presented with decreasing sensory and motor power of gradual progression in the lower extremities. He complained of radicular pain in both arm and lower extremities. Preoperative MR and CT images revealed central cervical stenosis

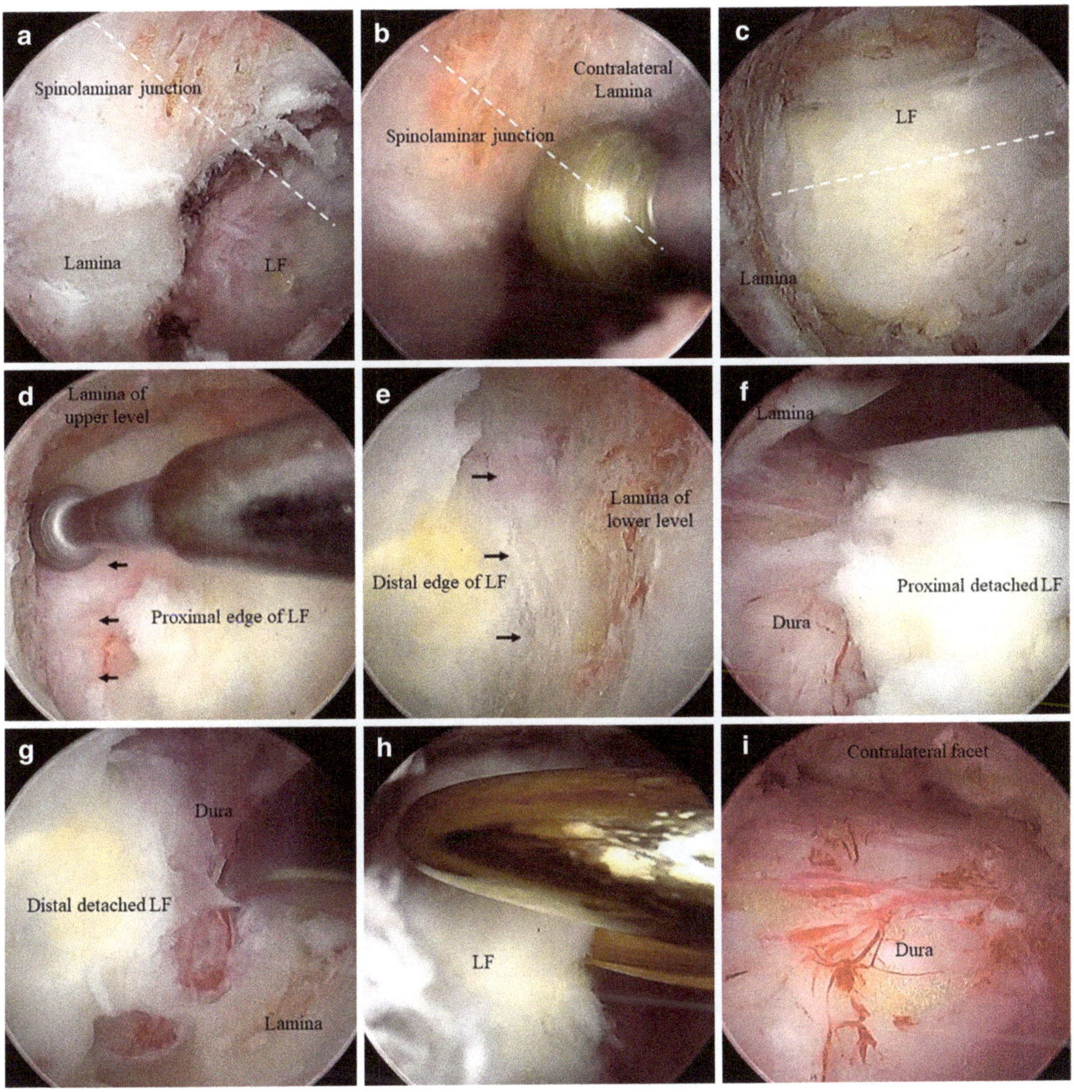

Fig. 17.3 Endoscopic view of surgical steps. Soft-tissue dissection and exposing the targeted lamina and interlaminar area (**a**). Drilling of spinolaminar junction and bilateral laminotomy (**b**). The bilateral interlaminar area was wholly exposed (**c**). Partial laminotomy along the inferior border of the upper lamina (**d**) and superior border of the lower lamina (**e**). Detached the LF from the upper and lower laminotomy sites (**f, g**). En bloc removal of the detached LF (**h**). A fully decompressed dural sac was found between the bilateral medial border of the facet joints (**i**)

with herniated disc compressing the spinal cord at the C5-C6-C7 levels. Instability was not found in the preoperative X-ray images (Fig. 17.5). We performed biportal endoscopic unilateral C5 laminotomy with bilateral decompression at the C5-C6 level through a left-sided approach (Video 17.2). The same procedures were performed at the C6-C7 level. Postoperative MR T2-weighted images showed adequate decompression of dural sac with well-preserved bilateral facet joints (Fig. 17.5). Postoperatively, symptoms of neurologic deficits and radicular pain were significantly improved.

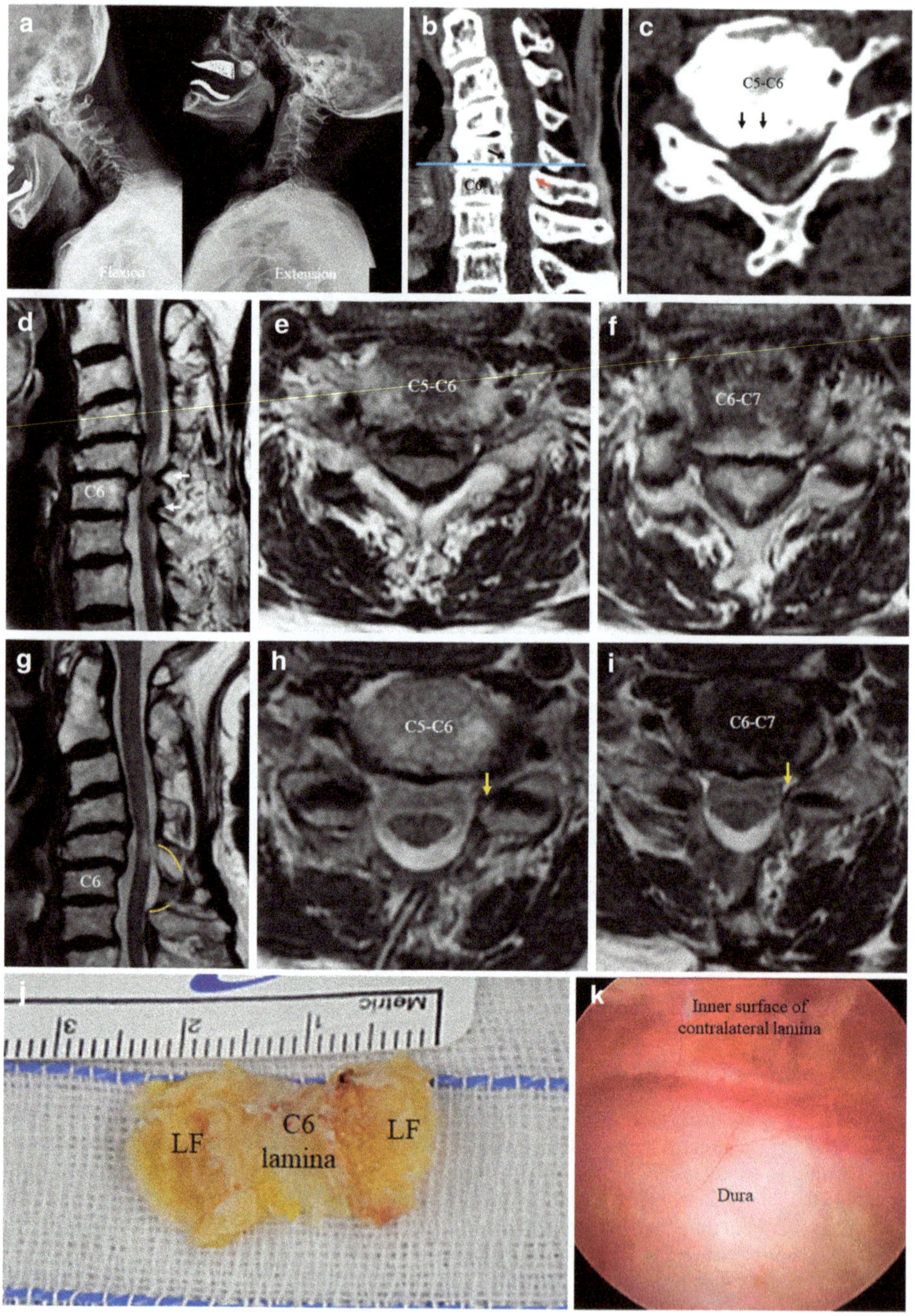

Fig. 17.4 An 88-year-old woman presented with motor weakness of insidious onset and gradual progression in the lower and upper extremities. There was no definite segmental instability on the preoperative dynamic X-ray images (**a**). Preoperative CT images showed narrowing of the spinal canal between the calcified herniated disc of the C5-C6 level (**b** and **c**, black arrows) and ventral part of the C6 lamina (**b**, red arrow). Preoperative MR images revealed central cervical stenosis at the C5-C6-C7 levels, which compressed the spinal cord secondary to ligamentum flavum hypertrophy (**d–f**, white arrows). Postoperative MR T2-weighted images showed adequate decompression of dural sac with well-preserved bilateral facet joints (**g–i**). The contralateral sublaminar bony drilling tract was found from the midline (**g**, yellow curved lines) to the medial border of the contralateral facet joint (**h** and **i**, yellow arrows). The extracted specimen is consisted of the C6 inner cortical bone and superiorly and inferiorly attached LF (**j**). The intraoperative view showed the fully decompressed dural sac (**k**)

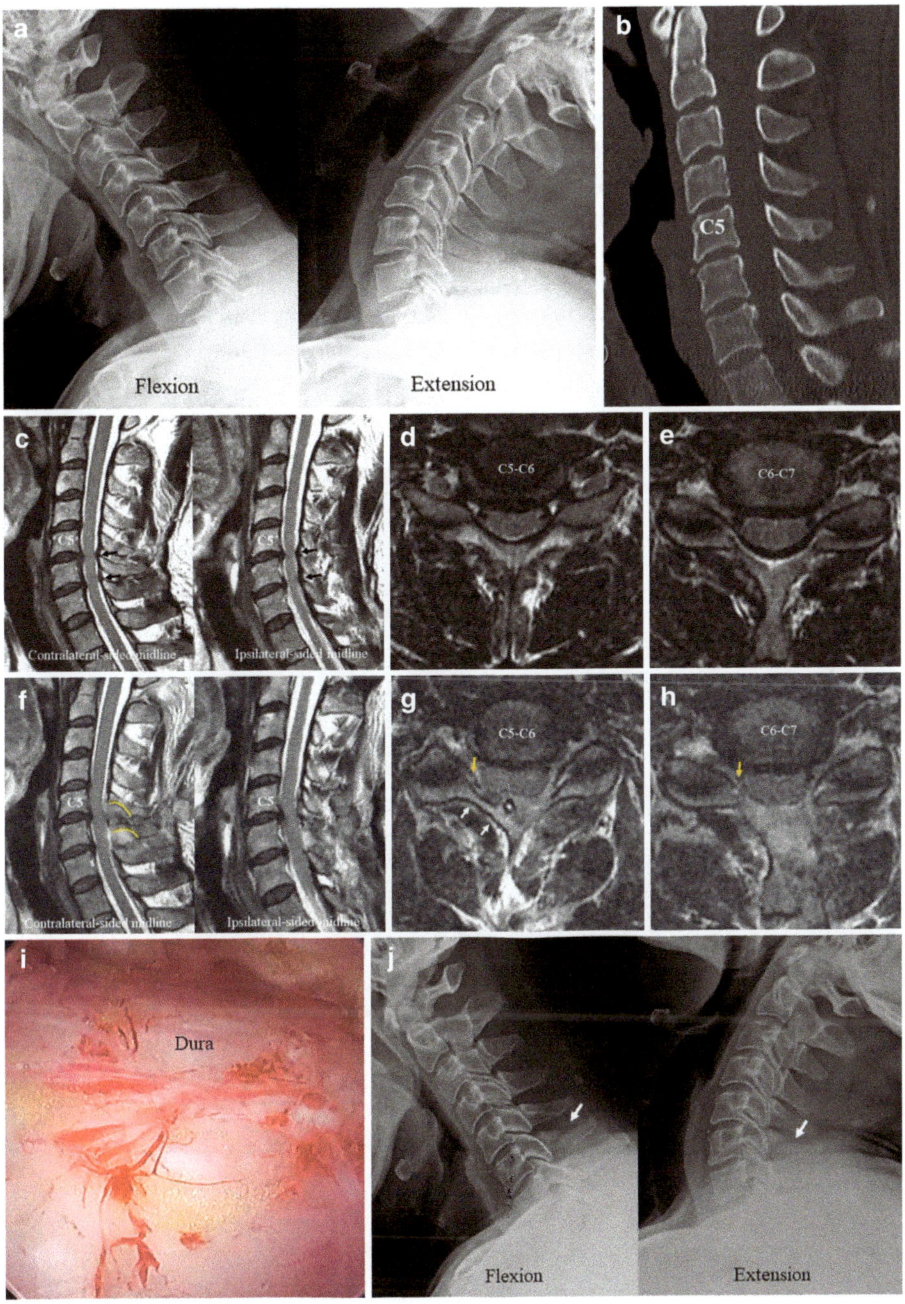

Fig. 17.5 A 45-year-old man presented with decreasing motor power and sensory of gradual progression in the lower extremities. There was no definite segmental instability on the dynamic X-ray images (**a**). Preoperative MR and CT images revealed central cervical stenosis (black arrows) with the herniated disc at the C5-C6-C7 levels (**b–e**). Postoperative MR images showed complete decompression of dural bilaterally (**f–h**). The tract of contralateral sublaminar bony drilling was found from the midline (**f**, yellow curved lines) to the medial border of the contralateral facet joint (**g** and **h**, yellow arrows) while preserving the contralateral outer cortical bone (**g**, white arrows). Intraoperative view showed the fully decompressed dural sac (**i**). Postoperative X-ray images showed delayed spinous process fracture (**j**, white arrows); however, he did not complain the mechanical neck pain

17.8 Complications and Their Management

A compressed spinal cord is vulnerable and may be injured with even slight pressure by the instruments. Intraoperative electrophysiological monitoring may be a good option for preventing iatrogenic dural injury. Continuous use of saline irrigation may increase the epidural pressure and cause nerve injury or irrigation [10]. We should keep the proper saline outflow by using the working cannula and carefully monitoring the outflow patency. Furthermore, the infusion pressure of saline should be maintained below 30 mmHg. A drainage catheter was inserted to prevent postoperative epidural hematoma, and the drainage bag was kept at negative pressure for approximately two days after surgery. Bony drilling over the LF is the essential technique during partial laminotomy. However, if we drill the lamina close to the detached LF, the high-speed drill can roll up the LF and dura simultaneously in a second (Fig. 17.6a, b). It may cause a sizeable dural tear and a severe spinal cord. If an incidental durot-

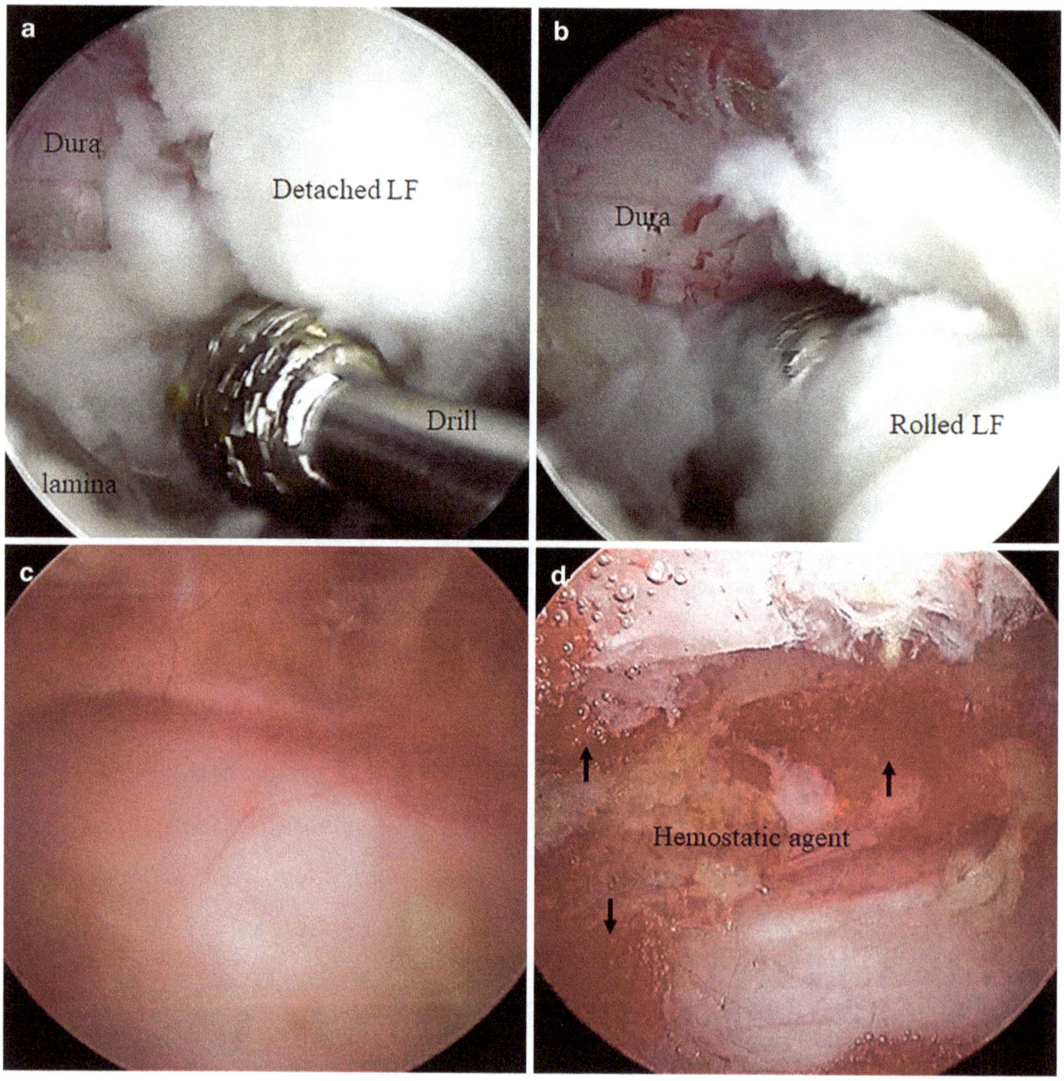

Fig. 17.6 Careful drilling is necessary during the laminotomy close to the detached LF using a high-speed unprotected drill (**a**). The spinning drill rolled up the LF and dura simultaneously (**b**). Blurred endoscopic view due to diffuse multifocal bleeding (**c**). Clear endoscopic view after use of foamy hemostatic agent (**d**)

omy occurs during operation, it can be repaired using a fibrin sealant patch or suture-less non-penetrating clips [11, 12]. If the primary dura repair fails, endoscopic surgery should be converted to open microscopic surgery for successful dural repair. The massive use of RF on the epidural vessels may induce spinal cord injury, and we recommend the foamy hemostatic agent for diffuse and multifocal epidural bleeding (Fig. 17.6c, d).

17.9 Surgical Tips and Pitfall

The compressed spinal cord is vulnerable and may be injured by even a slight pressure exerted by the instruments. Inserting instruments between the dura and LF before a detachment of the LF may compress the vulnerable spinal cord and induce spinal cord injury. Therefore, sufficient circumferential bony drilling along the hypertrophied LF is critical for safe neural decompression.

The LF protects the dura and spinal cord from the tearing injury during intimate inner cortical bone drilling, increased saline pressure, and thermal injury of RF. Therefore, en block removal of the LF after completion of bone drilling must be a critical technique for safe posterior cervical decompression surgery.

We recommend using the 3.0-mm or 3.5-mm diameter, water-proof diamond-type drill made for unilateral biportal endoscopic surgery rather than a cutting-type drill. Intimate laminotomy over the LF with cutting type drill has a high risk of dural injury and increases the use of punched for further removal before a detachment of LF. Punching of lamina over the hypertrophied LF may cause further compression of the spinal cord in the vulnerable state.

Blurred endoscopic view due to diffuse bleeding prohibits intimate bone drilling over LF. Meticulous bone bleeding control using the bone wax and the RF is essential for delicate and skillful instrument handling in the narrow working space.

Flexed neck position makes the working space wider between the adjacent laminas and induces easy access to the contralateral side with minimalized bone drilling of the spinolaminar junction area.

Some of the limitations of endoscopic posterior decompression in cervical spondylotic myelopathy include a technical difficulty with a steep learning curve of endoscopic techniques for surgeons accustomed to traditional open approaches, the limited direct field of view, and the narrowness of the working channel.

Acknowledgments None.

Conflicts of Interest The authors declare that they have no competing interests.

Consent to Participate Informed consent was obtained from all patients.

Consent to Publish Not applicable.

Data and/or Code Availability Not applicable.

Funding Statement This study did not receive grants or other financial and material support.

References

1. Heary RF, Mac Dowall A, Agarwal N. Cervical spondylotic myelopathy: a two decade experience. J Spinal Cord Med. 2018;42(4):1–9.
2. Hosono N, Yonenobu K, Ono K. Neck and shoulder pain after laminoplasty. A noticeable complication. Spine (Phila Pa 1976). 1996;21(17):1969–73.
3. Shiraishi T, Kato M, Yato Y, Ueda S, Aoyama R, Yamane J, et al. New techniques for exposure of posterior cervical spine through intermuscular planes and their surgical application. Spine (Phila Pa 1976). 2012;37(5):E286–96.
4. Lee BJ, Park JH, Jeon SR, Roh SW, Rhim SC, Jung SK. Posterior cervical muscle-preserving interspinous process approach and decompression: more minimally invasive and modified Shiraishi's selective laminectomy. World Neurosurg. 2020;133:e412–e20.
5. Zhang C, Li D, Wang C, Yan X. Cervical endoscopic laminoplasty for cervical myelopathy. Spine (Phila Pa 1976). 2016;41(Suppl 19):B44–51.
6. Shen J, Telfeian AE, Shaaya E, Oyelese A, Fridley J, Gokaslan ZL. Full endoscopic cervical spine surgery. J Spine Surg. 2020;6(2):383–90.
7. Park JH, Jun SG, Jung JT, Lee SJ. Posterior percutaneous endoscopic cervical foraminotomy and diskectomy with unilateral biportal endoscopy. Orthopedics. 2017;40(5):e779–e83.

8. Song KS, Lee CW. The Biportal endoscopic posterior cervical inclinatory foraminotomy for cervical radiculopathy: technical report and preliminary results. Neurospine. 2020;17(Suppl 1):S145–S53.
9. Kim J, Heo DH, Lee DC, Chung HT. Biportal endoscopic unilateral laminotomy with bilateral decompression for the treatment of cervical spondylotic myelopathy. Acta Neurochir. 2021;163(9):2537–43.
10. Hwa Eum J, Hwa Heo D, Son SK, Park CK. Percutaneous biportal endoscopic decompression for lumbar spinal stenosis: a technical note and preliminary clinical results. J Neurosurg Spine. 2016;24(4):602–7.
11. Heo DH, Ha JS, Lee DC, Kim HS, Chung HJ. Repair of incidental durotomy using sutureless nonpenetrating clips via biportal endoscopic surgery. Global Spine J. 2020.: 2192568220956606; https://doi.org/10.1177/2192568220956606.
12. Heo DH, Hong YH, Lee DC, Chung HJ, Park CK. Technique of biportal endoscopic transforaminal lumbar interbody fusion. Neurospine. 2020;17(Suppl 1):S129–s37.

Thoracic Unilateral Laminetomy for Bilateral Decompression by Unilateral Biportal Endoscopy

18

Man Kyu Park, Sang Kyu Son, and Seung Hyun Choi

18.1 Introduction

Conventional thoracic laminectomy is still the standard surgical approach in the treatment for thoracic spine pathology, including thoracic spinal stenosis or ossified ligamentum flavum (OLF) [1–3]. However, this procedure results in the removal of bony and musculoligamentous structures [3]. Hence, fusion surgery for the prevention of iatrogenic instability is often necessary, and it can also lead to postoperative back pain and complications [2, 4].

Unilateral biportal endoscopy (UBE) is a minimally invasive endoscopic spine surgery that is currently used to treat degenerative spinal diseases involving the cervical, lumbar, and thoracic spine [5–7]. The concept of unilateral laminectomy for bilateral decompression (ULBD) has been employed successfully by spine surgeons for treating lumbar spinal stenosis [8]. The application of ULBD by UBE is also being tried in treating thoracic spinal stenosis or OLF.

Thoracic ULBD by UBE can decrease postoperative instability and back pain by preserving the contralateral facet joint, lamina, and musculoligamentous structures. The main advantage of this technique lies in the availability of a clear and magnified surgical view during operation under endoscopy with continuous saline irrigation. Moreover, the independent movement of the surgical instruments and endoscope provides a wide view for operation with minimal facet violation. This can help achieve complete spinal cord decompression and improve neurological and functional outcomes while avoiding the complications related to conventional thoracic laminectomy.

In this chapter, we discuss the common indications for thoracic ULBD by UBE and the surgical techniques and tips for this procedure. We also focus on specific anatomical landmarks to highlight complication avoidance.

18.2 Indications and Contraindications

It is necessary to understand the indications for thoracic ULBD by UBE to obtain a better outcome.

Supplementary Information The online version contains supplementary material available at [https://doi.org/10.1007/978-981-16-8201-8_18].

M. K. Park · S. K. Son (✉)
Department of Neurosurgery, Parkweonwook Hospital, Busan, South Korea
e-mail: Bread0309@handmail.net

S. H. Choi
Department of Orthopedic Surgery, Parkweonwook Hospital, Busan, South Korea

D. H. Heo et al. (eds.), *Unilateral Biportal Endoscopic Spine Surgery*,
https://doi.org/10.1007/978-981-16-8201-8_18

The indications are as follows:

1. Thoracic spinal stenosis
2. OLF
3. Synovial cysts

Contraindications of thoracic ULBD by UBE are as follows:

1. Central disc herniation
2. Spinal tumor
3. Vascular malformations
4. Instability of the spinal column
5. High-grade deformity
6. Considering safety and technical difficulties, beginner UBE surgeons should exclude patients in cases of fused-type OLF, severe dural ossification, or severe thoracic stenosis.

18.3 Special Instruments

Most of the instruments used in thoracic ULBD by UBE are similar to other surgeries by UBE. Diamond drill and 1-mm Kerrison punch are necessary to perform thoracic ULBD by UBE.

18.4 Anesthesia and Position

After general anesthesia and intraoperative neurophysiological monitoring are performed, a patient is carefully placed in the prone position on a table. Satisfactory positioning is important to avoid abdominal compression. Abdominal compression may cause inadequate venous return and engorgement of the epidural venous plexus. Excessive intraoperative bleeding may lead to overuse of the radiofrequency (RF) probe and subsequent cord injury. Generally, the left-side approach is preferred for a right-handed surgeon. For right-handed surgeons, a left-side portal is used as the scopic portal for the endoscope and a right-side portal is used as a working portal for manipulation of the surgical instruments. An assistant on the opposite side of the operator holds the semi-tubular retractor.

18.5 Surgical Steps

18.5.1 Skin Marking and Making Portal

C-arm fluoroscopy is required to confirm the level of surgery. It is important to compare this count with preoperative images since one of the most common errors in thoracic spine surgery is performing it at a wrong spinal level. The docking point is identified using an anteroposterior (AP) view of C-arm fluoroscopy as the lower part of the cranial lamina. Two incisions are made approximately 2.5 cm apart, with the center being the lower part of the cranial lamina at the midline of the proximal and distal pedicles (Fig. 18.1a). In patients with obesity, the two incisions should be wider and located laterally from the midline. Serial dilators and endoscopic sheath are inserted to the docking point under C-arm guidance. Under C-arm fluoroscopy, serial dilators are inserted through the working portal, and a scopic sheath is introduced at the docking point through the scopic portal. The tip of the dilator and the endoscopic sheath make a triangulation above the docking point, and the locations of the portals are then confirmed on AP and lateral fluoroscopy. The muscle detacher is inserted and used to reach the inferior edge of the cranial lamina and the base of the spinous process. After positioning the endoscope and the semi-tubular retractor through each portal, the initial working space is made available under fluoloscopic guidance (Fig. 18.1b). The semi-tubular retractor is used to maintain the fluid output and to retract the paraspinal muscles. Care should be taken while placing the semi-tubular retractor so that fluid output is more crucial at the thoracic cord level, which is sensitive to pressure.

18.5.2 Bone Working (Video 18.1)

After confirming that both portals are placed correctly, the soft tissues are coagulated by the RF probe to expose the anatomical structure of the cranial lamina, the base of the spinous process, and the interlaminar space (Fig. 18.2a).

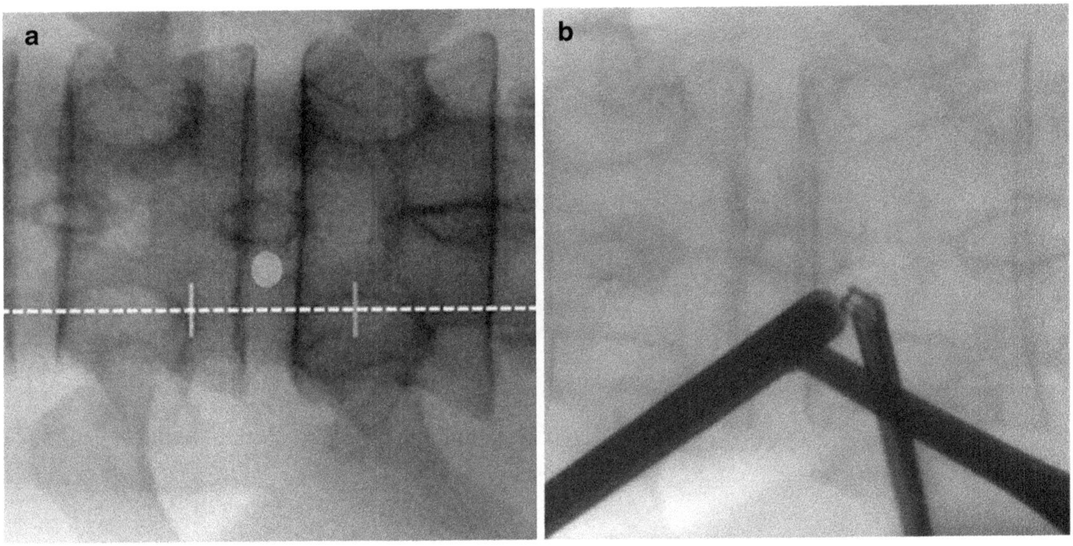

Fig. 18.1 Skin incision and docking point on the fluoroscopic anteroposterior view. The docking point (white circle) is the lower part of the cranial lamina. Two skin incisions (working portal: blue line, scopic portal: white line) are made about 2.5 cm apart, with the center being the lower part of the cranial lamina at the midline of the proximal and distal pedicles (dotted line) (**a**). The positioning the endoscope and surgical instruments with a semi-tubular retractor through each portal (**b**)

Subsequently, the outer cortex of cranial lamina is removed to expose the cancellous bone, and the round cutting burr is used to remove the cranial lamina down to the ligamentum flavum (LF) (Fig. 18.2b). Care should be taken not to compress the LF by burr or Kerrison punch. The base of the spinous processes is removed to make space for safe bone working, especially in contralateral decompression (Fig. 18.2c). The purpose of removing the base of the spinous process is to reduce compression of the spinal cord by the endoscope or surgical instruments when performing contralateral decompression (Fig. 18.3). After that, the midline gap of LF, which is the anatomical landmark of midline orientation, is identified (Fig. 18.2d). Based on this landmark, the extent of the bone working can be assessed by removing the base of the spinous process from the ipsilateral to the contralateral side as well as cranially and caudally underneath the spinous process. The cranial lamina is removed until the cranial attachment of the LF is exposed (Fig. 18.2e). Contact with the burr could bring serious complications to the spinal cord. Therefore, to avoid neural injury during thoracic ULBD by UBE, the LF is left as a protector until bone working is completed. After completing laminectomy wide enough to decompress both sides of the surgical segment while maintaining the LF, the medial aspect of the facet joint is partially removed (Fig. 18.2f). The lateral end of the laminectomy overlaps with the medial aspect of the facet joint, which should be preserved as far as possible for stability.

18.5.3 Removal of LF (Video 18.2)

After the finishing of bone working, the superficial layer of the LF is detached from the posterior surface of the caudal lamina using a freer elevator and pituitary forceps (Fig. 18.4a). Afterward, the junction between the medial margin of the superior articular process (SAP) and the caudal lamina is identified as a landmark for lateral decompression (Fig. 18.4b). Before the removal of these structures, a diamond burr is used to thin out the medial aspect of SAP and the upper portion of the caudal lamina, without which the Kerrison punch could compress the spinal cord underneath the bony structures (Fig. 18.4c, d). Once thinned out, the caudal lamina is partially

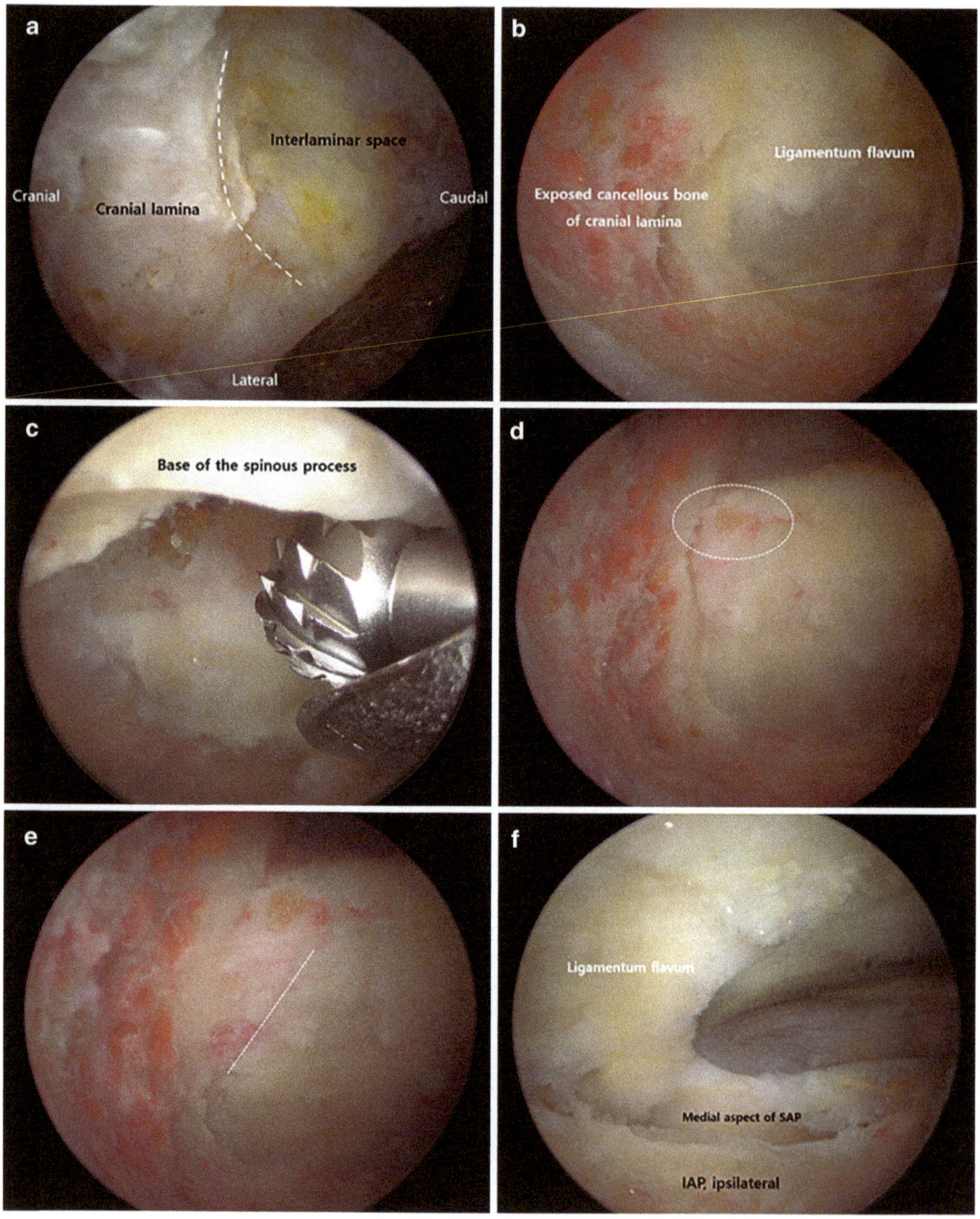

Fig. 18.2 Serial sequence endoscopic images of the bone working. The surgical anatomy is first noticed in the inferior edge of the cranial lamina (dotted line) and the interlaminar space (**a**). The outer cortex of cranial lamina is removed to expose the cancellous bone, and the round cutting burr is used to remove the cranial lamina down to the ligamentum flavum (**b**). The base of the spinous processes is removed to make space for safe bone working, especially in contralateral decompression (**c**). Anatomical landmark for midline orientation. Endoscopic view of midline gap of ligamentum flavum (white circle) (**d**). Anatomical landmark for cranial bone working. Dotted line indicates cranial end of the ligamentum flavum of ipsilateral side (**e**). Anatomical landmark for lateral bone working. The lateral end of the laminectomy overlaps with the medial aspect of the facet joint (**f**)

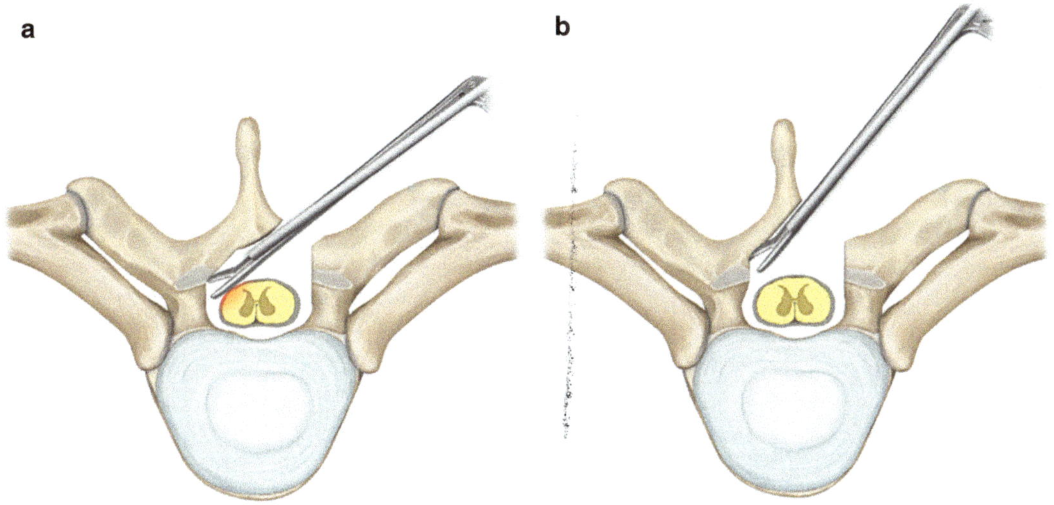

Fig. 18.3 Securing space for safe surgery in thoracic ULBD by UBE. If the base of the spinous process is not sufficiently removed, there is a possibility of cord injury caused by the instruments during contralateral decompression (**a**). The base of the spinous processes is removed to make space for safe bone working, especially in contralateral decompression (**b**)

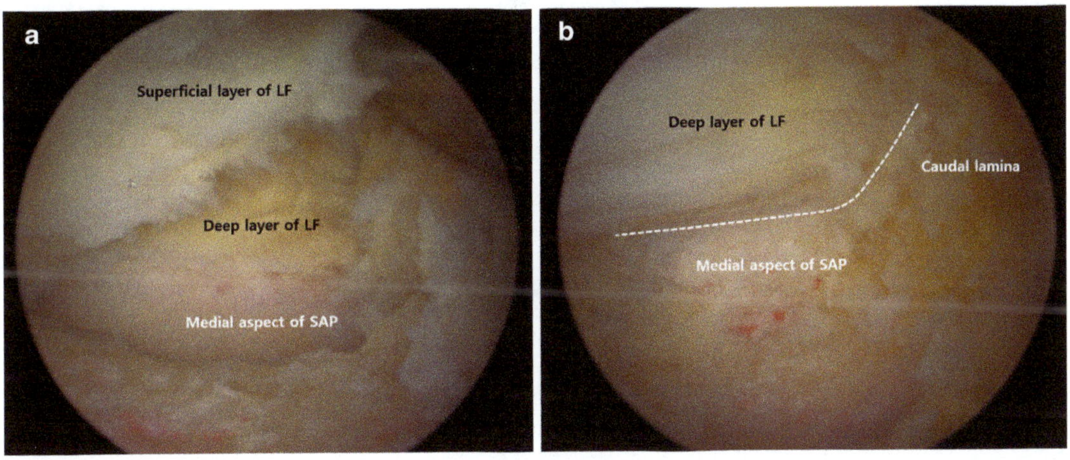

Fig. 18.4 Endoscopic images showing the sequential steps of removal of ligamentum flavum (LF). Detachment of the superficial layer of LF (**a**). Exposure of the upper portion of the caudal lamina and medial margin of the superior articular process at ipsilateral side (white dotted curved line) (**b**). A diamond burr is used to thin out the medial aspect of SAP and the upper portion of the caudal lamina (**c** and **d**). Once thinned out, the caudal lamina is partially removed with a freer elevator or 1-mm Kerrison punch that continues along the medial margin of the SAP and exposes the caudal end of the deep layer of LF (**e** and **f**). Because cord compression is usually not severe around the cranial part of the LF, the cranial side of the LF (white arrow) should be released after the detachment of the caudal part of LF (**g**). Exposure of the upper portion of the caudal lamina and medial margin of the SAP at contralateral side (white dotted curved line) (**h**). A diamond burr is used to thin out the medial aspect of SAP and the upper portion of the caudal lamina (**i**). Removal of the medial aspect of SAP and the upper portion of the caudal lamina (**j**). Coagulation of the cranial side of the LF (white arrow). Dotted line indicates midline (**k**). Detachment of the cranial side of the LF (white arrow) (**l**). The remaining medial aspects of SAP can be removed until the lateral margin of the thecal sac is confirmed, which is easily identified by epidural fat tissue (asterisk) (**m**). Confirmation of complete decompression (**n**)

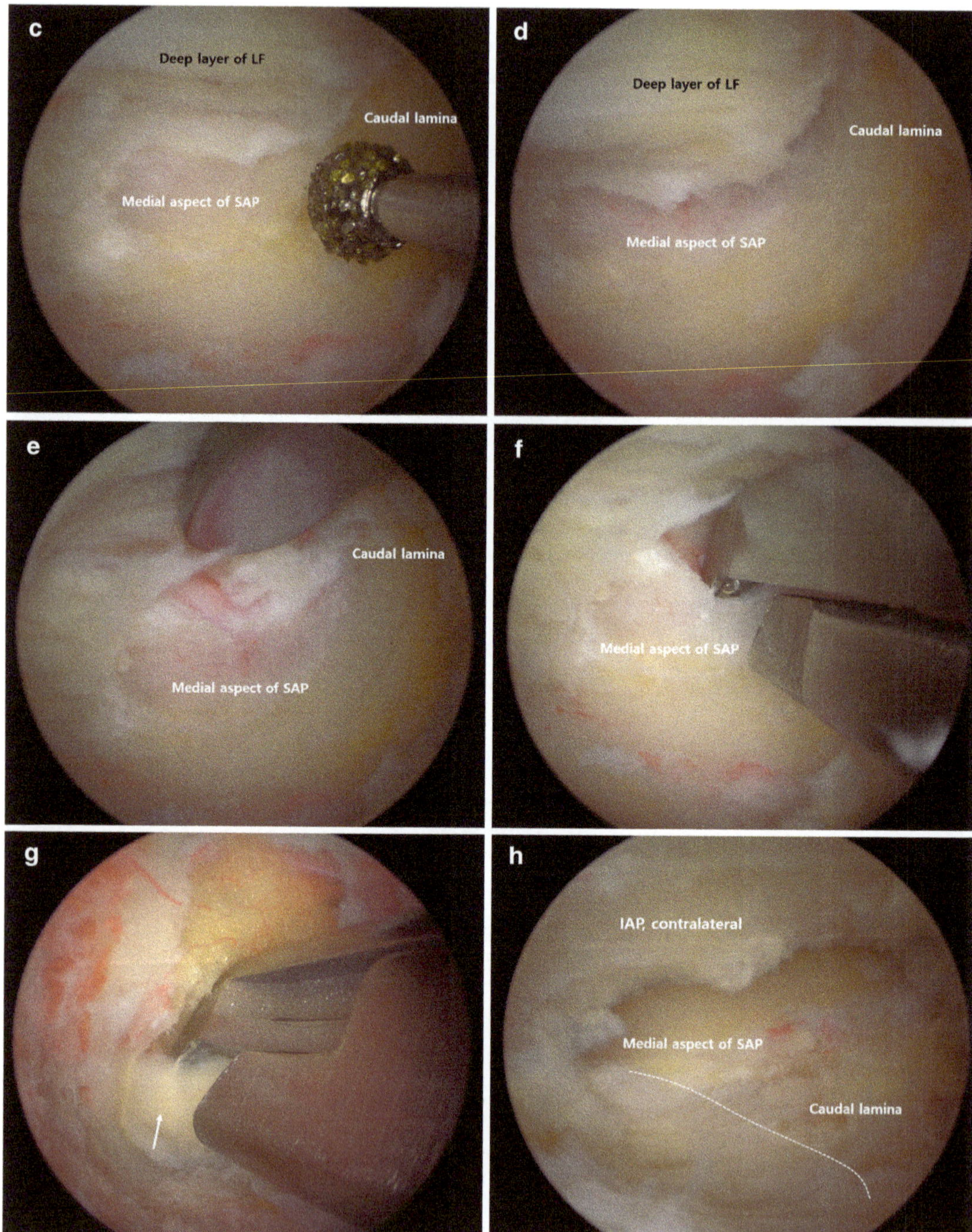

Fig. 18.4 (continued)

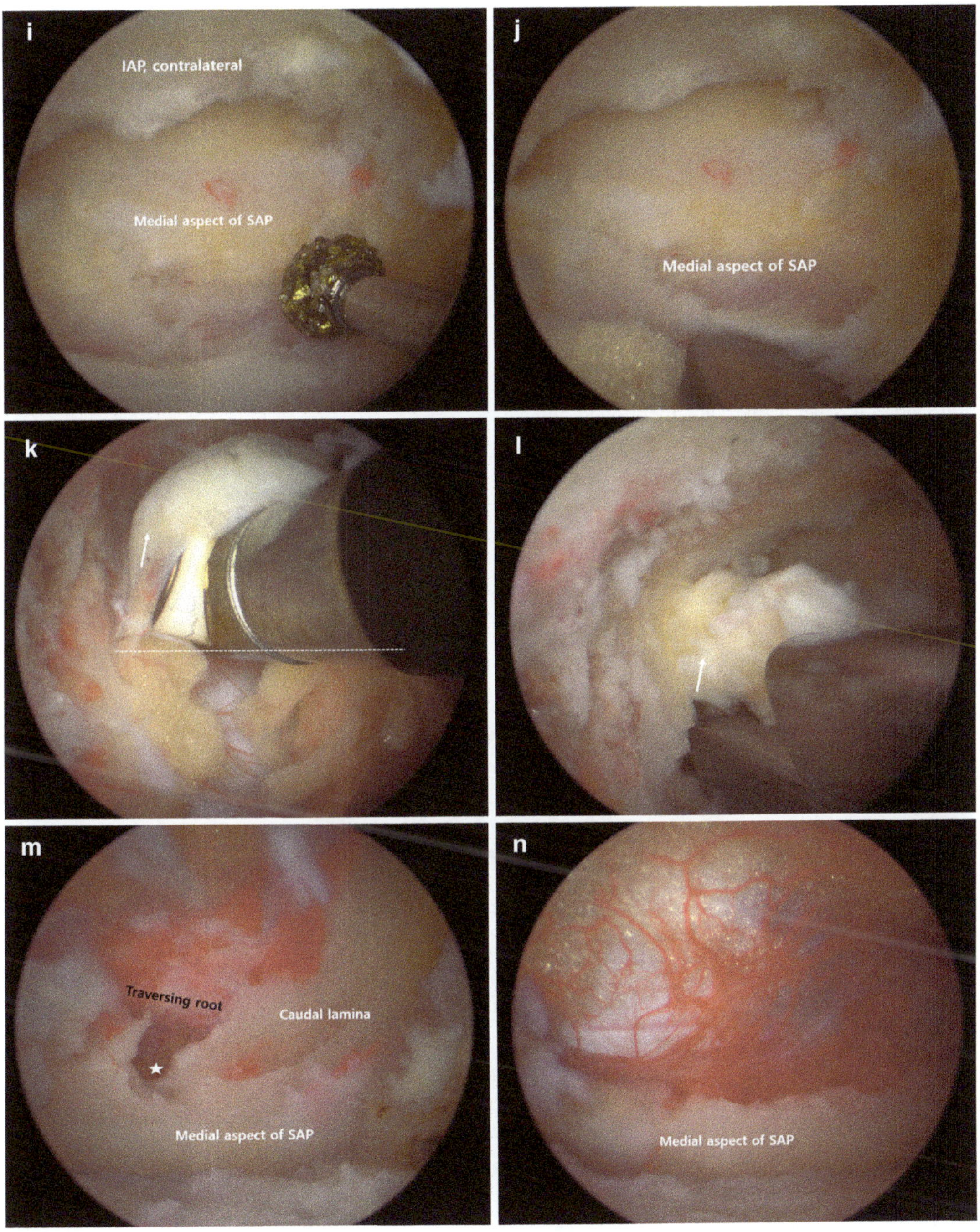

Fig. 18.4 (continued)

removed with a 1 mm Kerrison punch or freer elevator that continues along the medial margin of the SAP and exposes the caudal end of the deep layer of LF (Fig. 18.4e, f). Because cord compression is usually not severe around the cranial part of the LF, the cranial side of the LF should be released after the detachment of the caudal part of LF (Fig. 18.4g). This technique makes the *en block* removal of the deep layer of LF possible. Additionally, it should be noted that during the removal of the LF, there is often an adhesion between LF and dural matter that can access a plane below the LF.

The method for removing LF at the contralateral side is the same as mentioned above (Fig. 18.4h–l). Prior to the removal of LF at contralateral side, because of the abundance of epidural blood vessels around the cranial attachment of LF, the coagulation by RF probe is helpful for bleeding control (Fig. 18.4k). When removing the contralateral side of LF, the surgeon should pay attention not to compress the spinal cord with surgical instruments such as the Kerrison punch. In order to do this, the base of the spinous process should be sufficiently removed and the caudal lamina and medial aspect of SAP should be thinned out using a diamond drill (Fig. 18.3). The remaining medial aspects of SAP can be removed until the lateral margin of the thecal sac is confirmed, which is easily identified by epidural fat tissue (Fig. 18.4m). The lateral end of decompression is the medial aspect of the pedicle and the lateral margin of the thecal sac. The endpoint of decompression is spinal cord decompression, which can be confirmed with endoscopic guidance (Fig. 18.4n).

18.5.4 Removal of OLF (If Present) (Videos 18.3 and 18.4)

The removal of OLF can be organized as thinning-detaching-removing. After the removal of the nonossified LF, the underlying OLF can be identified (Fig. 18.5a). Basically, OLFs are thick and hard, and removing them with Kerrison punch is

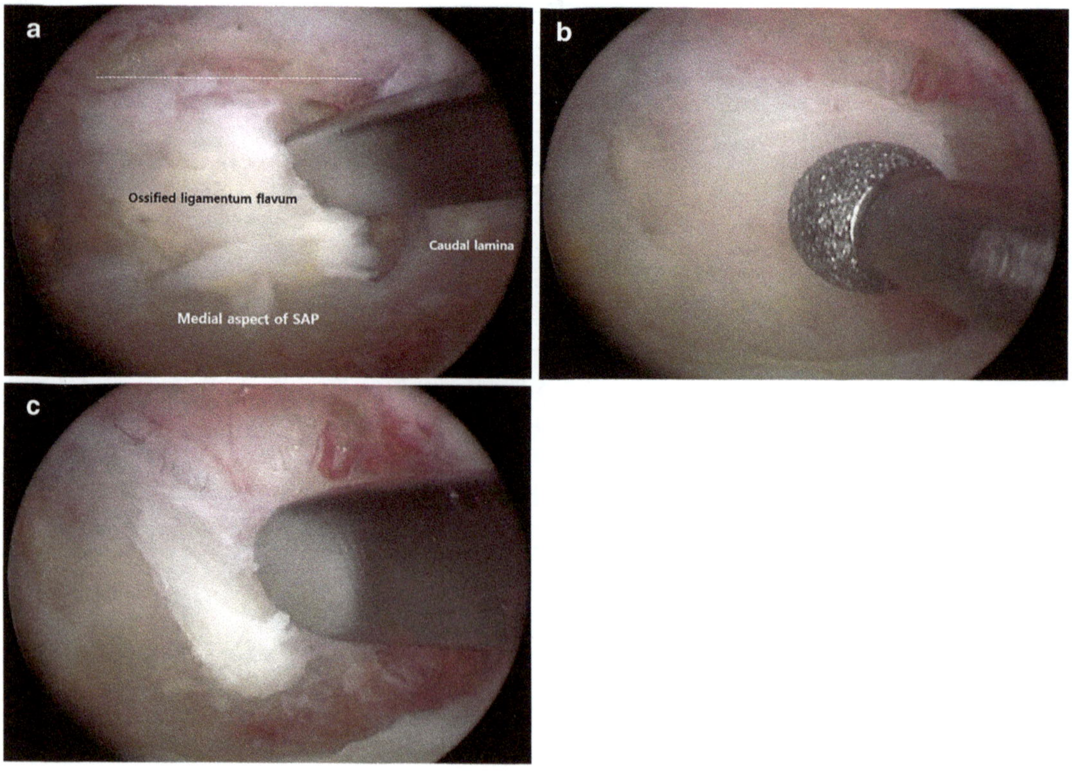

Fig. 18.5 Serial sequence endoscopic images of removal of ossified ligamentum flavum (OLF). Identification of the OLF. Dotted line indicates midline (**a**). The OLF is ground into a thin and translucent form using a diamond drill (**b**). The thinned-out OLF can be detached from the thecal sac using the freer elevator (**c**)

difficult and dangerous. Since the thoracic cord is particularly sensitive to compression, the OLF should be removed cautiously without unintended compression on the spinal cord. After the exposure of OLF, the OLF is ground into a thin and translucent form using a diamond drill (Fig. 18.5b). The thinned OLF should remain stable until the drilling is over as it protects the spinal cord from the diamond burr. The thinned-out OLF can be detached from the thecal sac using the freer elevator and removed gently piece by piece using small-sized pituitary forceps or a 1 mm Kerrison punch (Fig. 18.5c). If the removal of OLF fails due to severe adhesion or dural ossification, the OLF should be left as it is also known as the floating method. The complications that arise if dura tear occurs are described in detail later. Finally, free-floating dura mater is a sign of sufficient decompression under endoscopic guidance.

18.5.5 Postoperative Drain

After complete decompression, a Jackson–Pratt surgical drain (100 cc) is usually placed through the working portal to prevent postoperative hematoma. If the Jackson–Pratt surgical drain is inserted deeply, the tip of the drain could cause cord injury.

18.5.6 Postoperative Care

The patient may ambulate and be discharged the first day after the operation. Bedrest is needed if a dura tear occurs and is recommended for 5–7 days if lumbar drain is utilized. A postoperative MRI should be performed in 2 days to check for possible postoperative epidural hematoma and the degree of decompression.

18.6 Illustrated Cases

18.6.1 Case (1): Thoracic Spinal Stenosis

A 73-year-old woman exhibited neurologic symptoms in the bilateral lower extremities caused by compressive myelopathy because of thoracic spinal stenosis at T11-T12 for 12 months. She was treated conservatively for 2 months; however, her symptoms aggravated instead of improving. MRI scans revealed thoracic spinal stenosis at the T11-T12 level (Fig. 18.6a, b). The spinal cord was compressed by the bilateral hypertrophied LF at T11-T12. Postoperative MRI scans revealed adequate decompression of spinal cord at the T11-T12 level (Fig. 18.6c, d). The symptoms improved significantly. The patient had no symptoms of spastic paraparesis at the time of follow-up.

18.6.2 Case (2): OLF

A 61-year-old man presented with a 9-month history of spastic paraparesis. On preoperative MRI (Fig. 18.7a, b) and CT (Fig. 18.7c), we identified bilateral OLF, compressing the cord at the T9-T10 level. ULBD by UBE at T9–10 level was performed from the left side. The OLF was removed and the thecal sac was thoroughly decompressed. After surgery, the result was confirmed on postoperative MRI (Fig. 18.7d, e) and CT scan (Fig. 18.7f). At follow-up after 6 months, his physical strength in the lower extremities returned to 5 bilaterally, and he was able to walk long distances.

18.7 Complications and Their Management

18.7.1 Dural Tear (Video 18.5)

Small-sized dura tear can be treated with careful packing with fibrin collagen patch (TachoComb) and bed rest for 5–7 days. When dural tear occurs, the Jackson–Pratt surgical drain may be contraindicated or should be removed early as it may keep the dural tear patent. However, if the size of dural tear is larger than 10 mm, the dural defect should be repaired directly by a dural suture or by repair conversion under microscopic surgery.

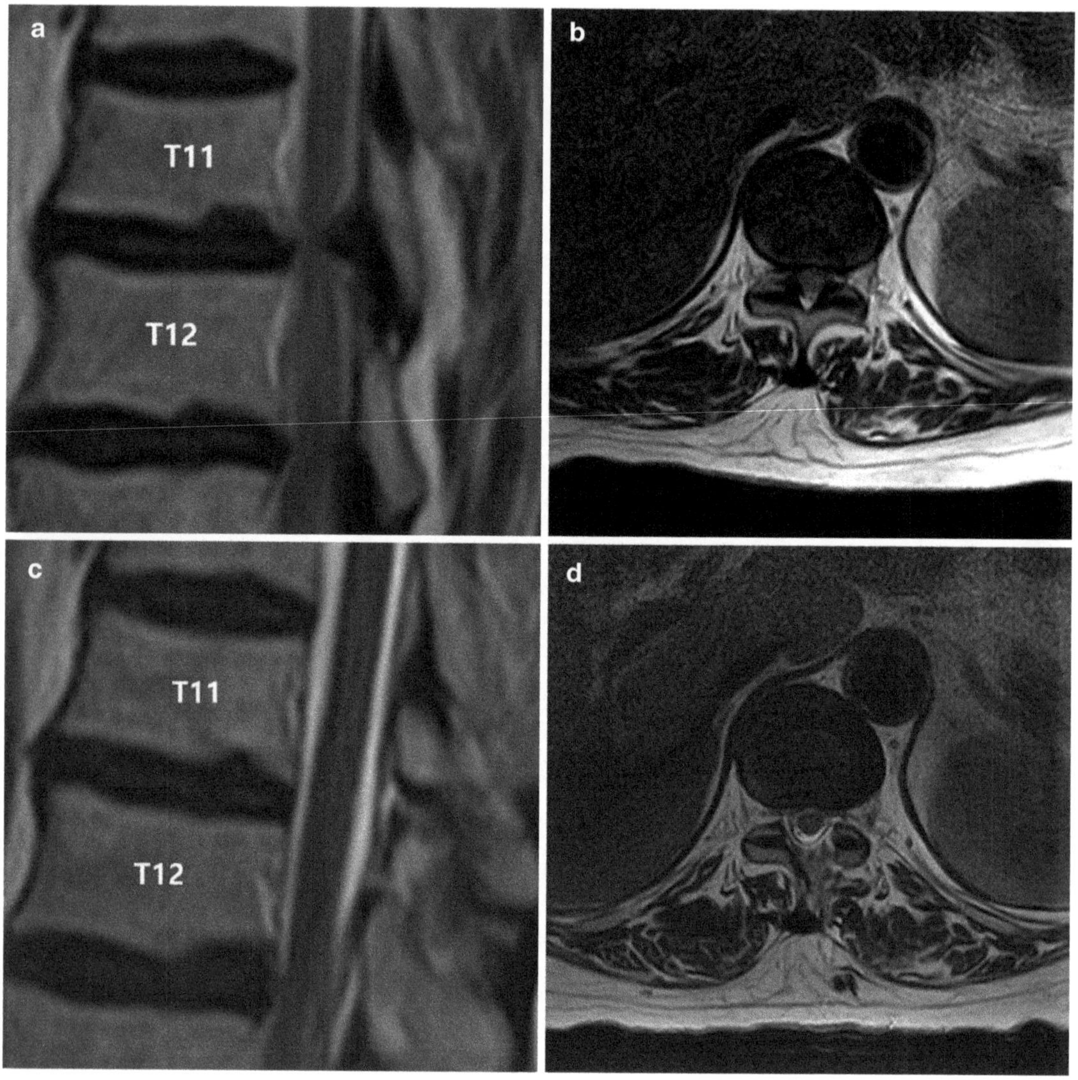

Fig. 18.6 Images of a 73-year-old woman with thoracic spinal stenosis at T11-T12 level. Preoperative MR images show thoracic spinal stenosis with bilateral hypertrophied LF at T11–12 level (sagittal: **a**, axial: **b**). Postoperative axial T2-weighted MRI show enough decompression with minimal facet violation (sagittal: **c**, axial: **d**)

18.7.2 Cord Injury

Care should be taken to avoid cord manipulation at all costs. Since the thoracic cord is particularly sensitive to compression, the thoracic decompression should be removed without inadvertent compression of the spinal cord. Therefore, to avoid cord injury during the bone working, the LF is left as a protector until bone working is completed. Additionally, it is important to sufficiently remove the base of the spinous process and to thin out bony structures or OLF using a diamond drill. If the removal of OLF is difficult due to severe adhesion or dural ossification, it is safe to leave OLF using the floating method. The RF probe should be used with much caution near neural structures. When manipulating an RF probe around the neural structures, surgeons should pay special attention to use it against neural structures with low power.

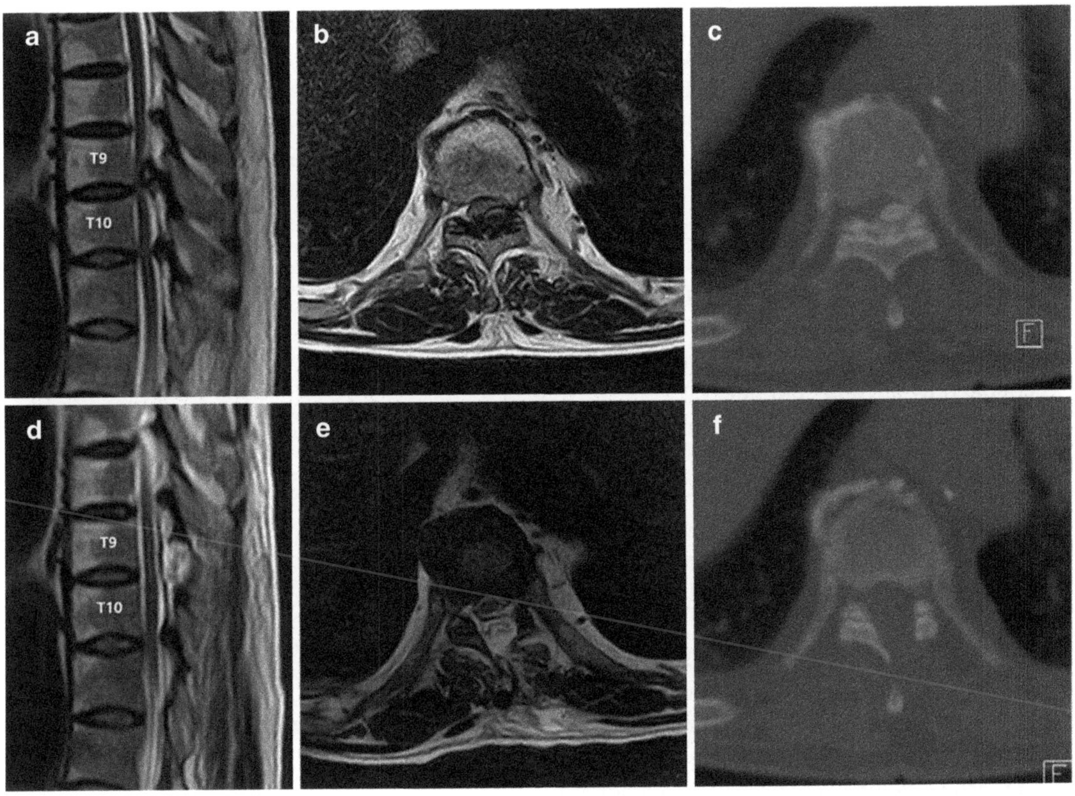

Fig. 18.7 Images of a 61-year-old man with OLF. Preoperative MRI and CT show bilateral OLF, compressing the cord at the T9-T10 level. (MRI sagittal: **a** and axial: **b**, CT axial: **c**). Postoperative axial T2-weighted MRI show well decompression of bilateral OLF (MRI sagittal: **d** and axial: **e**, CT axial: **f**)

18.7.3 Postoperative Hematoma

After decompression, bleeding from bone edges is thoroughly applied with bone wax, epidural veins are coagulated by a hook RF probe, and soluble hemostatic gauze (WoundClot) or Gelfoam is placed on the bleeding site in the epidural space. To prevent postoperative epidural hematoma, it is recommended to keep the Jackson–Pratt surgical drain (100 cc) in the working portal for 1 or 2 days.

18.8 Surgical Tips and Pitfall

The anatomy of the thoracic spine is different from that of the cervical and lumbar spine. The spinal canal is smaller in the thoracic spine, and the lamina is short, thick, broad, and overlapping. Also, the thoracic spinal cord has poor tolerance to compression as well as a limited amount of space to perform surgery [9]. Therefore, excessive compression of the spinal cord by surgical instruments may lead to spinal cord injury [4]. Thus, securing space for safe surgery is of utmost importance. In thoracic ULBD by UBE, surgeons are able to make enough space by undercutting the base of the spinous process and preserving the posterior bony and musculoligamentous structures.

Although UBE has gained widespread popularity in recent years, the adoption of UBE techniques on thoracic spine surgery can be challenging. Therefore, it is recommended to perform thoracic ULBD by UBE only when the surgeon has enough experience in performing lumbar decompression by UBE. This ensures that surgeons are familiar with the movement of the endoscope and the manipulation of surgical instruments and that the fluid output can be maintained well. Further, surgeons must keep in mind the anatomical landmark and the following surgical tips for thoracic ULBD by UBE to minimize potential complications.

1. A more lateral incision is recommended for patients with obesity.
2. The placement of semi-tubular retractor for fluid output requires more attention than lumbar surgery because the poor output of water at cord level is more likely to increase intracranial pressure and cord injury.
3. The diamond drill, fine Kerrison punch, and hook RF probe are invaluable tools.
4. Based on the midline gap of LF, the extent of the bone working can be accomplished by removing the base of the spinous process from the ipsilateral to the contralateral side as well as cranially and caudally by working entirely beneath the spinous process.
5. The cranial lamina is removed until the cranial attachment of the LF is exposed, and the junction between the medial edge of the SAP and caudal lamina is identified as a landmark for lateral decompression.
6. When performing contralateral decompression, special attention should be paid not to compress the spinal cord with surgical instruments such as the Kerrison punch. It is important to sufficiently remove the base of the spinous process and to thin out bony structures using a diamond drill.
7. Since it is dangerous to remove the OLF with a Kerrison punch, the OLF is drilled into a thin and translucent shape using a diamond drill.
8. The pathophysiology of OLF can lead to dural ossification, which is a technical challenge in UBE. If predictive signs of dural ossification are checked in preoperative images, we recommend the thinning and floating techniques. After floating of OLF, the dural opening should be completely sealed with a fibrin collagen patch.
9. Considering safety and technical difficulties, beginner UBE surgeons should exclude patients with fused-type OLF or severe thoracic stenosis as they may exhibit more severe clinical manifestations and poor prognosis.

References

1. Liao CC, Chen TY, Jung SM, Chen LR. Surgical experience with symptomatic thoracic ossification of the ligamentum flavum. J Neurosurg Spine. 2005;2(1):34–9.
2. Okada K, Oka S, Tohge K, Ono K, Yonenobu K, Hosoya T. Thoracic myelopathy caused by ossification of the ligamentum flavum. Clinicopathologic study and surgical treatment. Spine (Phila Pa 1976). 1991;16(3):280–7.
3. Palumbo MA, Hilibrand AS, Hart RA, Bohlman HH. Surgical treatment of thoracic spinal stenosis: a 2- to 9-year follow-up. Spine (Phila Pa 1976). 2001;26(5):558–66.
4. Yang Z, Xue Y, Zhang C, Dai Q, Zhou H. Surgical treatment of ossification of the ligamentum flavum associated with dural ossification in the thoracic spine. J Clin Neurosci. 2013;20(2):212–6.
5. Heo DH, Lee N, Park CW, Kim HS, Chung HJ. Endoscopic unilateral laminotomy with bilateral discectomy using biportal endoscopic approach: technical report and preliminary clinical results. World Neurosurg. 2020;137:31–7.
6. Park MK, Park SA, Son SK, Park WW, Choi SH. Clinical and radiological outcomes of unilateral biportal endoscopic lumbar interbody fusion (ULIF) compared with conventional posterior lumbar interbody fusion (PLIF): 1-year follow-up. Neurosurg Rev. 2019;42(3):753–61.
7. Kim J, Heo DH, Lee DC, Chung HT. Biportal endoscopic unilateral laminotomy with bilateral decompression for the treatment of cervical spondylotic myelopathy. Acta Neurochir. 2021;163(9):2537–43.
8. Ikuta K, Arima J, Tanaka T, Oga M, Nakano S, Sasaki K, et al. Short-term results of microendoscopic posterior decompression for lumbar spinal stenosis. Technical note. J Neurosurg Spine. 2005;2(5):624–33.
9. Dommisse GF. The blood supply of the spinal cord. A critical vascular zone in spinal surgery. J Bone Joint Surg Br. 1974;56(2):225–35.

www.ingramcontent.com/pod-product-compliance
Ingram Content Group UK Ltd.
Pitfield, Milton Keynes, MK11 3LW, UK
UKHW051318160826
14477UKWH00027B/692
* 9 7 8 9 8 1 1 6 8 2 0 3 2 *